ANGIOGENESIS AND DIRECT MYOCARDIAL VASCULARIZATION

CONTEMPORARY CARDIOLOGY

CHRISTOPHER P. CANNON, MD

SERIES EDITOR

ANGIOGENESIS AND DIRECT MYOCARDIAL REVASCULARIZATION

Edited by

ROGER J. LAHAM, MD

Beth Israel Deaconess Medical Center
Boston, MA

DONALD S. BAIM, MD

Brigham and Women's Hospital
Boston, MA

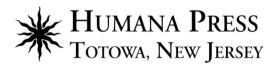

HUMANA PRESS
TOTOWA, NEW JERSEY

© 2005 Humana Press Inc.
999 Riverview Drive, Suite 208
Totowa, New Jersey 07512

humanapress.com

For additional copies, pricing for bulk purchases, and/or information about other Humana titles, contact Humana at the above address or at any of the following numbers: Tel.: 973-256-1699; Fax: 973-256-8341, E-mail: orders@humanapr.com; or visit our Website: www.humanapress.com

Production Editor: Tracy Catanese

Cover design by Patricia F. Cleary

Cover Illustration: Angiogenesis from bench to bedside: tube formation on in vitro matrigel (upper left) → CD31 staining showing increased capillary formation (upper right) → in vivo hind limb ischemia model with increased arterial collaterals (lower left) → cardiac magnetic resonance imaging to detect improvement in perfusion and function (lower right). This translational paradigm with agent discovery rapidly testing in vitro followed by animal models to investigate delivery modalities and efficacy leading to clinical testing with sensitive outcome measures should lead to functionally significant angiogenesis and myogenesis in patients with end-stage ischemic disease and heart failure.

This publication is printed on acid-free paper. ∞

ANSI Z39.48-1984 (American National Standards Institute) Permanence of Paper for Printed Library Materials.

Printed in the United States of America. 10 9 8 7 6 5 4 3 2 1
eISBN: 1-59259-934-6
Library of Congress Cataloging-in-Publication Data
Angiogenesis and direct myocardial revascularization / edited by Roger J. Laham.
    p. ; cm. -- (Contemporary cardiology)
  Includes bibliographical references and index.
  ISBN 1-58829-153-7 (alk. paper)
  1. Coronary heart disease. 2. Neovascularization.
  [DNLM: 1. Neovascularization, Physiologic. 2. Myocardial Revascularization--methods. WG 500 A5842 2005] I. Laham, Roger J. II.
Series: Contemporary cardiology (Totowa, N.J. : Unnumbered).
  RC685.C6A595 2005
  616.1'23--dc22

                                                                            2004026636

PREFACE

Si facile esset, iam factum sit.

Atherosclerotic disease remains the leading cause of death in the Western Hemisphere, and its prevalence continues to increase as the population ages. Despite progress in surgical and catheter-based revascularization, an ever increasing number of patients are either not candidates for these therapies or remain symptomatic despite prior revascularization and maximal ongoing medical treatment. Thus, it is clear that an alternative treatment strategy such as therapeutic angiogenesis and myogenesis is needed for these "no-option" patients.

The field of angiogenesis/myogenesis, however, has followed the same development pattern seen with other novel therapeutic interventions: early spectacular and "too-good-to-be-true" results leading to unrealistic expectations, followed by sobering complications and disappointments, only later maturing to cautious optimism when better understanding of the biological and logistic obstacles is achieved. We believe that this is such a time for therapeutic angiogenesis/myogenesis, putting behind us the early picture of angiogenesis as "an attempt to influence a process we do not understand, with the agents we do not know how to use and deliver, relying on the end-points we cannot assess." Unfortunately, this led to failure of early studies and a negative view of the field, at a time when we are finally developing a good understanding of the biology and therapeutic targets, have multiple available and well-studied therapeutic strategies, and have developed the necessary imaging to measure outcomes. From here, much work still needs to be done to eventually achieve functionally significant angiogenesis/myogenesis, but clearly we have turned at least the first developmental corner with the identification of novel therapeutic targets and pathways, the investigation of transcriptional factors, master switch molecules, cell-based approaches, chemokines, a better understanding of the effects of aging, endothelial dysfunction, and hypercholesterolemia in response to angiogenic stimuli, as well as a better understanding of delivery problems. Each development has brought us one step closer to our goal of helping patients with end-stage ischemic heart disease, peripheral vascular disease, and congestive heart failure.

Angiogenesis and Direct Myocardial Revascularization represents an interdisciplinary effort to balance the basic, preclinical, and clinical aspects in this field. The various sections are each written by pioneers and opinion leaders in angiogenesis/myogenesis. Their chapters reflect the latest developments in this rapidly evolving field, including the introduction of cell-based therapy for angiogenesis and myocardial repair. Wherever this field takes us, we hope that this book will be a useful waypoint, and that we can go forward balancing optimistic enthusiasm with a healthy dose of scientific skepticism, in order to finally realize the promise that such therapies may hold for patients with advanced cardiovascular disease.

Roger J. Laham, MD
Donald S. Baim, MD

CONTENTS

CONTRIBUTORS

BRIAN H. ANNEX, MD, *Division of Cardiology, Department of Medicine, Duke University School of Medicine, Durham, NC*

DONALD S. BAIM, MD, *Division of Cardiology, Brigham and Women's Hospital and Harvard Medical School, Boston, MA*

MUNIR BOODHWANI, MD, *Division of Cardiac Surgery, University of Ottawa Heart Institute, Ottawa, ON, Canada*

KWANG SOO CHA, MD, *Dong-A University Hospital, Busan, South Korea, and Minneapolis Heart Institute Foundation, Minneapolis, MN*

NICHOLAS A. CHRONOS, MD, *American Cardiovascular Research Institute, St. Joseph's Hospital of Atlanta, Atlanta, GA*

DAVID G. HARRISON, MD, *Division of Cardiology, Department of Medicine, Emory University School of Medicine, Atlanta, GA*

TIMOTHY D. HENRY, MD, *Minneapolis Heart Institute Foundation, Minneapolis, MN*

KEITH A. HORVATH, MD, *National Heart, Lung and Blood Institute, National Institutes of Health, Bethesda, MD*

ROGER J. LAHAM, MD, *Department of Medicine, Angiogenesis Research Center, Beth Israel Deaconess Medical Center and Harvard Medical School, Boston, MA*

CHU-PAK LAU, MD, *Cardiology Division, Department of Medicine, Queen Mary Hospital, The University of Hong Kong, Hong Kong, China*

PUI-YIN LEE, MBBS, *Cardiology Division, Department of Medicine, Queen Mary Hospital, The University of Hong Kong, Hong Kong, China*

DOUGLAS W. LOSORDO, MD, *Division of Cardiovascular Medicine, St. Elizabeth's Medical Center, Boston, MA*

KAPILDEO LOTUN, MD, *Division of Cardiovascular Medicine, St. Elizabeth's Medical Center, Boston, MA*

JIANG-YONG MIN, MD, *Cardiovascular Division, Department of Medicine, Beth Israel Deaconess Medical Center and Harvard Medical School, Boston, MA*

JAMES P. MORGAN, MD, PhD, *Cardiovascular Division, Department of Medicine, Beth Israel Deaconess Medical Center and Harvard Medical School, Boston, MA*

PETER OETTGEN, MD, *Division of Cardiology, Department of Medicine, Beth Israel Deaconess Medical Center and Harvard Medical School, Boston, MA*

JUSTIN D. PEARLMAN, MD, ME, PhD, *Advanced Cardiovascular Imaging Center, Dartmouth Hitchcock Medical Center, Lebanon, NH*

ERIK T. PRICE, MD, *Division of Cardiovascular Medicine, Stanford University Medical Center, Stanford, CA*

JAMAL S. RANA, MD, *Divisions of Cardiology and Cardiothoracic Surgery, Angiogenesis Research Center, Beth Israel Deaconess Medical Center and Harvard Medical School, Boston, MA*

MEHRDAD REZAEE, MD, PhD, *Division of Cardiovascular Medicine, Stanford University Medical Center, Stanford, CA*

AUDREY ROSINBERG, MD, *Divisions of Cardiology and Cardiothoracic Surgery, Angiogenesis Research Center, Beth Israel Deaconess Medical Center and Harvard Medical School, Boston, MA*

ROBERT S. SCHWARTZ, MD, *Minneapolis Heart Institute Foundation, Minneapolis, MN*

FRANK W. SELLKE, MD, *Division of Cardiothoracic Surgery, Beth Israel Deaconess Medical Center and Harvard Medical School, Boston, MA*

PINAK B. SHAH, MD, *Division of Cardiovascular Medicine, St. Elizabeth's Medical Center, Boston, MA*

HUNG FAT-TSE, MD, *Cardiology Division, Department of Medicine, Queen Mary Hospital, The University of Hong Kong, Hong Kong, China*

PIERRE VOISINE, MD, *Division of Cardiothoracic Surgery, Beth Israel Deaconess Medical Center and Harvard Medical School, Boston, MA*

RICHARD E. WATERS, MD, *Division of Cardiology, Department of Medicine, Duke University School of Medicine, Durham, NC*

JOANNA J. WYKRZYKOWSKA, MD, *Department of Medicine, Massachusetts General Hospital, Harvard Medical School, Boston, MA*

YONG-FU XIAO, MD, *Cardiovascular Division, Department of Medicine, Beth Israel Deaconess Medical Center and Harvard Medical School, Boston, MA*

AYSEGUL YEGIN, MD, *American Cardiovascular Research Institute, St. Joseph's Hospital of Atlanta, Atlanta, GA*

ALAN C. YEUNG, MD, *Division of Cardiovascular Medicine, Stanford University Medical Center, Stanford, CA*

COLOR PLATES

Color plates 1–6 appear in an insert following p. 116.

1 No-Option Patients
A Growing Problem

Roger J. Laham, MD
and Donald S. Baim, MD

CONTENTS

INTRODUCTION

Despite advances in preventive health care, medical management, interventional cardiology, and cardiovascular surgery, atherosclerotic disease remains the leading cause of morbidity and mortality in the Western Hemisphere. Cardiovascular disease accounted for 38.5% of all deaths or 1 of every 2.6 deaths in the United States in 2001. Cardiovascular disease mortality was about 60% of "total mortality," i.e., of over 2,400,000 deaths from all causes, cardiovascular disease was listed as a primary or contributing cause on about 1,408,000 death certificates. Since 1900, cardiovascular disease has been the number one killer in the United States every year except 1918 *(1)*. Treatment of coronary artery disease (CAD) includes risk factor modification, use of antiplatelet agents, medical therapy by decreasing myocardial oxygen demand and coronary vasodilation, and restoring myocardial perfusion using percutaneous coronary interventions (PCI) and coronary artery bypass grafting (CABG). Although significant advances have reduced the mortality

From: *Contemporary Cardiology: Angiogenesis and Direct Myocardial Revasularization*
Edited by: R. J. Laham and D. S. Baim © Humana Press Inc., Totowa, NJ

of cardiovascular disease, the number of cardiac interventions continues to grow: a total of 1.3 million inpatient cardiac catheterizations, 561,000 percutaneous transluminal coronary angioplasty (PTCA) procedures, and 519,000 coronary artery bypass procedures were performed in 2000 in the United States alone (1). This is because atherosclerotic disease is progressive and the effects of many cardiovascular procedures are not permanent. Finally, the cost of cardiovascular diseases and stroke in the United States in 2004 was estimated at $368.4 billion. This figure includes health expenditures and lost productivity resulting from morbidity and mortality.

In addition, ischemic heart disease remains the leading cause of congestive heart failure (CHF), which has reached epidemic proportion in the United States. Based on the 44-yr follow-up of the National Heart, Lung, and Blood Institute's (NHLBI) Framingham Heart Study, CHF incidence approaches 10 per 1000 population after age 65, with 22% of male and 46% of female myocardial infarction patients becoming disabled with heart failure. Hospital discharges for CHF rose from 377,000 in 1979 to 995,000 in 2001 (1).

A significant number of patients (5–21%) with ischemic heart disease are not optimal candidates for revascularization (PCI/CABG) or receive incomplete revascularizations with these procedures (2–6), and many have residual angina despite maximal medical therapy. Thus, an alternative treatment strategy is needed, and therapeutic angiogenesis may play that role by providing new venues for blood flow (7–18). Similarly, a significant number of patients with peripheral vascular disease (5%) have residual symptoms despite medical and surgical therapy and may benefit from such therapy (17,19–24). Furthermore, CHF is a progressive disease that results from irreversible myocyte loss and may benefit from strategies that would enable myocyte regeneration, i.e., myogenesis.

However, it is important first to define the target patient population for such therapies and to discuss available and experimental strategies that may provide relief to these patients, more commonly known as "no-option" patients. In this chapter we will concentrate on end-stage ischemic heart disease, since it is the most widely studied, and discuss therapeutic options not covered in this book.

NO-OPTION PATIENTS

An increasing number of patients are no longer candidates for percutaneous or surgical revascularization or have exhausted or failed these modalities. In a study of 500 patients at the Cleveland Clinic, 59 patients

Table 1
Conditions Resulting in No-Option Status

Condition	Incidence (%)
Recurrent in-stent restenosis	24
Prohibitive expected failure	28
Chronic total occlusion	29
Poor targets for coronary artery bypass grafting/ percutaneous coronary intervention	50
Saphenous graft total occlusion with patent left internal mammary artery graft to left anterior descending artery	28
Degenerated saphenous vein grafts	15
No conduits/calcified aorta	5
Comorbidities	3

(12%) were considered ineligible for PCI/CABG, a study commonly cited to describe this patient population (6,25,26). However, wide regional and institutional variability in treatment patterns of coronary disease including more or less aggressive revascularization practices contributes to different estimates of the magnitude of the problem, ranging from 5 to 21% of patients with CAD. Table 1 details the most common underlying reasons for residual unrevascularized yet ischemic myocardial territories.

Current management strategies for these patients are limited. Medications used concomitantly to help control symptoms include antiplatelet agents, nitrates, β-blockers, angiotensin-converting enzyme inhibitors, angiotensin II receptor blockers, and calcium channel blockers, and many patients continue to have symptoms on maximal medical therapy. The treatment of these patients is also a moving target since advances in interventional and surgical techniques have helped improve their quality of life. Most notably, the development of drug (e.g., sirolimus, paclitaxel)-eluting stents has all but solved the problem of recurrent restenosis (27–34).

ADVANCED REVASCULARIZATION STRATEGIES AND ANGIOGENESIS

The eligibility of patients for percutaneous or surgical revascularization is subject to wide geographic and institutional variability, highlighting differing practice patterns and offering patients referrals to advanced coronary revascularization centers. In addition, the development of various procedures such as endovascular cardiopulmonary bypass (35), rotational atherectomy for calcified undilatable lesions *(36,37)*, distal protection for vein graft interventions *(38–40)*, and chronic total occlusion wires and devices *(41)* has made possible the treatment of many patients previously deemed to be no-option. Figures 1–3 illustrate the advanced treatment of patients with undilatable lesions, chronic total occlusion, and degenerated vein grafts using rotational atherectomy, a frontrunner total occlusion catheter, and balloon distal protection. Thus, prior to considering experimental therapies in these patients, consideration of advanced intervention or referral to an aggressive revascularization program is warranted.

If all these options are exhausted, then patients are deemed truly without any options and alternative treatment strategies are needed. Therapeutic angiogenesis may provide a treatment strategy for these patients by providing new venues for blood flow. Angiogenesis is a complex process that involves stimulation of endothelial cell proliferation and migration, stimulation of extracellular matrix breakdown, attraction of pericytes and macrophages, stimulation of smooth muscle cell proliferation and migration, formation and "sealing" of new vascular structures, and deposition of new matrix *(7–12,15,16,42–45)*. It is likely that coordinated action of several mitogens and cascades is needed to achieve this process. Gradual occlusion of coronary arteries is frequently associated with development of collateral circulation in patients with atherosclerosis (Fig. 4) *(7–9,12,15–17,24,42,43,45–48)*. Although the existence of collateral circulation in such patients is associated with improved clinical outcomes, the net effect is rarely adequate to compensate fully for the flow lost as the result of the occlusion of native epicardial coronary arteries. The large number of revascularization procedures performed attests to the inadequacy of native collateralization. Myocardial ischemia is a potent angiogenic stimulus, and a number of growth factors have been isolated from ischemic myocardium, suggesting that these molecules may play a role in ischemia-induced angiogenesis. Among these growth factors, fibroblast growth factors (acidic [aFGF] and basic [bFGF]) and vascular endothelial growth factor (VEGF) are the most widely studied. Although often referred to as angiogenesis, the process of neovascularization can occur via three different mechanisms: vasculogenesis, angiogenesis, and arteriogenesis. Vasculogenesis is the formation of new vascular structures from stem cells during embryogenesis and may contribute to adult neovascularization *(49,50)*. Angiogenesis refers to the formation of thin-walled endothelium-lined structures lacking a smooth muscle layer from preexisting vessels (sprouting from postcapillary venules). For example, angiogenesis is the manner by which capillaries proliferate in healing wounds and along the border of

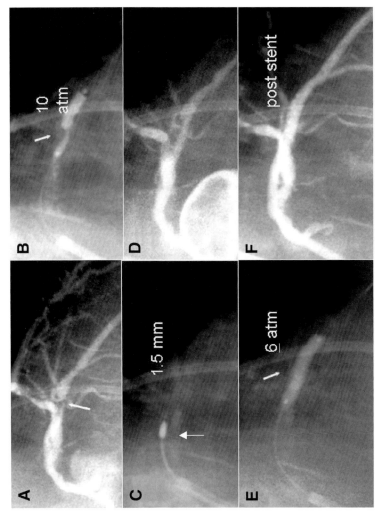

Fig. 1. Seventy-five-year-old patient with angina, severe left anterior descending disease, and a calcified aorta and coronary arteries. (A) Ninety percent left anterior descending disease (arrow). (B) Balloon inflated to 10 atm with inability to dilate lesion due to extensive calcification. (C) Rotational atherectomy using a 1.5-mm Burr (arrow). (D) Postatheretomy angiogram showing residual stenosis. (E, F) Dilatation with a balloon followed by stenting yields an excellent result.

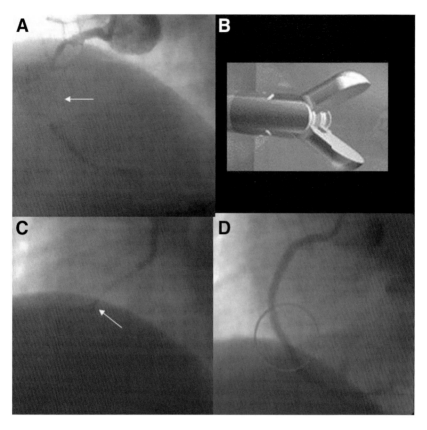

Fig. 2. Use of frontrunner (**B**) blunt dissection device for chronic total occlusion. (**A**) Angiography shows a chronically occluded right coronary artery, which could not be crossed using standard wires. (**C**) Frontrunner catheter (arrow) is used to cross the occlusion, which is stented (**D**), resulting in 0% residual stenosis.

myocardial infarctions. Arteriogenesis is the formation of vessels with a complete smooth muscle wall as seen in the development of angiographically visible collaterals in patients with advanced obstructive arterial disease. Arteriogenesis is believed to result from remodeling of existing collateral vessels as well as formation of new vessels (not well established). In addition, significant variability has been observed in intrinsic angiogenesis, with some patients having robust collaterals while others have none. The lack of an adequate angiogenic response may be related in part to reduced production of angiogenic factors or resistance to these factors. Comorbidities such as diabetes and hypercholesterolemia commonly accompany atherosclerotic occlusive disease.

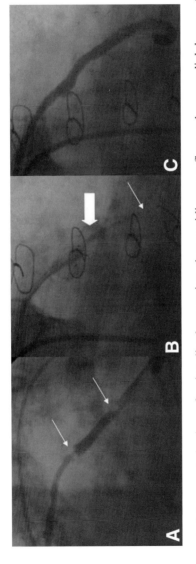

Fig. 3. Treatment of degenerated vein graft using distal protection, thus avoiding no reflow and myocardial damage. (**A**) Saphenous vein bypass graft to left circumflex with serial stenoses (arrows). (**B**) Distal protection balloon is used to occlude the graft (arrow), while a stent is placed and deployed (block arrow) followed by removal of debris and excellent angiographic result with normal flow (**C**).

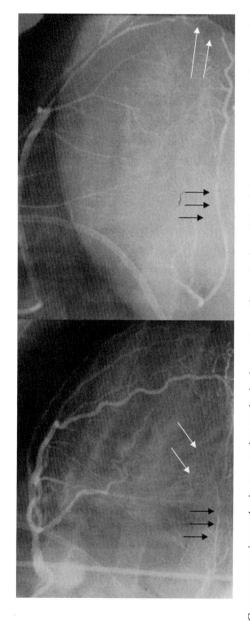

Fig. 4. Coronary angiography in two patients who had asymptomatic occlusion of the right coronary artery with extensive collaterals from the left coronary system. The right coronary artery (black arrows) fills by intramyocardial collaterals (left, white arrows) or large-bore epicardial collaterals (right, white arrows), underscoring the native collateralization process.

These conditions have been associated with decreased growth factor production *(51,52)*, and may contribute to the marginal results seen in clinical trials of therapeutic angiogenesis *(53)*.

Our group investigated the effect of endothelial dysfunction secondary to hypercholesterolemia on therapeutic angiogenesis. In a pig model of chronic myocardial ischemia, animals were fed either a high-cholesterol or a normal diet. Four weeks after placement of an ameroid constrictor on the left coronary circumflex artery, FGF-2 loaded in heparin alginate beads for slow release was implanted in the circumflex territory. The hypercholesterolemic group showed significant endothelial dysfunction and impaired angiogenesis manifest as decreased circumflex perfusion compared to the control, normal diet group. FGF receptor-1 expression was upregulated in the control group, but decreased in the hypercholesterolemic animals *(54)*. Decreased production of growth factors may contribute to a lack of compensatory neovascularization in some patients with ischemic cardiovascular disease.

A number of growth factors have been evaluated for their angiogenic potential including fibroblast growth factors, vascular endothelial growth factors, hepatocyte growth/scatter factor (HGF/SF), chemokines such as interleukin (IL)-8 and monocyte chemotactic protein (MCP)-1, growth factors involved in maturation of vascular tree such as angiopoietins and platelet-derived growth factor (PDGF) *(34,35)*, as well as transcription factors that stimulate expression of angiogenic cytokines and their receptors such as hypoxia-induced factor (HIF)-1α.

The problems that must be surmounted to achieve successful angiogenesis are detailed throughout the text, but they will be briefly discussed here. As with any biological therapy, the necessary steps are understanding the biology, developing therapeutic agents and vectors, site-specific delivery of therapeutic agents, and developing outcome measures to evaluate the benefits of the therapeutic intervention. Most of these will be discussed in separate chapters, but significant advances must be made in each step prior to achieving successful and functional angiogenesis. This problem is confounded by a very powerful placebo effect in this patient population, necessitating blinded studies and more powerful imaging and outcome measures to detect the small benefits expected with such therapies. All these will be discussed in detail in the ensuing chapters.

ALTERNATIVE TREATMENT STRATEGIES

For the sake of completeness, it is important to discuss three treatment modalities that could be offered to no-option patients with angina: spinal cord stimulation, extracorporeal counterpulsation, and metabolic modulation with ranolazine and trimetazidine.

Spinal Cord Stimulation

Spinal cord stimulation (SCS) has been proposed as a novel treatment strategy that may be effective in end-stage ischemic heart disease patients with intractable angina. The efficacy of spinal cord stimulation on the relief of otherwise intractable angina pectoris was studied in a 2-mo randomized study with 1-yr follow-up by quality-of-life parameters, cardiac parameters, and complications. Twenty-four patients were randomized to either an actively treated group A (12 patients received the device within a 2-wk period) or a control group B (10 patients had implantation after the study period). Spinal cord stimulation improved both quality-of-life and cardiac parameters. The latter included a trend towards reduction in ischemia after implantation of the device in both exercise testing with a treadmill (ETT) and 24-h ambulatory Holter recordings, with a concomitant improvement in exercise capacity *(55)*. Indices of ischemia were studied with and without SCS in 10 patients with otherwise intractable angina and evidence of myocardial ischemia on 48-h ambulatory electrocardiograph (ECG) recording. During SCS, the total ischemic burden of the entire group was significantly reduced from a median of 27.9 (1.9–278.2) before SCS to 0 (0–70.2) mm × min with SCS ($p < 0.03$) *(56)*.

The efficacy of SCS as a treatment for chronic intractable angina pectoris was further studied for 6 wk in 13 treated patients and 12 control patients with chronic angina. Assessments were exercise capacity and ischemia, daily frequency of anginal attacks and nitrate tablet consumption, and quality of life. Compared with control, exercise duration ($p = 0.03$) and time to angina ($p = 0.01$) increased; anginal attacks and sublingual nitrate consumption ($p = 0.01$) and ischemic episodes on 48-h electrocardiogram ($p = 0.04$) decreased. ST-segment depression on the exercise electrocardiogram decreased at comparable workload ($p = 0.01$). Anginal attacks and consumption of sublingual nitrates decreased ($p = 0.01$), perceived quality of life increased ($p = 0.03$), and pain decreased ($p = 0.01$) *(57)*. Nineteen consecutive patients implanted for spinal cord stimulation were studied. Annual admission rate after revascularization was 0.97/patient/yr, compared with 0.27 after spinal cord stimulation ($p = 0.02$). Mean time in hospital/patient/yr after revascularization was 8.3 vs 2.5 d after spinal cord stimulation ($p = 0.04$) *(58)*. A major unanswered question regarding SCS is whether its effect is predominantly the result of a placebo effect and whether it is indeed a revascularization strategy, or if it only provides symptomatic relief without any effects on survival, myocardial infarction, need for repeat revascularization, or left-ventricular function. These questions are being answered in a randomized Medtronic-sponsored study and in a planned ANS study.

Enhanced External Counterpulsation

Enhanced external counterpulsation (EECP) is an approved device for use in patients with disabling, chronic angina as well as heart failure. The device comprises inflatable cuffs that encompass the calf, thigh, and upper thigh and squeeze sequentially from low to high during diastole and then rapidly and simultaneously deflate at the onset of systole, with ECG gating. The arterial hemodynamics generated by EECP may simulate intra-aortic balloon pump counterpulsation with the generation of a retrograde arterial wave pulse. The usual course of treatment is 35 1-h sessions. This treatment modality has flourished on the fringes of mainstream academic cardiology, with most patients treated in the office setting, and has been supported by several registries and randomized clinical trials *(59–64)*. The International EECP Patient Registry (IEPR) was started in 1998 and fashioned on the basis of the NHLBI angioplasty registry in order to study the outcome of patients undergoing EECP *(64)*. This study investigated the long-term outcomes of EECP in relieving angina and improving the quality of life in a large cohort of patients with chronic angina pectoris. Seventy-three percent had a reduction by ≥ 1 angina class at the end of treatment, and 50% reported an improvement in quality-of-life assessment. However, there has been only one randomized, placebo-controlled trial to study the effect and safety of EECP in patients with chronic angina *(65)*. One hundred and thirty-nine patients were enrolled and had differing pressures applied to the cuffs, raising serious concerns about adequate blinding. Both groups had improvement in exercise duration, with the active group exercising longer (not statistically significant). The active group did show a statistically significant improvement in time to ST-segment depression. These effects were less impressive than were found for patients in the registry *(65)*. We believe that available data are not robust enough to support widespread use of EECP, but it remains an alternative yet unproven treatment strategy for no-option patients.

Metabolic Modulation

Considerable progress has been made over the last 25 yr in expanding the therapeutic options available in ischemic heart disease, including both pharmacological and interventional measures that improve symptoms and prognosis. However, many patients continue to experience intractable symptoms despite being on "optimal" medical therapy. In addition, an increasing number of patients, particularly elderly ones, are deemed unsuitable for coronary revascularization. A novel medical treatment would be particularly beneficial in relieving the significant morbidity that exists in this group.

The modes of action of most prophylactic antianginal agents involve hemodynamic changes, such as a reduction in systemic vascular resistance, coronary vasodilatation, or negative inotropism, thus improving the imbalance in myocardial oxygen supply and demand. Recently it has become apparent that certain antianginal treatments exert a primarily metabolic action and have little or no effect on coronary hemodynamics. These drugs have considerable potential as adjunctive therapy for angina, particularly in patients refractory to standard therapies, and may be a primary therapeutic option in certain circumstances. They generally do not adversely affect blood pressure, pulse rate, or left ventricular systolic function, offering a significant advantage in patients in whom conventional agents may induce symptomatic hypotension, inappropriate bradycardia, or worsening heart failure. The purpose of this review is to draw attention to some of these "metabolic" agents, while at the same time surveying the current level of evidence supporting their clinical use and mode of action. Two commonly used treatments for ischemic heart disease that also exert metabolic effects have been included (β-blockers and glucose–insulin–potassium).

Myocardial Metabolism

Under aerobic conditions, the predominant substrate used by the normal adult human heart are free fatty acids, accounting for 60–90% of the energy generated *(66–71)*. Carbohydrate metabolism, on the other hand, contributes only about 10–40% of energy generated by the healthy adult human heart *(66–71)*. Glucose taken up by the myocardial cell is either stored as glycogen or converted into pyruvate by glycolysis. Pyruvate is then oxidized within the mitochondria by pyruvate dehydrogenase into acetyl CoA.

In contrast to the adult heart, the fetal heart (which operates under hypoxic conditions) uses glucose as its predominant fuel. The energetic advantages of incremental glucose utilization arise from the fact that though fatty acid oxidation yields more ATP than glycolysis in aerobic conditions, this occurs at the expense of greater oxygen consumption. Fatty acids require approx 10–15% more oxygen to generate an equivalent amount of ATP when compared to glucose. Two drugs, trimetazidine (available in Europe) and ranolazine (studied in the United States and

Europe), are p-FOX inhibitors, which inhibit fatty acid metabolism and promote glycolysis, potentially making the heart more energy efficient. Several clinical trials have demonstrated the potential benefits of trimetazidine in ischemic heart disease *(66–69)*. However, a large, randomized, placebo-controlled trial recruiting 19,725 patients with acute myocardial infarction did not demonstrate short- or long-term mortality benefit *(72,73)*. More recently, a small, double-blind, randomized, placebo-controlled study demonstrated improved exercise capacity and ST-segment depression during post-myocardial infarction exercise testing *(74)*.

Ranolazine *(66,67,70,71)* is a substituted piperazine compound similar to trimetazidine. On the basis of recently completed phase 3 clinical trials, it appears to offer considerable potential.

The Monotherapy Assessment of Ranolazine in Stable Angina (MARISA) study *(75)* is a randomized, double-blind, crossover study that evaluated 191 patients with chronic stable angina given ranolazine as monotherapy following withdrawal of all other antianginal drugs. During follow-up ETT, patients had a significantly longer time to angina and 1-mm ST-segment depression while on ranolazine than with placebo.

The Combination Assessment of Ranolazine in Stable Angina (CARISA) trial *(70)* studied 823 patients with chronic stable angina on background antianginal therapy of either a β-blocker or calcium-channel blocker who were randomized to either ranolazine (750 or 1000 mg twice daily) or placebo. At follow-up ETT, patients randomized to ranolazine had a significantly increased duration of exercise, time to onset of ST-segment depression, and time to angina, while also reporting fewer weekly angina episodes when compared to the placebo group. There was a minor prolongation of QT interval in the ranolazine group. Both the MARISA and CARISA clinical trials offer encouraging data and indicate that ranolazine has a significant antianginal effect both as monotherapy and in combination with other antianginal agents. However, its long-term safety, particularly in relation to QT prolongation, remains to be established; in addition, enrollment in the pivotal CARISA study was predominantly in Eastern Europe, where the pattern of CAD treatment differs significantly from the US standard. Thus, metabolic antianginal therapies induce a shift from utilization by the myocardium of free fatty acid to predominantly glucose to increase ATP generation per unit oxygen consumption. These promising results have yet to be proven in large-scale clinical trials.

ACKNOWLEDGMENT

Supported in part by NIH grant HL 63609 (RJL).

REFERENCES

1. American Heart Association. AHA statistics. (http://www.americanheart.org/presenter.jhtml?identifier=4478).
2. McNeer JF, Conley MJ, Starmer CF, et al. Complete and incomplete revascularization at aortocoronary bypass surgery: experience with 392 consecutive patients. Am Heart J 1974;88(2):176–182.
3. Jones EL, Craver JM, Guyton RA, et al. Importance of complete revascularization in performance of the coronary bypass operation. Am J Cardiol 1983;51(1):7–12.
4. Atwood JE, Myers J, Colombo A, et al. The effect of complete and incomplete revascularization on exercise variables in patients undergoing coronary angioplasty. Clin Cardiol 1990;13(2):89–93.
5. de Feyter PJ. PTCA in patients with stable angina pectoris and multivessel disease: is incomplete revascularization acceptable? Clin Cardiol 1992;15(5):317–322.
6. Mukherjee D, Bhatt DL, Roe MT, Patel V, Ellis SG. Direct myocardial revascularization and angiogenesis—how many patients might be eligible? Am J Cardiol 1999;84(5):598–600, A8.
7. Laham RJ, Simons M, Tofukuji M, Hung D, Sellke FW. Modulation of myocardial perfusion and vascular reactivity by pericardial basic fibroblast growth factor: insight into ischemia-induced reduction in endothelium-dependent vasodilatation. J Thorac Cardiovasc Surg 1998;116(6):1022–1028.
8. Laham RJ, Simons M, Sellke F. Gene transfer for angiogenesis in coronary artery disease. Annu Rev Med 2001;52:485–502.
9. Laham RJ, Simons M. Growth Factor Therapy in Ischemic Heart Disease. In: Rubanyi G, ed. Angiogenesis in Health and Disease. New York: Marcel Decker, 2000:451–475.
10. Laham RJ, Post M, Sellke FW, Simons M. Therapeutic angiogenesis using local perivascular and pericardial delivery. Curr Interv Cardiol Rep 2000;2(3):213–217.
11. Laham RJ, Rezaee M, Post M, et al. Intracoronary and intravenous administration of basic fibroblast growth factor: myocardial and tissue distribution. Drug Metab Dispos 1999;27(7):821–826.
12. Laham RJ, Oettgen P. Bone marrow transplantation for the heart: fact or fiction? Lancet 2003;361(9351):11–12.
13. Laham RJ, Hung D, Simons M. Therapeutic myocardial angiogenesis using percutaneous intrapericardial drug delivery. Clin Cardiol 1999;22(1 Suppl 1):I-6–9.
14. Laham RJ, Garcia L, Baim DS, Post M, Simons M. Therapeutic angiogenesis using basic fibroblast growth factor and vascular endothelial growth factor using various delivery strategies. Curr Interv Cardiol Rep 1999;1(3):228–233.
15. Laham RJ, Chronos NA, Pike M, et al. Intracoronary basic fibroblast growth factor (FGF-2) in patients with severe ischemic heart disease: results of a phase I open-label dose escalation study. J Am Coll Cardiol 2000;36(7):2132–2139.
16. Laham R, Rezaee M, Post M, et al. Intrapericardial delivery of fibroblast growth factor-2 induces neovascularization in a porcine model of chronic myocardial ischemia. J Pharmacol Exp Ther 2000;292:795–802.
17. Isner JM. Angiogenesis for revascularization of ischaemic tissues [editorial]. Eur Heart J 1997;18(1):1–2.
18. Isner JM, Pieczek A, Schainfeld R, et al. Clinical evidence of angiogenesis after arterial gene transfer of phVEGF165 in patient with ischaemic limb. Lancet 1996;348(9024):370–374.
19. Asahara T, Bauters C, Zheng LP, et al. Synergistic effect of vascular endothelial growth factor and basic fibroblast growth factor on angiogenesis in vivo. Circulation 1995;92(9 Suppl):II365–371.

20. Baumgartner I, Rauh G, Pieczek A, et al. Lower-extremity edema associated with gene transfer of naked DNA encoding vascular endothelial growth factor. Ann Intern Med 2000;132(11):880–884.
21. Bauters C, Asahara T, Zheng LP, et al. Physiological assessment of augmented vascularity induced by VEGF in ischemic rabbit hindlimb. Am J Physiol 1994;267:H1263–1271.
22. Bauters C, Asahara T, Zheng LP, et al. Site-specific therapeutic angiogenesis after systemic administration of vascular endothelial growth factor. J Vasc Surg 1995;21(2):314–325.
23. Isner JM, Feldman LJ. Gene therapy for arterial disease. Lancet 1994;344(8938): 1653–1654.
24. Isner JM. Therapeutic angiogenesis: a new frontier for vascular therapy. Vasc Med 1996;1(1):79–87.
25. Hennebry TA, Saucedo JF. "No-pption" patients: a nightmare today, a future with hope. J Inv Cardiol 2004;17(2):93–94.
26. Rosinberg A, Khan TA, Sellke FW, Laham RJ. Therapeutic angiogenesis for myocardial ischemia. Expert Rev Cardiovasc Ther 2004;2(2):271–283.
27. Waugh J, Wagstaff AJ. The paclitaxel (TAXUS)-eluting stent: a review of its use in the management of de novo coronary artery lesions. Am J Cardiovasc Drugs 2004;4(4):257–268.
28. Doggrell SA. Sirolimus- versus paclitaxel-eluting stents in patients with stenosis in a native coronary artery. Expert Opin Pharmacother 2004;5(6):1431–1434.
29. Grube E, Gerckens U, Muller R, Bullesfeld L. Drug eluting stents: initial experiences. Z Kardiol 2002;91(Suppl 3):44–48.
30. Wong A, Chan C. Drug-eluting stents: the end of restenosis? Ann Acad Med Singapore 2004;33(4):423–431.
31. Serruys PW, Lemos PA, van Hout BA. Sirolimus eluting stent implantation for patients with multivessel disease: rationale for the Arterial Revascularisation Therapies Study part II (ARTS II). Heart 2004;90(9):995–998.
32. McClure S, Webb J. Drug-eluting stents and saphenous vein graft intervention. J Invasive Cardiol 2004;16(5):234–235.
33. Hoye A, Tanabe K, Lemos PA, et al. Significant reduction in restenosis after the use of sirolimus-eluting stents in the treatment of chronic total occlusions. J Am Coll Cardiol 2004;43(11):1954–1958.
34. Grube E, Buellesfeld L. Everolimus for stent-based intracoronary applications. Rev Cardiovasc Med 2004;5(Suppl 2):S3–8.
35. Reichenspurner H, Boehm DH, Welz A, et al. Minimally invasive coronary artery bypass grafting: port-access approach versus off-pump techniques. Ann Thorac Surg 1998;66(3):1036–1040.
36. Medina A, de Lezo JS, Melian F, Hernandez E, Pan M, Romero M. Successful stent ablation with rotational atherectomy. Catheter Cardiovasc Interv 2003;60(4):501–504.
37. Mauri L, Reisman M, Buchbinder M, et al. Comparison of rotational atherectomy with conventional balloon angioplasty in the prevention of restenosis of small coronary arteries: results of the Dilatation vs Ablation Revascularization Trial Targeting Restenosis (DART). Am Heart J 2003;145(5):847–854.
38. Lev E, Teplitsky I, Fuchs S, Shor N, Assali A, Kornowski R. Clinical experiences using the FilterWire EX for distal embolic protection during complex percutaneous coronary interventions. Int J Cardiovasc Intervent 2004;6(1):28–32.
39. Stone GW, Rogers C, Hermiller J, et al. Randomized comparison of distal protection with a filter-based catheter and a balloon occlusion and aspiration system during percutaneous intervention of diseased saphenous vein aorto-coronary bypass grafts. Circulation 2003;108(5):548–553.

40. Baim DS, Wahr D, George B, et al. Randomized trial of a distal embolic protection device during percutaneous intervention of saphenous vein aorto-coronary bypass grafts. Circulation 2002;105(11):1285–1290.
41. Tadros P. Successful revascularization of a long chronic total occlusion of the right coronary artery utilizing the frontrunner X39 CTO catheter system. J Invasive Cardiol 2003;15(11):3.
42. Laham RJ, Simons M, Pearlman JD, Ho KK, Baim DS. Magnetic resonance imaging demonstrates improved regional systolic wall motion and thickening and myocardial perfusion of myocardial territories treated by laser myocardial revascularization. J Am Coll Cardiol 2002;39(1):1–8.
43. Laham RJ, Simons M. Basic fibroblast growth factor protein for coronary artery disease. In: Handbook of Myocardial Revascularization and Angiogenesis. New York: Martin Dunitz Ltd, 1999:175–187.
44. Laham RJ, Mannam A, Post MJ, Sellke F. Gene transfer to induce angiogenesis in myocardial and limb ischaemia. Expert Opin Biol Ther 2001;1(6):985–994.
45. Laham R, Sellke F, Pearlman J. Magnetic resonance blood-arrival maps provides acccurate assessment of myocardial perfusion and collaterization in therapeutic angiogenesis. Circulation 1998;98:I–373.
46. Folkman J, Shing Y. Angiogenesis. J Biol Chem 1992;267:10931–10934.
47. Folkman J. Angiogenic therapy of the human heart. Circulation 1998;97(7):628–629.
48. Folkman J. Therapeutic angiogenesis in ischemic limbs. Circulation 1998;97(12): 1108–1010.
49. Asahara T, Murohara T, Sullivam A, et al. Isolation of putative progenitor endothelial cells for angiogenesis. Science 1997;275:964–967.
50. Asahara T, Isner JM. Endothelial progenitor cells for vascular regeneration. J Hematother Stem Cell Res 2002;11(2):171–178.
51. Rivard A, Silver M, Chen D, et al. Rescue of diabetes-related impairment of angiogenesis by intramuscular gene therapy with adeno-VEGF. Am J Pathol 1999;154(2):355–363.
52. Couffinhal T, Silver M, Kearney M, et al. Impaired collateral vessel development associated with reduced expression of vascular endothelial growth factor in ApoE -/- mice. Circulation 1999;99(24):3188–3198.
53. Simons M, Bonow RO, Chronos NA, et al. Clinical trials in coronary angiogenesis: issues, problems, consensus: an expert panel summary. Circulation 2000;102(11):E73–86.
54. Ruel M, Wu GF, Khan TA, et al. Inhibition of the cardiac angiogenic response to surgical FGF-2 therapy in a swine endothelial dysfunction model. Circulation 2003;108(Suppl 1):II335–340.
55. de Jongste MJ, Staal MJ. Preliminary results of a randomized study on the clinical efficacy of spinal cord stimulation for refractory severe angina pectoris. Acta Neurochir Suppl (Wien) 1993;58:161–164.
56. de Jongste MJ, Haaksma J, Hautvast RW, et al. Effects of spinal cord stimulation on myocardial ischaemia during daily life in patients with severe coronary artery disease. A prospective ambulatory electrocardiographic study. Br Heart J 1994;71(5):413–418.
57. Hautvast RW, DeJongste MJ, Staal MJ, van Gilst WH, Lie KI. Spinal cord stimulation in chronic intractable angina pectoris: a randomized, controlled efficacy study. Am Heart J 1998;136(6):1114–1120.
58. Murray S, Carson KG, Ewings PD, Collins PD, James MA. Spinal cord stimulation significantly decreases the need for acute hospital admission for chest pain in patients with refractory angina pectoris. Heart 1999;82(1):89–92.

59. Linnemeier G, Rutter MK, Barsness G, Kennard ED, Nesto RW. Enhanced external counterpulsation for the relief of angina in patients with diabetes: safety, efficacy and 1-year clinical outcomes. Am Heart J 2003;146(3):453–458.
60. Linnemeier G, Michaels AD, Soran O, Kennard ED. Enhanced external counterpulsation in the management of angina in the elderly. Am J Geriatr Cardiol 2003;12(2):90–96.
61. Humphreys DR. Treating angina with EECP therapy. Nurse Pract 2003;28(2):7.
62. Blazing MA, Crawford LE. Enhanced external counterpulsation (EECP): enough evidence to support this and the next wave? Am Heart J 2003;146(3):383–384.
63. Michaels AD, Accad M, Ports TA, Grossman W. Left ventricular systolic unloading and augmentation of intracoronary pressure and Doppler flow during enhanced external counterpulsation. Circulation 2002;106(10):1237–1242.
64. Michaels AD, Linnemeier G, Soran O, Kelsey SF, Kennard ED. Two-year outcomes after enhanced external counterpulsation for stable angina pectoris (from the International EECP Patient Registry [IEPR]). Am J Cardiol 2004;93(4):461–464.
65. Arora RR, Chou TM, Jain D, et al. The multicenter study of enhanced external counterpulsation (MUST-EECP): effect of EECP on exercise-induced myocardial ischemia and anginal episodes. J Am Coll Cardiol 1999;33(7):1833–1840.
66. Lee L, Horowitz J, Frenneaux M. Metabolic manipulation in ischaemic heart disease, a novel approach to treatment. Eur Heart J 2004;25(8):634–641.
67. Pauly DF, Pepine CJ. Ischemic heart disease: metabolic approaches to management. Clin Cardiol 2004;27(8):439–441.
68. Slavov S, Djunlieva M, Ilieva S, Galabov B. Quantitative structure-activity relationship analysis of the substituent effects on the binding affinity of derivatives of trimetazidine. Arzneimittelforschung 2004;54(1):9–14.
69. Feola M, Biggi A, Francini A, et al. Trimetazidine improves myocardial perfusion and left ventricular function in ischemic left ventricular dysfunction. Clin Nucl Med 2004;29(2):117–118.
70. Chaitman BR, Pepine CJ, Parker JO, et al. Effects of ranolazine with atenolol, amlodipine, or diltiazem on exercise tolerance and angina frequency in patients with severe chronic angina: a randomized controlled trial. JAMA 2004;291(3):309–316.
71. Louis AA, Manousos IR, Coletta AP, Clark AL, Cleland JG. Clinical trials update: The Heart Protection Study, IONA, CARISA, ENRICHD, ACUTE, ALIVE, MADIT II and REMATCH. Impact of Nicorandil on Angina. Combination Assessment of Ranolazine in Stable Angina. ENhancing Recovery in Coronary Heart Disease Patients. Assessment of Cardioversion Using Transoesophageal Echocardiography. AzimiLide post-Infarct surVival Evaluation. Randomised Evaluation of Mechanical Assistance for Treatment of Chronic Heart failure. Eur J Heart Fail 2002;4(1):111–116.
72. Marzilli M, Mariani M. About EMIP-FR and reperfusion damage in AMI: a comment to the comment. Eur Heart J 2001;22(11):973–975; author reply 978.
73. Effect of 48-h intravenous trimetazidine on short- and long-term outcomes of patients with acute myocardial infarction, with and without thrombolytic therapy; a double-blind, placebo-controlled, randomized trial. The EMIP-FR Group. European Myocardial Infarction Project—Free Radicals. Eur Heart J 2000;21(18):1537–1546.
74. Guler N, Eryonucu B, Gunes A, Guntekin U, Tuncer M, Ozbek H. Effects of trimetazidine on submaximal exercise test in patients with acute myocardial infarction. Cardiovasc Drugs Ther 2003;17(4):371–374.
75. Chaitman BR, Skettino SL, Parker JO, et al. Anti-ischemic effects and long-term survival during ranolazine monotherapy in patients with chronic severe angina. J Am Coll Cardiol 2004;43(8):1375–1382.

2

Transcriptional Regulation of Angiogenesis

Peter Oettgen

CONTENTS

From: *Contemporary Cardiology: Angiogenesis and Direct Myocardial Revasularization*
Edited by: R. J. Laham and D. S. Baim © Humana Press Inc., Totowa, NJ

INTRODUCTION

Until recently, the transcription factors necessary for regulating vascular development were largely unknown. This is in sharp contrast with other developmental processes, such as hematopoiesis and myogenesis, in which several cell- or tissue-specific transcription factors have been identified. Vascular development requires the differentiation of endothelial cells from pluripotent stem cells. Progress in identifying the molecular mechanisms underlying vascular development has lagged considerably, in large part the model systems for studying vascular blood vessel development are more limited. The identification of several vascular-specific genes involved in vasculogenesis and the genomic regulatory regions required for directing their expression over the past decade has facilitated the identification of the transcriptional mechanisms required for vascular-specific gene expression. Targeted disruption of additional transcription factors that have been associated with vascular defects led to the elucidation of a role for these factors in vascular development. Angiogenesis, the development of additional blood vessels from a primary vascular network, may recapitulate many of the molecular events occurring during vascular development.

ANIMAL MODELS OF VASCULAR DEVELOPMENT

One of the major difficulties in identifying the specific transcription factors involved in regulating vascular-specific gene expression, particularly as it relates to blood vessel development, is the difficulty in isolating either embryonic or extraembryonic blood vessels during mouse embryogenesis. Because the process of blood vessel development is highly conserved over evolution, the use of alternate model systems has permitted easier access to studying blood vessel development. Two animal models that have been particularly useful for these studies are the developing zebrafish and chicken. Both have the advantages of allowing direct visualization of blood vessels. Two genes that have been identified in zebrafish and appear to be critical early regulators for initiating vascular development are *cloche* and *spade tail (1)*. Similarly, the stem cell leukemia transcription factor, SCL, was also shown to promote vasculogenesis, hematopoiesis, and endothelial differentiation when expressed ectopically in zebrafish mesoderm *(2)*. The ETS transcription factor Fli-1 has also been shown to be enriched in the developing blood vessels of zebrafish embryos *(3)*. As an alternative model of blood vessel development, several investigators have used the developing chicken because of the easier access to developing blood vessels, particularly in the extraembryonic chorioallantoic membrane.

These blood vessels can be microdissected at different stages of development, facilitating the determination of whether specific genes are upregulated or enriched in developing blood vessels. This approach was used to identify which of the members of the ETS transcription factor family are upregulated during blood vessel development. A novel role for the ETS factor E74-like factor (ELF)-1 in vascular development was identified using this approach *(4)*. *In situ* hybridization and immunohistochemical experiments confirmed the enriched expression of this factor in extraembryonic and embryonic blood vessels of the developing chicken embryo *(4)*. The ETS factor ETS-1 has also been shown to be enriched in the developing blood vessels of the chicken, and antisense oligonucleotides have been shown to inhibit angiogenesis when delivered to the chicken chorioallantoic membrane *(5)*.

CONSERVATION OF TRANSCRIPTION FACTORS INVOLVED IN VASCULAR DEVELOPMENT

One potential criticism of using nonmammalian models to identify the transcription factors involved in regulating blood vessel development is that the same factors may not be evolutionarily conserved. Arguing against this is the fact that studies in the chicken and zebrafish have demonstrated that the factors not only are conserved with regard to protein sequence, but also show a similar enriched expression pattern during vascular development. For example, the helix–loop–helix transcription factor, SCL, is expressed in developing blood vessels and in the vasculature of both the developing mouse and zebrafish *(2,6)*. The ETS factor ELF-1, which has previously been identified for its role for T-cell specific gene expression, has also been shown to be a strong transactivator of the *Tie1* and *Tie2* genes and is highly enriched in developing blood vessels of the developing chicken embryo. The overall homology between the chicken and human ELF-1 protein is 80% *(4)*. Similarly, the ETS factor Fli-1 has recently been shown to be a critical regulator of blood vessel development, not only in zebrafish, but also in the mouse *(3,7)*. *In situ* hybridization studies of the developing mouse have also demonstrated that ETS-1 is expressed in developing blood vessels associated with tumor angiogenesis *(8)*. Targeted disruption of Fli-1 in mice results in a loss of vascular integrity accompanied by bleeding and embryonic lethality at d 11.5 *(7)*. Expression of the *Tie2* gene is also down regulated in these mice. The expression of two GATA factors, GATA-2 and GATA-3, has recently been examined in human fetal tissues. Both factors are enriched in the developing dorsal aorta at 5 wk of age *(9)*.

TRANSCRIPTIONALLY MEDIATED HYPOXIA RESPONSES DURING ANGIOGENESIS AND LATER STAGES OF BLOOD VESSEL DEVELOPMENT

After the development of a primary vascular network, the developing embryo requires the formation of additional blood vessels or angiogenesis. This process is largely driven by hypoxia, which serves as a stimulus for the release of angiogenic growth factors. One of the main classes of transcription factors that promote this process is the basic helix–loop–helix (bHLH) PAS domain family. A prototype member of this family is the arylhydrocarbon-receptor nuclear translocator (ARNT) *(10)*. ARNT forms a heterodimeric complex with another PAS transcription factor, hypoxia-induced factor (HIF)-1α *(11)*. In response to oxygen deprivation, these transcription factors stimulate the expression of such angiogenic factors as vascular endothelial growth factor (VEGF) *(12)*. Targeted disruption of the ARNT gene results in embryonic lethality by d 10.5 *(13)*. Although a primary vascular network forms, the predominant defective angiogenesis occurs in the yolk sac and branchial arches, and overall growth of the embryos is stunted. These defects are similar to those observed in VEGF or tissue factor-deficient mice *(14,15)*. Thus, although the primary vascular network develops, the angiogenic responses to hypoxia are severely impaired. Similar findings are observed in HIF-1α knockout mice in which embryonic lethality occurs by d 10.5 as a result of cardiac and vascular malformations *(16)*. Although neither of these transcription factors is expressed in a vascular-specific way, their roles in angiogenesis and vascular development are primarily related to their ability to stimulate the production of angiogenic factors such as VEGF in response to hypoxia. A third member of this family of transcription factors, endothelial PAS domain protein 1 (EPAS1), was recently identified *(17)*. EPAS is predominantly expressed in endothelial cells and can also heterodimerize with ARNT. Targeted disruption of the EPAS gene has been evaluated by two different groups, resulting in two different phenotypes *(18,19)*. Tian et al. *(18)* detected abnormalities in catecholamine homeostasis in EPAS–/– mice and no distinct abnormalities in blood vessel formation, whereas Peng et al. *(19)* identified vascular defects at later stages of embryogenesis during vascular remodeling in their EPAS–/– mice. The differences in the phenotype cannot be attributed to differences in targeting construct, since both groups disrupted the expression of the bHLH domain, but were more likely attributed to differences in the strain of the mice or subtle differences in the embryonic stem (ES) cells used. Although the formation of a primary vascular network or vasculogenesis occurs, later defects in vascular remodeling are observed during large vessel formation associated with hemorrhaging and the inability of the vessels to fuse properly. This suggests that all three of these PAS family members play a similar role in facilitating later stages of vascular remodeling and angiogenesis in the developing embryo.

Modulation of the function of HIF-1α is also achieved by interaction with other proteins. The transcriptional adapter proteins p300 and CREB-binding protein (CBP) form a multiprotein/DNA complex together with HIF-1α on the promoters of the VEGF and erythropoietin genes to promote expression of these genes in response to hypoxia *(20)*. CBP-deficient mice exhibit abnormalities in both vasculogenesis and angiogenesis *(21)*. In contrast, the von Hippel–Lindau tumor suppressor protein (pVHL) has been shown to promote proteolysis of HIF-1α through ubiquitylation under normoxic conditions. Defective VHL function is associated with cancers that exhibit dysregulated angiogenesis and upregulation of hypoxia inducible genes *(22)*.

The signaling mechanisms by which hypoxia activates HIF-1α are beginning to be elucidated. The catalytic subunit of PI3-kinase, p110, plays a pivotal role in the induction of HIF-1 activity in response to hypoxia *(23)*. Both induction of VEGF gene expression and HIF-1α activity in response to hypoxia could be blocked by the addition of a PI3-kinase inhibitor. Further support of this concept comes from experiments in which VEGF gene expression and HIF-1 activity is induced by cotransfection of p110. Other studies have recently demonstrated that HIF-1α activity may also be modulated by the mitogen-activated protein kinases p42 and p44 *(24)*.

INDUCTION OF ANGIOGENESIS IN THE SETTING OF INFLAMMATION

In addition to hypoxia, inflammation is a potent stimulus of angiogenesis. Inflammation is associated with the release of inflammatory cytokines such as interleukin (IL)-1 β or tumor necrosis factor (TNF)-α. These inflammatory cytokines have been shown to promote the induction of a number of angiogenic growth factors including VEGF, growth factor (FGF), and, more recently angiopoietin-1 (AP-1). The classic transcription factor involved in mediating several inflammatory responses is nuclear factor (NF)-κB. One of the main sources of VEGF in the setting of inflammation is the macrophage. The induction of VEGF in response to inflammatory cytokines in the macrophage has recently been shown to be largely dependent on the activation of NF-κB *(25)*. The regulatory elements responsible for AP-1 gene induction do not contain classical NF-κB sites used for personal communication. In contrast, we have identified a role for the Ets factor ESE-1 as a transcriptional mediator of AP-1 induction in the setting of inflammation. We have previously shown that ESE-1 is induced in a number of cell types in response to inflammatory cytokines and interacts with NF-κB to regulate several genes, including nitric oxide synthase (26). This suggests that the molecular mechanisms by which angiogenic growth factors are activated at the transcriptional level may be very different from those in the setting of hypoxia and that each angiogenic factor is independently regulated at the transcriptional level.

TARGETED DISRUPTION AND OVEREXPRESSION STUDIES OF ADDITIONAL TRANSCRIPTION FACTORS

An alternative approach that has resulted in the identification of other transcription factors required for blood vessel development is through targeted disruption. In many cases this has unexpectedly resulted in determining a novel role for a particular factor in blood vessel development. An example is targeted disruption of the AP-1 transcription factor family member Fra1, which leads to abnormalities in extraembryonic vascularization (27). The zinc finger transcription factor, lung krueppel-like factor (LKLF), is expressed in a variety of vascular and nonvascular cell types. However, targeted disruption of this transcription factor leads to abnormalities in later stages of blood vessel development (28). Although the early events of both angiogenesis and vasculogenesis were normal in LKLF-deficient mice, they develop abnormalities in the smooth muscle architecture of the tunica media, leading to aneurysmal dilatation of the blood vessels with eventual blood vessel rupture. Diminished numbers of endothelial cells, pericytes, and extracellular matrix deposition are also seen. The transcription factor Tfeb, a bHLH transcription factor, was recently shown to be required for vascularization of the placenta (29). The homeobox gene *Hox D3* is induced in endothelial cells in response to basic fibroblast growth factor (bFGF), and antisense oligonucleotides to *Hox D3* block the ability of bFGF to induce urokinase plasminogen activator (uPA). Overexpression of *Hox D3* increases integrin expression in endothelial cells (30). Another homeobox transcription factor that may contribute to both hematopoeisis and endothelial differentiation is hhex. Overexpression of this factor in zebrafish embryos leads to enhanced endothelial and erythroid differentiation (31).

ENDOTHELIAL DIFFERENTIATION

One of the first steps during vascular development is the differentiation of endothelial cells from pluripotent stem cells. This process initially involves the expression of other endothelial-specific markers such as CD31(PECAM-1). VE-cadherin is associated with the differentiation of these cells into mature endothelial cells. The specific transcription factors that mediate these events have not yet been identified. However, because there are conserved binding sites for several of the transcription factors involved in hematopoiesis in the regulatory regions of vascular-specific genes, it is suggested that members of the same transcription factor families are also involved in the process of endothelial differentiation.

Several studies have recently suggested the existence of a common precursor for both endothelial cells and cells of hematopoietic origin. The possible existence of a common precursor was originally suggested because of the close association of hematopoietic cells and endothelial cells in the developing embryos in the so-called blood islands. Hematopoietic and endothelial cells coexpress a number of genes. One of the earliest markers expressed on cells of endothelial and hematopoietic origin is the VEGF receptor *flk-1*. Further support for the existence of the hemangioblast comes from differentiation of pluripotent embryonic stem cells along endothelial and hematopoietic lineages *(32,33)*. When individual blast colonies are allowed to differentiate further, they form adherent cells that express more endothelial-specific markers such as PECAM-1 and Tie2, whereas many of the nonadherent cells presumed to be hematopoietic origin express such genes as β-*H1* and β*major* consistent with cells derived from the erythroid lineage. Furthermore, when Flk-1-positive cells were isolated from ES cells and allowed to differentiate in vitro, they could be sorted into cells of both endothelial and hematopoietic origin by flow cytometry using surface markers specific for endothelial or hematopoietic cells *(34)*. Some of the specific transcription factors required for endothelial differentiation have recently been identified. The vascular defects seen in mice with targeted disruption of the immediate-early gene *Fra1* were partially attributed to a marked reduction in the number of endothelial cells. The defects were mainly seen in the placenta with severely impaired vascular development leading to embryonic lethality between E10.0 and E10.5 *(27)*. The zinc finger transcription factor Vezf1 is expressed solely in vascular endothelial cells and their precursors *(35)*. Endothelial-specific expression of Vezf1 was also observed in endothelial cells of the developing dorsal aorta, the branchial arch artery, and endocardium and co-localized with Flk-1 expression.

ENDOTHELIAL TUBE FORMATION

Following their differentiation from pluripotent stem cells, endothelial cells migrate and form primitive tubes. The bHLH transcription factor *HESR1* has recently been shown to be upregulated during endothelial tube formation *(36)*. Overexpression of this gene in endothelial cells results in downregulation of Flk-1, which may result in inhibiting endothelial cell proliferation by diminishing endothelial responsiveness to VEGF. Antisense oligonucleotides directed against HESR1 were able to block the formation of capillary tubes. The homolog of this factor in zebrafish is called gridlock and is a critical mediator of the development of arteries such as the aorta but not of veins *(37)*. The homeobox gene *HOX B3* has recently been shown to be involved in facilitating capillary morphogenesis *(38)*. Overexpression of this factor in the chicken chorioallantoic membrane leads to increased capillary vascular density, and antisense oligonucleotides inhibit endothelial tube formation of microvascular endothelial cells cultured on extracellular matrix. Another transcription factor involved in endothelial tube formation is nuclear receptor peroxisome proliferator-activated receptor (PPAR)-γ. In contrast to *HESR1* and *HOX B3*, ligand activation of this transcription factor blocks endothelial tube formation and endothelial proliferation *(39)*.

SMOOTH MUSCLE CELL DIFFERENTIATION

After initial endothelial tube formation, vessel maturation requires the subsequent recruitment of surrounding mesenchymal cells and their differentiation into vascular smooth muscle cells. This process involves the interaction of endothelial cells with mesenchymal cells and the release of specific growth factors such as platelet-derived growth factor (PDGF) *(40,41)*. A number of transcription factors have also been shown to be critical for smooth muscle differentiation (Table 1). One such family is the MADS-box transcription factor family. Two members of this family, SMAD5 and MEF2C, are important in vascular development and in smooth muscle cell differentiation *(42,43)*. Targeted disruption of SMAD5 leads to vascular defects resulting in embryonal lethality at d 10.5–11.5. The defects included enlarged blood vessels with diminished numbers of vascular smooth muscle cells. The absence of SMAD5 results in apoptosis of mesenchymal cells and marked reduction in the differentiation of mesenchymal cells into vascular smooth muscle cells *(43)*. Similarly, the targeted disruption of MEF2C leads to abnormalities in smooth muscle cell differentiation and the inability of endothelial cells to form into vascular structures *(42)*. LKLF is a member of the krueppel-like family of zinc finger transcription factors. Targeted dis-

Table 1
Transcription Factors, Their Families, and Their Roles

Transcription factor (ref.)	Family	Role
AML-1 (53)	CBF	Angiogenesis
ELF-1 (4)	ETS (wHTH)	Tie2 gene regulation
Ets-1 (5)	ETS (wHTH)	Angiogenesis
Fli-1 (7)	ETS (wHTH)	Vascular development, Tie2 gene regulation
NERF2 (48)	ETS (wHTH)	Tie2 gene regulation
TEL (49)	ETS (wHTH)	Yolk sac angiogenesis
MEF2 (42)	MADS box	Vascular development, smooth muscle cell differentiation
SMAD5 (43)	MADS box	Smooth muscle differentiation, angiogenesis
SCL/tal-1 (6)	bHLH	Vascular development
dHAND (45)	bHLH	Vascular smooth muscle differentiation
Tfeb (29)	bHLH-Zip	Placental vascularization
HESR1, gridlock (36,37)	bHLH	Aorta development, endothelial tube formation
EPAS (18,19)	PAS-bHLH	Angiogenesis
HIF-1a (16)	PAS-bHLH	Angiogenesis
ARNT (13)	PAS-bHLH	Angiogenesis
Fra1 (27)	bZip	Endothelial differentiation
Vezf1 (35)	Zinc finger	Endothelial differentiation
LKLF (28)	Zinc finger	Vascular smooth muscle differentiation
HOXD3 (30)	Homeobox	Endothelial response to angiogenic factors
COUP-TFII (54)	Nuclear receptor	Yolk sac angiogenesis

See text for abbreviations.

ruption of this gene leads to vascular defects. Most notably, there is a reduction in the number of differentiated smooth muscle cells and pericytes. These defects result in aneurysmal dilatation of the large vessels and eventual rupture with intra-amniotic hemorrhage (28). A similar phenotype was recently reported for mice lacking the cytoplasmic domain of Ephrin B2, suggesting that signaling through ephrin B2 may involve activation of LKLF or similar transcription factors during later stages of blood vessel development (44). The bHLH transcription factor dHAND has recently been shown to be crucial for yolk sac vascular development. In dHAND null mice, endothelial cell differentiation and recruitment of surrounding mesenchymal cells occurs normally. However, the mesenchymal cells fail to differentiate into vascular smooth muscle cells *(45)*. One of the genes that was shown to be downregulated in these mice was the $VEGF_{165}$ receptor neuropilin, suggesting that dHAND may be a critical mediator of the VEGF signaling pathway.

OVERLAPPING TRANSCRIPTIONAL MECHANISMS BETWEEN THE HEMATOPOIETIC AND ENDOTHELIAL LINEAGES

One of the most recent findings regarding the transcriptional regulation of vascular development was the determination that the transcription factor SCL/tal-1, which was originally thought to play a role strictly in hematopoiesis, also appears to be critical for embryonic blood vessel development. Targeted disruption of this gene leads to embryonic lethality by d 9.5 as a result of an absence of yolk sac erythropoiesis *(46)*. However, it was unclear whether this gene might also contribute to nonhematopoietic pathways at later stages of development. By performing transgenic experiments in which the GATA-1 promoter is used to restore SCL gene expression in hematopoietic lineages in SCL–/– mice, the mice develop striking abnormalities in yolk sac angiogenesis *(6)*. This suggests that certain transcription factors may be critical for both the normal development of hematopoietic cells and blood vessels and that there may be a common stem cell precursor for both lineages. The most striking defects were a disorganized array of capillaries and absence of normal vitelline blood vessel formation. Although the larger vitelline blood vessels were not present, a smaller network of interconnecting vessels did exist. The architecture of these vessels revealed normal-appearing endothelial cells as well as the smooth muscle cells or pericytes that constituted the outer lining of the blood vessels. The expression of a number of vascular-specific genes including *Tie-1*, *Tie-2*, *Flk-1*, and *Flt-1* also appeared normal. Members of the ETS transcription factor family that were originally described for their role in lymphoid development have now also been shown to regulate vascular specific genes. The ETS factor *NERF* was originally identified for its role in regulating the expression of B-cell-specific genes such as the tyrosine kinase *blk (47)*. The *NERF* gene is expressed as at least three isoforms, *NERF1a*, *NERF1b*, and *NERF2*. Whereas *NERF2* is a potent transactivator, the *NERF1* isoforms have a truncated transactivation domain and act as natural dominant negative forms of *NERF2*. These isoforms are differentially expressed in different cell types. Whereas *NERF1a* and *1b* are expressed in B-cells, *NERF2* is highly expressed in endothelial cells and is a strong transactivator of the endothelial-specific *Tie1* and *Tie2* genes *(48)*. Similarly, the related ETS factor *ELF-1*, which was originally shown to regulate T-cell-specific genes, was also shown to be enriched in developing blood vessels of the chicken *(4)*. The ETS factor *Tel* was originally identified for its role as a proto-oncogene in the development of human leukemias. Targeted disruption of this factor led to defects not only in hematopoiesis, but also in extraembryonic angiogenesis *(49)*.

Another mechanism for providing cell type specificity, even though the particular factor may be expressed in several cell types, is through differential expression of functionally different isoforms of the transcription factor in different cell types. The ETS transcription factor *NERF*, for example, which was originally identified as being important in B-cell function by regulating the B-cell-specific tyrosine kinase *blk*, has also subsequently been shown to regulate the *Tie2* tyrosine kinase in endothelial cells *(47,48)*. The *NERF* gene has multiple isoforms that are differentially expressed in B-cells compared with endothelial cells *(48)*.

TEMPORAL AND SPATIAL ASPECTS
OF VASCULAR DEVELOPMENT

Differentiating cells migrate to the proper location in the correct spatial and temporal organization to form specific structures such as organs or tissues. Blood vessel development similarly involves the correct spatial organization of differentiating endothelial and vascular smooth muscle cells. Endothelial differentiation is an early event followed by the formation of primitive tubes. The subsequent recruitment of surrounding mesenchymal cells and their differentiation into vascular smooth muscle cells is a later event leading to the formation of stable blood vessels. Growth factors including PDGF, bFGF, VEGF, AP-1, and transforming growth factor (TGF)-β are key mediators of these events, promoting the proliferation and migration of cells. Several of the transcription factors described above are key regulators of the expression of either growth factors or their receptors or mediators of the cellular responses to these growth factors. A summary of the temporal role for these transcription factors is shown in Fig. 1. One of the earliest transcription factors required for the differentiation of a pluripotent stem cell into a hemangioblast is *SCL/tal-1 (50)*. Knockout studies suggest that two transcription factors that may be required for differentiation or survival of endothelial cells early in development are Fra1 and Vezf1 *(27,35)*. Another early step in the differentiation of endothelial cells is the expression of VEGF receptors that promote not only the

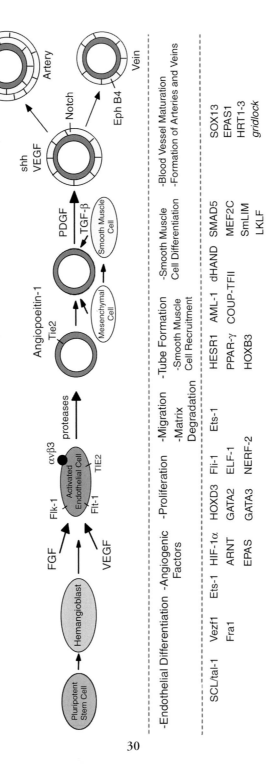

Fig 1. The role of transcription factors during different stages of vascular development.

30

differentiaion but also the proliferation of endothelial cells. Regulation of the VEGF receptor's gene expression is mediated by the Ets transcription factors, GATA factors, and bHLH factor dHAND *(45,51,52)*. The expression of VEGF is largely mediated by the PAS domain family of transcription factors, including HIF-1α, EPAS, and ARNT, in response to hypoxia. The next stage of blood vessel development involves the proliferation and migration of endothelial cells and their formation into primitive tubes. Endothelial tube formation is regulated at least in part by the transcription factors HESR1 and PPAR-γ *(36,39)*. Maturation of primitive endothelial tubes into mature blood vessels requires the recruitment of surrounding mesenchymal cells or pericytes and their differentiation into vascular smooth muscle cells. This process is largely mediated by the angiopoietins and the Tie2 receptor. *Tie2* gene expression has been shown to be regulated by the ETS factors NERF, ELF-1, and Fli-1 *(4,7,48)*. One of the key regulators of AP-1 expression is the transcription factor AML1. Targeted disruption of this factor led to abnormalities in angiogenesis that could be rescued by administration of AP-1 *(53)*. Another transcription factor that also appears to regulate AP-1 levels is the nuclear receptor *COUP-TFII (54)*. Targeted disruption of this gene is associated with angiogenic defects and marked reductions in the level of AP-1. The differentiation of mesechymal cells into vascular smooth muscle cells is also a highly orchestrated process. Members of the MADS-box factors such as SMAD5 and MEF2C mediate the effects of TGF-β, thereby promoting endothelial mesenchymal interactions and smooth muscle cell differentiation. Crucial gaps in our understanding of the role of specific transcription factors in this process include the lack of identification of transcriptional mediators that mediate endothelial responses to growth factors such as VEGF and AP-1. The list of factors mentioned above likely represents only a small subset of the factors required for vascular development. Several additional factors likely exist for the different stages of vascular development.

CLINICAL IMPLICATIONS

The identification of the genomic regulatory regions and the specific transcription factors required for vascular-specific gene expression has several implications regarding the potential treatment of several diseases. First, the identification of vascular-specific fragments allows the possibility of delivering genes and their protein products specifically to blood vessels. The Tie1 promoter has been used not only to direct the expression of the β-galactosidase gene in an endothelial-specific fashion but has also been used to express growth hormone *(55)*. Although these experiments were performed in transgenic animals, they could similarly be used in viral vectors to direct endothelial-specific gene expression. Potential therapeutic uses of these vectors include the expression of modulators of inflammation or cell growth in diseases such as the restenosis associated with angioplasty, vasculopathy related to cardiac transplantation, and chronic inflammation associated with atherosclerosis. An example of a protein that has been successfully used to treat restenosis is the Fas ligand, which promotes cell death *(56)*. However, if this gene was expressed in nonvascular cells, it could lead to significant adverse effects. In addition to inflammatory conditions, a vascular-specific promoter might also be used to block vascular growth during tumor growth, since most endothelial cells are not actively proliferating. The identification of transcription factors that may serve as master switches of endothelial differentiation or angiogenesis may also allow the use of these factors to be used in a therapeutic manner or serve as a therapeutic target for blocking angiogenesis. The ability of two transcription factors to direct angiogenesis was recently shown in two studies. In the first study the delivery of the early response gene transcription factor egr-1 in a wound-healing model enhanced the degree of angiogenesis and promoted normal healing *(57)*. Similarly, the administration of a constitutively active form of the transcription factor HIF-1α augmented the angiogenic response by expression of this transcription factor in vivo in a rabbit model of hindlimb ischemia *(58)*. The fact that several other transcription factors have been shown to be enriched during blood vessel development or that the targeted disruption of these genes is associated with significant vascular defects, as described above, suggests that these factors may also be used therapeutically to promote angiogenesis. Alternatively, several of these newly identified transcription factors could serve as targets for inhibiting blood vessel development or angiogenesis. Drugs used to augment or interfere with the function of these factors could enhance the development of angiogenesis in diseases such as ischemic heart disease, where the development of new blood vessel development may be beneficial. Downregulation or blockade of the function of these factors might also be effective in inhibiting the angiogenesis that promotes such diseases as cancer, rheumatoid arthritis, or diabetic retinopathy.

SUMMARY

Angiogenesis requires the carefully orchestrated proliferation and migration of endothelial cells, followed by their formation into primitive tube-like structures. Maturation of these primitive tubes into fully developed blood vessels requires the recruitment of surrounding pericytes and their differentiation into vascular smooth muscle cells. Many of the events that occur during angiogenesis recapitulate events that occur during embryonic blood vessel development. More recently, it has also been shown that endothelial progenitors can be mobilized from the bone marrow to active sites of angiogenesis, thereby providing another source of endothelial cells. Two of the main stimuli that promote angiogenesis are hypoxia and inflammation. Transcription factors have been shown to serve as master switches for regulating a number of developmental processes, such as vascular development, and similarly act to orchestrate angiogenesis. The purpose of this review is to provide an update on the progress that has been made in our understanding of the transcriptional regulation of angiogenesis over the past few years. Ultimately, a better understanding of the molecular mechanisms underlying angiogenesis may provide insights into novel and better therapeutic approaches to promote angiogenesis in the setting of ischemic heart disease.

REFERENCES

1. Thompson MA, Ransom DG, Pratt SJ, et al. The cloche and spadetail genes differentially affect hematopoiesis and vasculogenesis. Dev Biol 1998;197:248–269.
2. Gering M, Rodaway AR, Gottgens B, Patient RK, Green AR. The SCL gene specifies haemangioblast development from early mesoderm. EMBO J 1998;17:4029–4045.
3. Brown LA, Rodaway AR, Schilling TF, et al. Insights into early vasculogenesis revealed by expression of the ETS-domain transcription factor Fli-1 in wild-type and mutant zebrafish embryos. Mech Dev 2000;90:237–252.
4. Dube A, Thai S, Gaspar J, et al. Elf-1 is a transcriptional regulator of the Tie2 gene during vascular development. Circ Res 2001;88:237–244.
5. Wernert N, Stanjek A, Hugel A, Giannis A. [Inhibition of angiogenesis on the chicken chorioallantoic membrane by Ets 1 antisense oligodeoxyribonucleotides]. Verh Dtsch Ges Pathol 1999;83:212–215.
6. Visvader JE, Fujiwara Y, Orkin SH. Unsuspected role for the T-cell leukemia protein SCL/tal-1 in vascular development. Genes Dev 1998;12:473–479.
7. Hart A, Melet F, Grossfeld P, et al. Fli-1 is required for murine vascular and megakaryocytic development and is hemizygously deleted in patients with thrombocytopenia. Immunity 2000;13:167–177.
8. Vandenbunder B, Wernert N, Stehelin D. [Does oncogene c-ets 1 participate in the regulation of tumor angiogenesis?]. Bull Cancer 1993;80:38–49.
9. Minegishi N, Ohta J, Yamagiwa H, et al. The mouse GATA-2 gene is expressed in the para-aortic splanchnopleura and aorta-gonads and mesonephros region. Blood 1999;93:4196–4207.
10. Burbach KM, Poland A, Bradfield CA. Cloning of the Ah-receptor cDNA reveals a distinctive ligand-activated transcription factor. Proc Natl Acad Sci USA 1992;89:8185–8159.
11. Wang GL, Jiang BH, Rue EA, Semenza GL. Hypoxia-inducible factor 1 is a basic-helix-loop-helix-PAS heterodimer regulated by cellular O_2 tension. Proc Natl Acad Sci USA 1995;92:5510–5514.

12. Forsythe JA, Jiang BH, Iyer NV, et al. Activation of vascular endothelial growth factor gene transcription by hypoxia-inducible factor 1. Mol Cell Biol 1996;16:4604–4613.

13. Maltepe E, Schmidt JV, Baunoch D, Bradfield CA, Simon MC. Abnormal angiogenesis and responses to glucose and oxygen deprivation in mice lacking the protein ARNT. Nature 1997;386:403–407.

14. Carmeliet P, Ferreira V, Breier G, et al. Abnormal blood vessel development and lethality in embryos lacking a single VEGF allele. Nature 1996;380:435–439.

15. Carmeliet P, Mackman N, Moons L, et al. Role of tissue factor in embryonic blood vessel development. Nature 1996;383:73–75.

16. Kotch LE, Iyer NV, Laughner E, Semenza GL. Defective vascularization of HIF-1alpha-null embryos is not associated with VEGF deficiency but with mesenchymal cell death. Dev Biol 1999;209:254–267.

17. Tian H, McKnight SL, Russell DW. Endothelial PAS domain protein 1 (EPAS1), a transcription factor selectively expressed in endothelial cells. Genes Dev 1997;11:72–82.

18. Tian H, Hammer RE, Matsumoto AM, Russell DW, McKnight SL. The hypoxia-responsive transcription factor EPAS1 is essential for catecholamine homeostasis and protection against heart failure during embryonic development. Genes Dev 1998;12:3320–3324.

19. Peng J, Zhang L, Drysdale L, Fong GH. The transcription factor EPAS-1/hypoxia-inducible factor 2alpha plays an important role in vascular remodeling. Proc Natl Acad Sci USA 2000;97:8386–8391.

20. Arany Z, Huang LE, Eckner R, et al. An essential role for p300/CBP in the cellular response to hypoxia. Proc Natl Acad Sci USA 1996;93:12969–12973.

21. Oike Y, Takakura N, Hata A, et al. Mice homozygous for a truncated form of CREB-binding protein exhibit defects in hematopoiesis and vasculo-angiogenesis. Blood 1999;93:2771–2779.

22. Cockman ME, Masson N, Mole DR, et al. Hypoxia inducible factor-alpha binding and ubiquitylation by the von Hippel-Lindau tumor suppressor protein. J Biol Chem 2000;275:25733–25741.

23. Mazure NM, Chen EY, Laderoute KR, Giaccia AJ. Induction of vascular endothelial growth factor by hypoxia is modulated by a phosphatidylinositol 3-kinase/Akt signaling pathway in Ha-ras-transformed cells through a hypoxia inducible factor-1 transcriptional element. Blood 1997;90:3322–3331.

24. Richard DE, Berra E, Gothie E, Roux D, Pouyssegur J. p42/p44 mitogen-activated protein kinases phosphorylate hypoxia-inducible factor 1alpha (HIF-1alpha) and enhance the transcriptional activity of HIF-1. J Biol Chem 1999;274:32631–32637.

25. Kiriakidis S, Andreakos E, Monaco C, Foxwell B, Feldmann M, Paleolog E. VEGF expression in human macrophages is NF-kappaB-dependent: studies using adenoviruses expressing the endogenous NF-kappaB inhibitor IkappaBalpha and a kinase-defective form of the IkappaB kinase 2. J Cell Sci 2003;116:665–674.

26. Rudders S, Gaspar J, Madore R, et al. ESE-1 is a novel transcriptional mediator of inflammation that interacts with NF-kappa B to regulate the inducible nitric-oxide synthase gene. J Biol Chem 2001;276:3302–3309.

27. Schreiber M, Wang Z, Jochum W, Fetka I, Elliott C, Wagner EF. Placental vascularisation requires the AP-1 component fra1. Development 2000;127:4937–4948.

28. Kuo CT, Veselits ML, Barton KP, Lu MM, Clendenin C, Leiden JM. The LKLF transcription factor is required for normal tunica media formation and blood vessel stabilization during murine embryogenesis. Genes Dev 1997;11:2996–3006.

29. Steingrimsson E, Tessarollo L, Reid SW, Jenkins NA, Copeland NG. The bHLH-Zip transcription factor Tfeb is essential for placental vascularization. Development 1998;125:4607–4616.

30. Boudreau N, Andrews C, Srebrow A, Ravanpay A, Cheresh DA. Induction of the angiogenic phenotype by Hox D3. J Cell Biol 1997;139:257–264.

31. Liao W, Ho C, Yan YL, Postlethwait J, Stainier DY. Hhex and scl function in parallel to regulate early endothelial and blood differentiation in zebrafish. Development 2000;127:4303–4313.

32. Kennedy M, Firpo M, Choi K, et al. A common precursor for primitive erythropoiesis and definitive haematopoiesis. Nature 1997;386:488–493.

33. Choi K, Kennedy M, Kazarov A, Papadimitriou JC, Keller G. A common precursor for hematopoietic and endothelial cells. Development 1998;125:725–732.

34. Nishikawa SI, Nishikawa S, Hirashima M, Matsuyoshi N, Kodama H. Progressive lineage analysis by cell sorting and culture identifies FLK1+VE-cadherin+ cells at a diverging point of endothelial and hemopoietic lineages. Development 1998;125:1747–1757.

35. Xiong JW, Leahy A, Lee HH, Stuhlmann H. Vezf1: a Zn finger transcription factor restricted to endothelial cells and their precursors. Dev Biol 1999;206:123–141.

36. Henderson AM, Wang SJ, Taylor AC, Aitkenhead M, Hughes CC. The basic helix-loop-helix transcription factor HESR1 regulates endothelial cell tube formation. J Biol Chem 2001;276:6169–6176.

37. Zhong TP, Rosenberg M, Mohideen MA, Weinstein B, Fishman MC. gridlock, an HLH gene required for assembly of the aorta in zebrafish. Science 2000;287:1820–1824.

38. Myers C, Charboneau A, Boudreau N. Homeobox B3 promotes capillary morphogenesis and angiogenesis. J Cell Biol 2000;148:343–351.

39. Xin X, Yang S, Kowalski J, Gerritsen ME. Peroxisome proliferator-activated receptor gamma ligands are potent inhibitors of angiogenesis in vitro and in vivo. J Biol Chem 1999;274:9116–9121.

40. Hirschi KK, Rohovsky SA, D'Amore PA. PDGF, TGF-beta, and heterotypic cell-cell interactions mediate endothelial cell-induced recruitment of 10T1/2 cells and their differentiation to a smooth muscle fate. J Cell Biol 1998;141:805–814.

41. Hirschi KK, Rohovsky SA, Beck LH, Smith SR, D'Amore PA. Endothelial cells modulate the proliferation of mural cell precursors via platelet-derived growth factor-BB and heterotypic cell contact. Circ Res. 1999;84:298–305.

42. Lin Q, Lu J, Yanagisawa H, et al. Requirement of the MADS-box transcription factor MEF2C for vascular development. Development 1998;125:4565–4574.

43. Yang X, Castilla LH, Xu X, et al. Angiogenesis defects and mesenchymal apoptosis in mice lacking SMAD5. Development 1999;126:1571–1580.

44. Adams RH, Diella F, Hennig S, Helmbacher F, Deutsch U, Klein R. The cytoplasmic domain of the ligand ephrinB2 is required for vascular morphogenesis but not cranial neural crest migration. Cell 2001;104:57–69.

45. Yamagishi H, Olson EN, Srivastava D. The basic helix-loop-helix transcription factor, dHAND, is required for vascular development. J Clin Invest 2000;105:261–270.

46. Shivdasani RA, Mayer EL, Orkin SH. Absence of blood formation in mice lacking the T-cell leukaemia oncoprotein tal-1/SCL. Nature 1995;373:432–434.

47. Oettgen P, Akbarali Y, Boltax J, Best J, Kunsch C, Libermann TA. Characterization of NERF, a novel transcription factor related to the Ets factor ELF-1. Mol Cell Biol 1996;16:5091–5106.

48. Dube A, Akbarali Y, Sato TN, Libermann TA, Oettgen P. Role of the Ets transcription factors in the regulation of the vascular-specific Tie2 gene [see comments]. Circ Res. 1999;84:1177–1185.

49. Wang LC, Kuo F, Fujiwara Y, Gilliland DG, Golub TR, Orkin SH. Yolk sac angiogenic defect and intra-embryonic apoptosis in mice lacking the Ets-related factor TEL. EMBO J 1997;16:4374–4383.

50. Porcher C, Liao EC, Fujiwara Y, Zon LI, Orkin SH. Specification of hematopoietic and vascular development by the bHLH transcription factor SCL without direct DNA binding. Development 1999;126:4603–4615.

51. Wakiya K, Begue A, Stehelin D, Shibuya M. A cAMP response element and an Ets motif are involved in the transcriptional regulation of flt-1 tyrosine kinase (vascular endothelial growth factor receptor 1) gene. J Biol Chem 1996;271:30823–30938.

52. Kappel A, Schlaeger TM, Flamme I, Orkin SH, Risau W, Breier G. Role of SCL/Tal-1, GATA, and ets transcription factor binding sites for the regulation of flk-1 expression during murine vascular development. Blood 2000;96:3078–3085.

53. Takakura N, Watanabe T, Suenobu S, et al. A role for hematopoietic stem cells in promoting angiogenesis. Cell 2000;102:199–209.

54. Pereira FA, Qiu Y, Zhou G, Tsai MJ, Tsai SY. The orphan nuclear receptor COUP-TFII is required for angiogenesis and heart development. Genes Dev 1999;13:1037–1049.

55. Iljin K, Dube A, Kontusaari S, et al. Role of ets factors in the activity and endothelial cell specificity of the mouse Tie gene promoter. FASEB J 1999;13:377–386.

56. Sata M, Perlman H, Muruve DA, et al. Fas ligand gene transfer to the vessel wall inhibits neointima formation and overrides the adenovirus-mediated T cell response. Proc Natl Acad Sci USA 1998;95:1213–1217.

57. Bryant M, Drew GM, Houston P, Hissey P, Campbell CJ, Braddock M. Tissue repair with a therapeutic transcription factor. Hum Gene Ther 2000;11:2143–2158.

58. Vincent KA, Shyu KG, Luo Y, et al. Angiogenesis is induced in a rabbit model of hindlimb ischemia by naked DNA encoding an HIF-1alpha/VP16 hybrid transcription factor. Circulation 2000;102:2255–2261.

3 Preclinical Models and Experience to Date

Aysegul Yegin, MD
and Nicolas A. Chronos, MD

CONTENTS

INTRODUCTION

In the last decade, therapeutic angiogenesis in cardiovascular diseases has been extensively investigated using a variety of animal models. Recently, there have been great efforts to begin such research in human trials. There is still, however, an ongoing need for continued preclinical investigations to illuminate the complexity of angiogenic agents. Therapeutic modalities including autologous stem cell transplantation, targeted protein delivery, prolonged protein half-life, and various combination therapies are only some of the areas that require further investigation.

From: *Contemporary Cardiology: Angiogenesis and Direct Myocardial Revasularization*
Edited by: R. J. Laham and D. S. Baim © Humana Press Inc., Totowa, NJ

This chapter presents a current update of preclinical angiogenesis studies using animal models. A number of important studies have been completed, each addressing many unknowns and providing further guidance for future studies. Our goal is to provide scientists with the necessary information to design future studies and better understand completed studies. The primary role of today's scientist is to be able to evaluate results in an objective manner and to develop angiogenic solutions for those cardiac patients who are unresponsive to conventional therapies.

ANIMAL MODEL SELECTION CRITERIA

Each animal model has its own strengths and weaknesses. Selecting the best model to study a particular human disease depends on the extent to which the experimental animal system mimics the disease. The major points to consider when selecting models for preclinical angiogenesis studies include (1) the experimental advantages of one species over another; (2) the reproducibility characteristics of the model in the laboratory; and (3) the potential for that particular model to produce the desired angiogenic response without major limiting side effects. Secondary issues influencing the model selection are experimental goals, available expertise/equipment/technology, and the study budget. An ideal animal model for angiogenesis studies should have the following characteristics *(1)*:

1. Small, yet easily implemented and maintained
2. Coronary anatomy and innate collateral circulation similar to humans
3. Collateral development in the virtual absence of infarction
4. Consistent, regional abnormalities in left-ventricular (LV) perfusion and function
5. Easily assessed in response to simple interventions

Although this optimal model may not always be attainable, models should strive to reflect the "ideal" based on the above criteria and following the basic knowledge of anatomy, physiology, and function (Table 1).

Anatomy of Coronary Circulation

The anatomy of the porcine coronary circulation is analogous to a human's, with three major coronary arteries. In contrast, dogs have essentially a two-vessel system, with a nondominant right coronary artery supplying only the right ventricle, as is the case in the vast majority of animals.

Pre-Existing Interconnecting Arterioles and Collateral Circulation

Collateral vessels develop from pre-existing interconnecting arterioles, but not all species are endowed with a sufficient number to react

Table 1
Comparison of Characteristics of Pig and Dog Models in Angiogenesis Studies

Model	Pre-existing interconnecting arterioles	Infarct type with coronary ligation	Coronary system	Innate collateral circulation	Response to ameroid constrictor	Preference in angiogenesis studies
Pig	Few	Transmural	3-coronary system	Very limited endocardial	Small capillary size vessels	High
Dog	Numerous	Nontransmural	2-coronary system	Numerous epicardial	Large muscular arteries	Low

rapidly to critical coronary stenosis. Morphological studies of coronary vessels in different species have shown that while rats, rabbits, and pigs have anatomical end arteries with no arteriolar connections, dogs and cats are well endowed with these vessels and guinea pigs hearts exhibit a truly abundant arteriolar network *(2)*. The normal human heart has fewer interconnecting arterioles than a dog heart *(3,4)*. Pigs have a very limited innate collateral circulation, with only sparse endocardial connections; however, dogs have numerous, generally epicardial, innate anastomoses, which are thought to have greater potential for development than those of pigs *(5)*. This difference has resulted in a preference for the pig model for angiogenesis studies.

The canine ameroid model is characterized by the development of large, muscular collateral arteries with limited new capillary growth and is the ideal model to study neoarteriogenesis *(6)*. In contrast, neovascularization in response to ischemia in the pig ameroid model consists mainly of small vessels about the size of capillaries that lack an arterial coat. These vessels mostly develop around areas of focal necrosis *(7)*, although they can be found throughout the ischemic territory. The low pressure in the collateral system is perhaps one of the reasons why these vessels remain thin-walled but do not leak. Another explanation could be that porcine myocardium does not have an efficient smooth muscle-recruiting mechanism such as the angiopoietin-tie-2 system *(8)*.

MODELS OF MYOCARDIAL ISCHEMIA

Collateral vessels develop in response to a gradually developing high-grade coronary stenosis or occlusion growing at the interface between normal and ischemic tissue. These vessels may be sufficient to preserve wall motion and prevent or reduce ischemia at rest or during stress.

Enhancing this process by delivering angiogenic factors to promote neovascularization may therefore be a useful therapeutic strategy *(9)*.

Myocardial Ischemia or Infarction

Reversible myocardial ischemia and myocardial infarction are fundamentally different pathophysiological events. Following an abrupt interruption of coronary perfusion, there is a limited time for myocyte survival (hours) compared to the time required for vascular development (days). It is unlikely that angiogenic mechanisms can importantly affect the initial events in myocardial infarction. It is also unclear if these mechanisms can alter the healing response to myocardial infarction. Various experimental models that cause acute myocardial infarction (AMI) through direct coronary occlusion, circulatory embolization with microspheres, or inorganic mercury/thrombus have limited applicability to studies of collateral development. Therefore, the preferred approach to study coronary collateral development involves chronic models of intermittent or progressive coronary occlusion *(10)*.

Ameroid Constrictor Model

An ameroid constrictor model was initially used by Litvak in the 1950s *(11)* and extensively characterized by Schaper and colleagues in the 1960s and 1970s *(6)*. This model has been used to investigate chronic collateral structure/function and remains a useful tool in preclinical angiogenesis studies. Ameroid constrictors are implanted mostly in larger animals, primarily dogs and pigs.

STRUCTURE AND MECHANISM OF FUNCTION

There are different types and sizes of ameroid constrictors. The device is usually placed around the left circumflex coronary artery (LCX) via left lateral thoracotomy through the fourth intercostal space under general anesthesia (Fig. 1). The ameroid constrictor is a C-shaped device consisting of a hygroscopic material encased in an inflexible stainless steel outer ring. When implanted around an artery, the inner hygroscopic material swells over a period of days to weeks. Because the outward movement is limited by the steel sleeve, swelling is directed inward, causing arterial compression. Ameroids generally cause complete coronary occlusion within 2–3 wk (Fig. 2). The common perception that ameroids cause gradual coronary occlusion leading to myocardial ischemia with eventual collateral development may be an oversimplification. It should be noted that they may also cause mechanical trauma, which can lead to endothelial damage, platelet aggregation and/or throm-

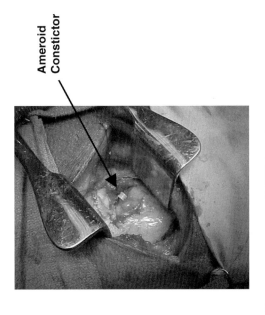

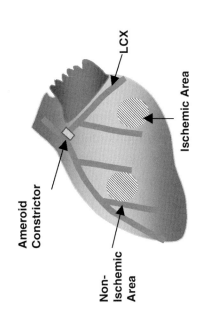

Fig 1. Ameroid constrictor implanted around left circumflex coronary artery (LCX) in swine.

41

LCX Occlusion

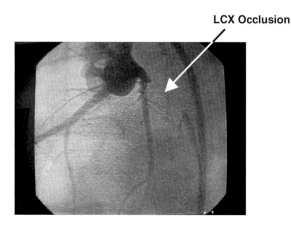

Fig 2. Coronary angiography indicating 100% left circumflex artery (LCX) occlusion 4 wk after implantation of an ameroid constrictor in Yucatan pig.

bus formation, and foreign body reaction with local scar formation *(6)*. The degree to which ameroid devices cause ischemia is dependent on general coronary artery topography, the location of the constrictor along the coronary artery (i.e., proximal vs distal), its placement relative to side branches, the extent of pre-existing collaterals, the animal's level of activity, and genetic/species differences.

In swine, gradual occlusion of the coronary artery over 7–14 d is accompanied by the rapid development of collateral vessels and <2% infarction of the "at-risk" vascular bed *(12,13)*. Pigs implanted with ameroid constrictors have collateral-dependent myocardium distal to the occlusion. The collateral vessels function adequately at rest, and usually ischemia is not observed. However, during stress conditions, such as feeding, treadmill exercise, or rapid atrial pacing, the collateral-dependent myocardium becomes ischemic. This remains stable for at least 6 mo, and the animals show stable, stress-induced ischemia with no further evidence of collateral formation *(14)*.

White and colleagues extensively quantified the development of the coronary collateral circulation in the pig using the ameroid model *(15)*. They described the ameroid occluder to cause gradual occlusion resulting in small uniform infarcts and minimal contractile dysfunction. Yucatan minipigs, approx 7 mo old, were used in their study. The ameroid occluder (2–2.5 mm) was placed around the LCX near its origin. There was a total of four subgroups, including sham-operated and 3-wk, 8-wk, and 16-wk groups, each interval representing the period after placement of the ameroid. The coronary collateral circulation was evaluated by injection of multiple colors of a silicone polymer into the coronary arteries and the aorta. Overall, intercoronary and extracardiac collaterals (originating from bronchial and internal mammary arteries) were quantified. Comparison of the preexisting collateral flow in the LCX region $(0.06 \pm 0.01$ mL/min/g) with the collateral flow in the endocardium of the 3-wk ameroid group $(0.86 \pm 0.08$ mL/min/g) indicated a 14-fold increase in collateral-dependent flow in the ameroid group. There were differences in the endocardial and epicardial blood flows between the sham and ameroid animals. Under resting conditions, blood flow values in the sham and 16-wk animals were slightly higher in the endocardium than in the epicardium. However, blood flow values in the endocardial region of the 3- and 8-wk ameroid groups were lower than the epicardial region. Only the 3-wk group experienced a relative underperfusion of the endocardial region during nonvasodilated conditions. Endocardial blood flow showed a decrease in the 3-wk group, but then increased in the 8- and 16-wk groups. The investigators observed a relative underperfusion only in the 3-wk group, and only in the endocardial region. Normal blood flow was maintained in the occluded region by 8 wk after ameroid implantation. Most of the collateral development occured by 3 wk, and further collateral growth was minimal after this time. In addition, extracardiac collateral flow, which contributed 30–40% of the total collateral flow, was found to be higher in the epicardium than in the endocardium. By 16 wk after ameroid implantation, the extracardiac collaterals showed moderate smooth muscle development, whereas the intercoronary collaterals developed primarily in the midmyocardial and endocardial regions.

Recently, use and function of the porcine ameroid constrictor model for therapeutic angiogenesis was investigated by Radke et al. *(16)*. The group studied a total of 94 animals with ameroid constrictor placed around the LCX. An extensive evaluation, including echocardiography, coronary angiography, and blood flow measurements, was performed at 26 ± 5 d after ameroid placement. Complete LCX occlusion was observed in 36% of animals, with demonstrated ischemia of the lateral wall at rest and under stress. By applying an additional set of angiographic criteria (TIMI < 2 flow in LCX, or collateral flow Rentrop class >1), another 29% of animals were identified to have myocardial ischemia under stress conditions. The researchers reported that echocardiographic parameters of regional and global myocardial function were not associated with myocardial blood flow or ischemia level. No relation was found between the collateral formations as assessed by angiography, echocardiography, or blood flow parameters. The investigators concluded that the ameroid constrictor model is not an optimal prerequisite for establishing the pathophysiology of chronic myocardial ischemia.

ADVANTAGES OF THE DEVICE

Advantages include:

1. Provides slow and progressive coronary artery occlusion, mimicking chronic ischemia
2. Simple development of arterial occlusion after implantation around a coronary artery

DISADVANTAGES OF THE DEVICE

Disadvantages include:

1. The occlusion process may be influenced by vascular tone, platelet aggregability, thrombogenicity, inflammation, and fibrosis.
2. A variety of angiogenic growth factors and anti-inflammatory/ antithrombotic/antiplatelet agents may directly affect the process of ameroid-induced coronary occlusion, which could impact the dynamics of collateral expansion. Basic fibroblast growth factor (bFGF)-2 has been shown to be a nitric oxide-dependent vasodilator and possibly a coronary vasodilator as well, a property that might affect the process of ameroid-induced coronary occlusion in vivo.
3. A variable amount of infarction (mostly subendocardial), as well as sudden death in a significant fraction of animals, occurs *(6)*. The production of scar tissue and the variation in its extent affect the overall variability of the ameroid model, because scarring profoundly affects the parameters used to assess collateral function including vascular density, cell proliferation, myocardial perfusion, and function. Since the effect of the angiogenic intervention being assessed may be modest, even limited LV scarring may have the potential to confound the assessment of collateral function. Therefore, larger sample sizes are required to overcome variability and achieve statistical significance.

RABBIT MODEL OF AMEROID CONSTRICTOR

Operschall et al. recently developed a novel ameroid device in rabbits *(17)*. In this model, ameroid material simply rides on the epicardial surface, and a nonabsorbable suture material, threaded twice through the ameroid and the subjacent epicardium, is used to entrap the underlying LCX. Because the suture penetrates the myocardium deep to the circumflex, the artery is not subject to the trauma of direct dissection. A Doppler flow probe is used both to localize the artery and adjust the baseline tension in the suture. Using coronary cineangiography and corrosion casts, the investigators demonstrated total arterial occlusion/severe stenosis in eight animals after 21 d. Mortality rate was 22%, with a number of these animals sustaining large infarctions. In surviving rabbits, infarct size was fairly substantial. Perfusion in the risk area reduced at d 7 and progressively increased on d 14 and 21. On d 21, endocardial perfusion was approximately half that of sham-operated rabbits, whereas epicardial perfusion was equivalent. Although the feasibility of the model was demonstrated, an apparent disadvantage was the propensity for infarcts. Suggested potential solutions included implanting the constrictor more distally or using less hygroscopic ameroid material that swells more slowly. This model, when better characterized, may have a potential to provide investigators with a small-animal model of chronic, single-vessel coronary occlusion.

Intermittent Occlusion Model

It has been demonstrated that brief and repetitive total coronary occlusions provide a potent stimulus for coronary collateral development *(18)*. To create this model, the coronary artery is subjected to repetitive proximal occlusions through a periodic inflation of a chronically implanted hydraulic balloon occluder. Sonomicrometer crystals embedded in the myocardium are used to assess regional LV function in the territory of the instrumented coronary artery.

The steps leading to collateral development are as follows: (1) initial coronary occlusions cause significant LV dysfunction in the territory of the occluded artery; (2) as collateral expansion progresses, the degree of LV dysfunction associated with each occlusion diminishes until the lack of LV dysfunction in response to coronary occlusion signals the development of an adequate collateral supply; and (3) the rapidity of collateral development is inversely related to the number of coronary occlusions required before the changes in regional LV function in response to balloon occlusion are abolished. This model has been criticized owing to alternations between total arterial occlusion and complete patency being artificial and unable to mimic the pathophysiology of human coronary disease. However, the principal advantage of this model is the invariability of myocardial infarction, as coronary occlusion is predictably followed by reperfusion, avoiding irreversible injury. The major disadvantages of the model are its technical complexity and labor-intensiveness, which may explain the lack of wide acceptance.

Variation of Vineberg Direct Arterial Implantation Procedure

Vineberg pioneered a palliative treatment for ischemic heart disease in which an internal mammary artery (IMA) and its intercostal branches were transected and tunneled directly into the myocardium with the supposition that anastomoses would form between the implanted artery and the coronary circulation *(19)*. The operation was used clinically for a number of years prior to the advent of coronary artery bypass grafting

(CABG) surgery. By combining the ameroid model with the Vineberg operation, a systemic artery can be brought into contact with the coronary circulation in a collateral-dependent area. This artery has the potential to develop collateral circulation in communication with the myocardium and can be implanted with an infusion pump to administer angiogenic agents and enhance the development of systemic-to-coronary anastomoses. This model is unique because it can be used in patients with severe multivessel disease and no patent feeder artery. Its main disadvantage is variability in the extent of internal mammary-to-coronary anastomoses.

Minimally Invasive Coronary Stenosis Model for Imaging

Recently, a minimally invasive method of coronary stenosis has been developed in swine to investigate myocardial perfusion in magnetic resonance imaging (MRI) and single photon emission computed tomography (SPECT) studies *(20)*. *The aim is to overcome the shortcomings of the open chest and pericardium models such as the impact on normal cardiac mechanics, coronary autoregulation, and the required period for the development of significant stenosis.* Coronary stenosis was developed in a closed-chest model by using a biocompatible and relatively nonthrombogenic, radiolucent, and MRI-compatible coronary flow-reduction device. Pigs were implanted with a coronary flow-reduction fitting in the left anterior descending artery (LAD). These fittings were turned from a nylon rod, tapered from a maximum outer diameter of 3 mm, and drilled to a specific inner diameter depending on the degree of required coronary stenosis. The flow-reducing fittings were advanced to a wedge position in the proximal LAD with an angioplasty catheter via carotid artery approach. Perfusion determined by contrast-enhanced MRI at peak dipyridamole stress was compared with that obtained by ^{99m}Tc-sestamibi SPECT. Radiolabeled microspheres were injected at rest, after stenosis implantation, and at peak pharmacological stress to assess the coronary lesion severity. There was significant coronary stenosis (80–90%) in 7 animals and mild stenosis (60%) in 4 animals out of 11 animals studied. It was concluded that this new technique for creating angioplasty-guided coronary stenosis may be a less invasive alternative to open-chest techniques such as hydraulic occluders and ameroid constrictors.

Cryothermia-Induced Myocardial Infarction Model

A rat cryothermia-induced myocardial infarction model was used to study microvascularization and ventricular function after local alginate-encapsulated angiogenic growth factor treatment in rat model by Huwer et al. *(21)*. After exposing the hearts of Sprague-Dawley rats through a left lateral thoracotomy, cryothermia was induced to the LV wall using a 5-mm cryoprobe cooled to $-120°C$, and 0.2 mL of calcium-algineate beads were injected into the cryoinjured tissue. The beads contained 0.4 µg bFGF, 0.1 µg vascular endothelial growth factor (VEGF), or 4.2 µg epidermal growth factor (EGF). Four weeks later the chest was reopened and the formation of microvessels within the myocardial lesion, hemodynamics, and LV function were evaluated. The results of the study indicated that although the functional capillary density did not improve, there was a significant increase in the number of microvessels larger than capillaries. The increased number of microvessels within the infarcted tissue only marginally improved the LV function. The same group earlier investigated angiogenesis and microvascularization after cryothermia-induced myocardial infarction using intravital fluorescence microscopic techniques in rat model *(22)*. A standardized cryolesion was induced to the right ventricle by freezing for 5 min to $-160°C$. Myocardial angiogenesis and microvascularization were analyzed quantitatively on d 7 or 28. Seven days after cryothermia, the central area of the injured myocardium indicated a complete lack of capillary perfusion, while the periphery of the lesion revealed a heterogeneous capillary perfusion pattern with a density of 301 ± 39 cm^{-1}. Adjacent myocardial tissue showed intact capillary perfusion (density: 563 ± 44 cm^{-1}) comparable with that of sham-operated controls. After 28 d, the area lacking capillary perfusion was found to be significantly reduced, still surrounded by a heterogeneously perfused area of myocardial tissue, indicating partial restitution of capillary perfusion. Although at d 7 capillary perfusion was completely shut down within the central zone of the cryolesions, perfusion of microvessels larger than capillaries was maintained, but with a markedly lower density when compared with that of sham controls. After 28 d, the number of these larger-sized microvessels increased significantly with values of density even higher compared with those observed in controls, indicating new vessel formation. The results of this work indicated partial restitution and function of the microvascular network within infarcted myocardial tissue, which may serve as an appropriate prerequisite for successful application of novel therapeutic strategies to improve myocardial function.

Microembolization Model

This model is created by injecting microspheres into a discrete vascular bed. The diameter of the beads can be selected to correspond to approximate the diameter of vessels ranging from arteries to capillaries. In time, repeated administration of smaller microspheres, referred to as "repetitive microembolization," has become the method of choice. Microspheres can produce regional ischemia that is less severe than a complete blockage at a more proximal point. They are administered via catheters while the animal is under general anesthesia. The microspheres (usually ~15 μm in diameter) can be made of glass, polystyrene, or other plastics. The microembolization model has been used in studies measuring both short- and long-term capillary growth (23–25). Dogs and pigs are the most animals commonly used for this model. This model is quite flexible since the bead size, frequency, and quantity of injection can be altered. Smaller size beads and repetitive embolizations are more likely to produce significant and chronic LV dysfunction and mimic human coronary atherosclerosis.

Myocardial Infarction (Ligation) Model

This is a rather simplistic model that guarantees the onset of ischemia. Coronary ligation produces transmural infarction in pigs and smaller animals and nontransmural infarctions in dogs (26). Although it can be used in dogs and rats, pigs will not survive this procedure. The appearance of myocardium can be complicated by cell death, myocyte hypertrophy, and fibroblastic growth; however, border areas and nonischemic myocardium are easier to interpret. This model and the baseline data provided by Li et al. (27) can be useful in angiogenesis studies.

HINDLIMB ISCHEMIA MODEL

This model is created by dissection, ligation, and complete excision of a portion of the femoral artery in one hindlimb. As a result, the distal limb becomes entirely dependent on collateral arteries. Advantages of this technique are as follows:

1. Relatively simple surgical technique
2. Easy-to-measure indices of collateral development such as blood pressure ratios between ischemic and normal limbs, pressure gradients across obliterated portions of the femoral artery, etc.
3. Readily defined zones of collateral development and easily harvested samples

This model has been used in multiple angiogenesis studies that investigated the outcome of angiogenic gene and protein therapies in rats and rabbits (28,35,43). Other groups have studied various cell therapy strategies including autologous bone marrow-derived mononuclear cells, endothelial progenitor cells, and peripheral leukocytes/platelets in rat and rabbit models of hindlimb ischemia (46,49,50,55).

Table 2
Preclinical Angiogenesis Studies Investigating Growth
Factor Proteins Using Various Animal Models

Species	Investigator/ref.	Agent
Pig	Battler et al., 1993 (31)	FGF-2
	Harada et al., 1994 (70)	FGF-2
	Lopez et al., 1997 (71)	FGF-2
	Sato et al., 2000 (72)	FGF-2
	Laham et al., 2000 (73)	FGF-2
Dog	Yanagisawa-Miwa et al., 1992 (32)	FGF-2
	Banai et al., 1994 (34)	VEGF
	Unger et al., 1994 (74)	FGF-2
	Lazarous et al., 1995 (75)	FGF-2
	Uchida et al., 1995 (76)	FGF-2
	Shou et al., 1997 (77)	FGF-2
	Villanueva et al., 2002 (78)	VEGF-121
Rabbit	Baffour et al., 1992 (79)	FGF-2
	Takeshita et al., 1994 (80)	VEGF
Rat	Edelman et al., 1992 (81)	FGF-2

EXPERIENCE IN PROTEIN THERAPY

To date, the angiogenic potency of a number of growth factors, including FGF, VEGF, and hepatocyte growth factor (HGF), has been investigated using various animal models (14). Some of these studies are listed in Tables 2 and 3. Although preclinical evidence of in vivo efficacy has been obtained for all of the major angiogenic growth factors, studies of FGF-2 and VEGF-A are the most extensive to date (29). FGF-2 belongs to the FGF family, which includes 22 members. The ability of FGF-2 to induce angiogenesis in mature tissues was suggested by studies that documented significantly higher vessel counts following intracoronary injections in the setting of acute coronary thrombosis in dogs and pigs (30–32). These studies were followed by a more detailed evaluations of therapeutic efficacy of FGF-2 using an ameroid constrictor model to create chronic myocardial ischemia accompanied by myocardial hibernation in the affected coronary territory with limited subendocardial infarction (15,33). Most of these studies indicated an increase in collateral blood flow or a tendency toward the preservation of ventricular function under strain. However, there are many questions to be answered, such as the range of peptide concentrations necessary for a measurable effect and the timing of administration during the process of collateralization.

Table 3

Preclinical Studies of Angiogenesis Using Different Animal Models, Growth Factors, and Methodologies

Investigator/ref.	Species, ischem-ia-infarct model	Angiogenic agent/route of delivery	Histopathological assessment	Evaluation of perfusion and function
Yanagisawa-Miwa et al., 1992 (32)	Dog	FGF-2 Intracoronary (IC)	Arteriole/capillary count	
Battler et al., 1993 (31)	Pig beads	FGF-2 (slow-release)	Immunohistochemistry	Serial echocardiography
Harada et al., 1994 (70)	Pig, ameroid	FGF-2 Extraluminal administration by beads	% volume of infarcted LV	Colored microspheres—flow, echocardiography
Uchida et al. 1995 (76)	Dog	FGF-2 (30 μg)/heparin sulfate (3 mg) Transcatheter intrapericardial	Vessel count	
Yang et al., 1996	Rat	IV/VEGF (250 μg/kg)		HR, MAP, CO, SV, LVt dp/dt, hematocri
Lopez et al., 1997 (71)	Pig, ameroid	FGF-2 (10 μg/100 μg) Heparin-alginate microspheres	LCX-LAD sections: neointima formation	Coronary angiography, echocardiography colored microspheres—flow
Lopez et al., 1998	Pig, ameroid	IC Local/IC bolus infusion/ epicardial osmotic delivery system: VEGF (20 μg)		Coronary angiography, colored microspheres—flow, MRI (function, perfuison, infarct size)
Laham et al., 2000 (73)	Pig, ameroid	Single intrapericardial (IP): Heparin (3 mg)/Heparin (3 mg) + FGF-2 (30 μg)/FGF-2 (200 μg)/ FGF-2 (2 μg)	Macroscopy and histology (number of capillaries)	Coronary angiography, colored microspheres—flow, MRI (global and re-gional function, perfusion)
Villnanueva et al., 2002 (78)	Dog, ameroid	C: VEGF-121 (108 μg)/ ISC: VEGF-121 (1 mg)	Immunohistochemistry, arteriole count	Myocardial contrast echocardiography, radio-labeled microspheres—flow

VEGF was studied by Unger's group in the dog model *(34)* in which the injections were made into the peripheral stump of the occluded LAD. The results indicated significantly higher microsphere counts in the collateral dependent bed at d 24 and 38, but not at d 31. Although VEGF is known to be a specific mitogen for endothelial cells, capillary density remained unchanged, but the number of muscular distribution vessels increased in the collateral-dependent region. The authors suggested that VEGF-activated endothelium might have produced platelet-derived growth factor (PDGF). Although 2 wk of daily injections of high VEGF concentrations were needed to achieve a relatively modest effect in Unger's model, Isner's group *(35)* showed that a single intra-arterial dose of VEGF had a beneficial effect on hindlimb collaterals in the rabbit. The primary findings indicated an increase in calf blood pressure, visual angiographic scores, and capillary density. Angiograms showed corkscrew-type collaterals suggestive of muscular arteries, which is somewhat unexpected for an endothelium-specific mitogen.

Unger et al. concluded that bFGF exerted its most convincing action at the time of presumed closure of the ameroid. This may be reflecting the tendency of the FGF receptors to downregulate under physiological conditions. A pathological stimulus is required to upregulate them again. However, this view is not shared by Baird et al., who suggest that the bioavailability of the growth factor is of exclusive importance *(36)*.

UPDATE IN GENE THERAPY

Intramyocardial Injection Via Thoracotomy

Mack et al. *(37)* investigated the direct intramyocardial injection of an adenovirus encoding an angiogenic gene in porcine myocardial ischemia (ameroid) model. Regional function (echocardiography) and perfusion (radionuclide imaging) were assessed 3 wk after proximal LCX ameroid placement. Adenovirus encoding VEGF-121 (Ad.VEGF-121) or adenovirus vector was administered by needle into the ventricular wall at 10 injection sites (each with 10^8 plaque-forming units [pfu]). At 4 wk, both regional function and perfusion during stress were improved in Ad.VEGF-121-treated animals. The results of this study indicated that gene transfer by relatively low amounts of adenovirus results in positive improvements.

Patel et al. *(38)* used the porcine ameroid model of stress-induced myocardial ischemia to determine what toxic effects might result from intramyocardial injection of Ad.VEGF-121 at 21 d after LCX ameroid placement. The dose used per injection site was 10^8 or 10^9 pfu. Echocardiography, blood analysis, survival, and myocardial/liver histology were evaluated at 3 and 28 d after vector administration. Minimal inflammation and necrosis were observed in the hearts of animals that received gene transfer. The mild myocardial inflammation and necrosis observed was statistically significant and dose-related, with increased amounts in the animals that received 10^9 pfu per site. This amount of adenovirus is 75% less than the dose associated with marked inflammation as reported by other investigators (39).

Catheter-Based Transendocardial Injection

Kornowski et al. (40) used the porcine ameroid model of regional stress-induced myocardial ischemia to evaluate the effects of transendocardial delivery of Ad.VEGF-121. Using an electromagnetic-based catheter guidance system, recombinant adenovirus encoding Ad.VEGF-121 or lacZ was injected at two to six sites at a dose of 1×10^{10} virus particles (vp) per site through a retractable needle. The injection sites exhibited VEGF-121 expression comparable to that obtained by transepicardial Ad.VEGF-121 gene transfer with thoracotomy. Transgene expression was observed to be adjacent to the site of injection, and 5–10% of injections showed no detectable gene transfer, possibly as a result of systemic delivery of the vector. This study showed that the approach could be used for gene transfer. However, there were no data regarding histological changes in the heart, regional myocardial perfusion, function, or angiogenesis.

Intramyocardial/Intramuscular Injection

Tio et al. (41), using the porcine ameroid model, investigated whether intramyocardial injection of a plasmid vector encoding VEGF-165 increases regional myocardial blood flow (MBF). Microspheres were used to assess regional blood flow at rest and during adenosine infusion. Gene transfer was achieved by minimally invasive thoracotomy and needle insertion into the wall of the heart in which four injections delivering a total of 200 μg of plasmid in a volume of 2.0 mL (0.5 mL per injection site) were performed 3–4 wk post ameroid placement. The results demonstrated the feasibility of thoracotomy to administer the plasmid and also showed increased plasma VEGF levels. In addition, the investigators observed an increase in LCX blood flow during adenosine infusion after gene transfer. The actual degree of gene transfer with this method was substantially less than that achieved with other vectors and routes of delivery, and the results indicated that small amounts of transgene protein can have physiologically positive effects.

Recently, the angiogenic potential of human HGF gene transfer was recently studied in the normal and infarcted rat myocardium (42). HGF or control vectors were injected into rat hearts via thoracotomy. Transfection of the HGF gene resulted in increased immunoreactive HGF and PCNA-positive endothelial cells compared with control vector. HGF gene transfer, in both normal and infarcted myocardium, activated the angiogenic transcription factor, etc. Reduced HGF concentration in infarcted hearts increased to normal levels 4 d after HGF gene transfer. Angiogenesis was assessed by a light microscopic analysis following perfusion–fixation. In both normal and infarcted tissue, HGF-treated animals exhibited greater numbers of vessels per section than animals that had received injections of control vector. Surface myocardial blood flow assessed by laser Doppler at thoracotomy revealed higher values for HGF-treated normal and infarcted rats compared to controls. This was a study that documented angiogenesis in a blinded and controlled manner.

The feasibility of gene therapy using HGF to treat peripheral arterial disease (PAD) in diabetic rats was also investigated *(43)*. Intramuscular injection of hemagglutinating virus of Japan (HVJ)-liposome was used to transfect the human HGF gene into the diabetic rat hindlimb model. A significant increase in blood flow as assessed by laser Doppler imaging and increased capillary density accompanied the detection of human HGF protein. The degree of natural recovery of blood flow was significantly greater in nondiabetic rats than in diabetic rats. In an in vitro culture system, the molecular mechanisms of how diabetes delayed angiogenesis were also studied. High D-glucose treatment of endothelial cells resulted in a significant decrease in matrix metalloproteinase (MMP)-1 protein and ets-1 expression in human aortic endothelial cells. Similarly, high D-glucose significantly decreased the mRNA and protein of HGF in endothelial cells. The investigators concluded that intramuscular injection of human HGF plasmid induced therapeutic angiogenesis in a diabetic rat ischemic hindlimb model as a potential therapy for PAD. It has been suggested that the delay of angiogenesis in diabetics is due to downregulation of MMP-1 and ets-1 through a decrease in HGF by high D-glucose.

Intrapericardial Delivery

Lazarous and colleagues explored the effects on collateral vessel development following intrapericardial delivery of an adenovirus encoding VEGF-165 (Ad.VEGF-165) using the ameroid model of ischemia in dogs *(44)*. Ten days after ameroid placement, Ad.VEGF165 (6×10^9 pfu), an adenovirus encoding lacZ (6×10^9 pfu), or control was injected into the pericardial space through an indwelling catheter placed at the initial thoracotomy. Twenty-eight days later, maximal MBF was measured using the microsphere technique. Gene expression was abundant in pericardium and epicardium but not evident in the midmyocardium or endocardium. VEGF expression was detectable in fluid samples from the pericardial space, with a peak occurring 3 d after gene transfer with subsequent decline. Plasma VEGF was not increased. Maximal myocardial blood flow was equivalent in all groups and unchanged by VEGF gene transfer. Thus, despite sustained increased amounts of VEGF produced and released into the pericardial space and gene transfer in pericardium and epicardium, increased myocardial blood flow did not occur. Ad.VEGF-165 gene transfer was associated with large pericardial effusions, requiring drainage and resulting in death due to pericardial tamponade in one animal. The authors suggested that large pericardial effusions might be a result of the effect of VEGF on permeability.

Intracoronary Delivery

Giordano et al. *(45)* used the porcine ameroid model to perform an intracoronary injection of a recombinant adenovirus expressing a human fibroblast growth factor (Ad.FGF-5). The study compared the efficacy of intracoronary Ad.FGF-5 and intracoronary adenovirus encoding lacZ, both at 2×10^{11} vp, in the treatment of already existing stress-induced regional myocardial ischemia. Two weeks after gene transfer, regional abnormalities in stress-induced function and perfusion were examined by transthoracic echocardiography. Improved function and perfusion were associated with evidence of angiogenesis. This report documented successful treatment of abnormalities in myocardial blood flow and function following gene transfer. Although capillary angiogenesis was documented, evidence for increased numbers of larger caliber vessels was not reported, thus limiting study results.

In brief, previous animal studies have proven the feasibility of enhancing angiogenesis by delivering various factors to the myocardium via different routes. It is still not known which is the most effective and safe delivery strategy to induce therapeutic angiogenic responses in ischemic myocardium. With intracoronary injection, during its first pass a significant amount of the angiogenic factor will not be taken up from the vascular compartment by the heart and will be delivered to other tissues. Therefore, it may be preferable to deliver the angiogenic agent directly into the target tissue. These studies indicate that the model, vector, and route of administration are the major critical elements of success in angiogenesis studies.

CELL THERAPY STUDIES

Since the initial encouraging work utilizing gene and protein therapies, various studies are currently being conducted to look at the possi-

Table 4
Preclinical Studies of Angiogenesis Using Various Animal Models and Cell Types

Investigator/ref.	Animal model	Injury model	Cell type/location of delivery
Asahara et al., 1997 (46)	Mouse + rabbit	Hindlimb ischemia	EPC/iv injection
Tomita et al., 1999 (47)	Adult rat	Cryoinjury	Autologous BMC/scar
Kobayashi et al., 2000 (48)	Rat	LAD ligation	Autologous BMC/ischemic area
Schatteman et al., 2000 (49)	Diabetic rat	Hindlimb ischemia	CD34+ cells/intramuscular
Shintani et al., 2001 (50)	Rabbit	Hindlimb ischemia	Autologous BMC/ischemic area
Orlic et al., 2001 (51)	Rat	Coronary ligation	BMC/ischemic area
Fuchs et al., 2001 (52)	Pig	LCX ameroid	Autologous BMC/intra-myocardial
Kim et al., 2001 (53)	Rat	Cryoinjury	EPC/scar
Kocher et al., 2001 (54)	Rat	LAD ligation	CD34+ cells/ischemic area
Kobayashi et al., 2002 (55)	Rat	Hindlimb ischemia	Peripheral leukocytes and platelets/scar
Hamano et al., 2002 (56)	Dog	LAD ligation	Autologous BMC/normal, marginal, infarct areas

EPC, endothelial progenitor cells; BMC, bone marrow cells; LAD, left anterior descending artery; LCX, left circumflex artery.

bility of a more natural angiogenic agent—cells. Different cell types, including allogeneic vs autologous, and different cell sources, such as skeletal muscle, bone marrow, and peripheral blood, are under swift investigation. Some examples of recent cell therapy studies in various animal models are given in Table 4 (46–56).

NONINVASIVE IMAGING TECHNIQUES

There has been a tremendous improvement in the imaging techniques utilized for evaluation of therapeutic angiogenesis strategies. Recently, important trends have been observed in the use of noninvasive and high-tech approaches such as MRI. In the past, the identification of collateral circulation has been limited because of the insensitivity of utilized techniques. One of these techniques is conventional angiography, which is capable of identifying only vessels larger than 180 μm in diameter. This limits detection to a subset of epicardial collateral vessels, making it impossible to detect smaller intramyocardial vessels.

Demonstrating physiological improvements in myocardial perfusion or function is critically important in therapeutic angiogenesis studies. Currently, MRI appears to be the most promising and sensitive imaging modality *(57)*. Nuclear imaging techniques (e.g., SPECT, positron emission tomography [PET]) and x-ray angiography have been used to assess changes in perfusion and anatomical appearance, respectively. There have been concerns related to SPECT's sensitivity and spatial resolution in detecting subtle improvement in perfusion. On the other hand, with PET imaging, attenuation correction significantly improves image quality and has the potential to detect subtle changes in blood flow and flow reserve. However, the limited availability and expense of PET are some factors preventing its application *(58)*. New MRI techniques are able to identify early changes in vivo and are more sensitive in detecting the effects of new vessel growth than x-ray angiography or nuclear imaging *(59)*. Cardiac magnetic resonance (CMR), with its higher sensitivity and specificity indices in identifying coronary artery disease (CAD), has not been extensively used in earlier trials of angiogenic therapies. Using CMR as a noninvasive test that assesses myocardial function and perfusion in one session may considerably lower the cost of such trials *(60)*.

COLLATERAL-SENSITIVE MRI IN SWINE
MODEL OF CHRONIC ISCHEMIA

The novel technique of collateral-sensitive MRI appears promising as a noninvasive quantitative measure of the progress of collateral development. Recently, the ability of collateral-sensitive MR imaging to examine the presence and quantify the extent of neovas- cularization has been investigated in chronic ischemic porcine myocardium *(61)*. In pigs with vascular occluders, the extent of collaterals was determined with collateral sensitive imaging and correlated with measurements by three-dimensional (3D) computed tomography (CT), coronary blood flow distribution (microspheres), and histological examination. The presence of intramyocardial collateral microvessels was accurately determined with collateral-sensitive MRI. The histological slices stained with anti-von Willebrand factor antibody to determine new vessel development demonstrated the presence of typical thin-walled intramyocardial collateral microvessels in the areas depicted with the dark flare but not in the nonischemic myocardium. The comparison of two studies demonstrated that thallium imaging had no predictive value for coronary collateral microvessels.

Advantages of this technique include:

1. Depicts small areas of neovascularization
2. Provides quantitative assessment of extent of neovascularization
3. Enables serial noninvasive studies of collateral development

Disadvantages of this technique include:

1. Is not useful in determining the time of arrival of the contrast agent in the LV
2. Identifies new vessels that are much smaller than the image resolution, owing to the signal flare of magnetic susceptibility, which could result in an overestimation of the extent of collateral development

The extent of collateral territory determined with collateral-sensitive MRI was compared to that determined with the ex vivo images acquired with elastic-match 3D CT after intracoronary contrast agent injection. There was a remarkable visual identity between both sets of images, and quantitative analysis of the territory extent also demonstrated a close correlation between the two techniques. Similarly, the extent of collateral perfusion determined with collateral-sensitive MRI was comparable to that determined with coronary microspheric data, demonstrating a close correlation between the techniques. The presence of a dark flare signal detected with collateral-sensitive MRI was associated with the histological evidence of intramyocardial collateral microvessels (the extent corresponding to the anatomical extent of intramyocardial neovascularization), suggesting that the latter is responsible for this effect. The increase in dark flare area in the VEGF-treated animals was comparable to the control group, further supporting the technique's sensitivity to the extent of collateral perfusion. The signal at collateral-sensitive MRI is not obscured by LV filling with magnetic susceptibility contrast agent, does not obscure myocardial signal, and is not influenced by variations in ventricular wall thickness.

Catheter-Based Endomyocardial Injections With Real-Time MRI in Swine

Technological advances in MRI allow for rapid image acquisition and display. Lederman et al. recently tested the feasibility of targeted LV mural injections using real-time MRI (rtMRI) in swine *(62)*. They used a 1.5T MRI scanner customized with a fast reconstruction engine, transfemoral guiding catheter-receiver coil, MRI-compatible needle, and tableside consoles. It was concluded that percutaneous endomyocardial delivery is feasible with the aid of rtMRI, which permits precise 3D localization of injection within the LV wall.

ELECTROMECHANICAL LV MAPPING/INJECTION SYSTEM

Angiogenesis can be induced by direct injection of growth factors into ischemic myocardium during open-heart surgery. Catheter-based transendocardial injection of angiogenic factors may provide equivalent benefit without need for surgery. The feasibility of catheter-mediated direct injection of an Ad.vector inducing gene expression in the ventricle has been previously demonstrated *(63)*. Recently, electromechanical mapping and a percutaneous approach has been used to deliver proangiogenic transgenes into the pig myocardium *(64)*. This includes a new guidance system utilizing magnetic fields and catheter-tip sensors to locate the position in space and reconstruct 3D LV electromechanical maps without using fluoroscopy.

Structure and Mechanism of Function

An electromechanical mapping system includes the following parts:

1. A location pad containing three coils generating ultralow magnetic field energy
2. A stationary reference catheter with a miniature magnetic field sensor located on the body surface
3. A navigation sensor mapping catheter with a deflectable tip and electrodes providing endocardial signals
4. A workstation for information processing and 3D LV reconstruction

One advantage of this approach is that it precisely localizes gene transfer and directs it towards the most ischemic myocardial regions. The mapping catheter is introduced retrograde across the aortic valve into the LV. The initial three points outlining the boundaries of the LV (apex, aortic outflow, and mitral inflow) are acquired with fluoroscopic guidance. The mapping process proceeds after stabilizing the catheter tip on the endocardial surface as evidenced by a local activation time, location, loop, and cycle length stability parameters. Once all endocardial regions are represented on the map, an injection catheter replaces the mapping catheter. The needle is controlled by a handle mechanism located proximal to the standard deflection handle. Standard manual operation of the syringe attached to the injection handle delivers the agent to the myocardium. The exact catheter-tip location, orientation, and injection sites are indicated in real time on the LV map, and local electrical and location signals are traced to assure catheter stability and optimal endocardial contact. Arrhythmia is evaluated from the LV mapping catheter data during mapping and by electrocardiographic recording after injection.

A study by Vale et al. *(64)* was designed to test the feasibility of myocardial angiogenic gene expression using a novel catheter-based transendocardial injection system. In 12 pigs, the catheter was used to inject 0.1 mL of methylene-blue (MB) dye, and 8 pigs had myocardial injections of adenoviral vector (1×10^{10} particles per site) containing the LacZ transgene. Ten pigs underwent catheter-based transendocardial injection, and six pigs were injected using a transepicardial approach with the gene encoding adenovirus vascular endothelial growth factor-121 (Ad.VEGF-121, 1×10^{10} viral particles $\times$ 6 sites) and sacrificed at 24 h. Injection sites were identified with ultraviolet light by coinjection of fluorescent beads. Tissue staining was 7.1 ± 2.1 mm in depth and 2.3 ± 1.8 mm in width. No animal had pericardial effusion or tamponade. Gross pathology showed positive staining in injected zones, and histology confirmed positive myocyte staining. Ad.VEGF-121 injected sites showed high levels of VEGF-121 production, which were of similar magnitude whether injected via transendocardial or transepicardial delivery.

This less invasive catheter-based system offers a similar gene-delivery efficiency and, thus, may have clear advantages when compared to a surgically based transepicardial injection approach. Importantly, the VEGF-121 results showed much greater expression at the site of injection, with a significant drop-off of VEGF production even 1 cm from the injection site. This study showed that the catheter-based approach for gene delivery makes possible equivalent gene transfection efficiency and gene expression compared with a surgically based transepicardial injection approach.

ANIMAL MODELS FOR ANGIOGENESIS: DEPENDABLE BASIS FOR HUMAN STUDIES?

Studies using small and large animal models of ischemia have shown that significant development, the both in cardiac and peripheral circulation, can be achieved through the administration of angiogenic factors. Obviously, it would be premature to expect that the encouraging results obtained in animals will necessarily be observed in humans *(65)*. There are a number of points to be considered in translating the results of the preclinical studies into the clinical arena:

1. Animals do not have atherosclerotic vascular disease. The presence of such disease may adversely affect the response to growth factors.
2. Patients in angiogenesis trials are typically older, whereas a typical animal in a preclinical study is usually a young adult or is still growing. A limited amount of data suggest that angiogenic potential and responsiveness to therapeutic angiogenesis decreases with age *(66–68)*.

3. A number of commonly used medications can potentially interfere with angiogenic response.

4. Laboratory animals represent an unselected population, whereas a typical patient in therapeutic angiogenesis trials has been selected because he or she demonstrated a failure to develop adequate collateral circulation and/or respond to prior therapeutic interventions, also known as a "no-option" patient.

All of these factors combined suggest that a lack of response in a large animal study should translate into a lack of response in a clinical trial. Similarly, a positive animal study does not guarantee a positive outcome in a patient trial *(69)*.

SUMMARY AND CONCLUSIONS

Preclinical efforts have moved therapeutic angiogenesis forward in two major areas. The first and most important area attempts to answer the question, 'how do we treat,' which includes other questions such as 'which animal model,' 'which route,' and 'what dose.' The second area, which has emerged more recently, attempts to answer the question, 'how do we capture the treatment effect.' Obviously, without the most precise assessment tools, it may not be possible to clearly understand if the field is moving on the right track. Furthermore, we need to investigate and decide upon the best time points at which to use these tools for the most accurate results. On the other hand, given the differences and complexity of the pathophysiology and progress of human cardiovascular diseases compared to relatively simplistic animal models, translation of these results to clinical practice may not be as fast or easy as originally believed.

REFERENCES

1. Unger EF. Experimental evaluation of coronary collateral development. Cardiovasc Res 2001;49:497–506.
2. Schaper W. Experimental infarcts and the microcirculation. In: Hearse DJ, Yellon DM, eds. Therapeutic Approaches to Myocardial Infarct Size Limitation. Raven, New York, NY: 1984:79–90.
3. Baroldi G, Scomazzoni G. Coronary circulation in the normal and the pathologic heart. Office of the Surgeon General, Department of the Army, 1967.
4. Baroldi G, Radice F, Schmid G, et al. Morphology of acute myocardial infarction in relation to coronary thrombosis. Am Heart J 1974;87:65–75.
5. Cohen MV. Coronary Collaterals, Clinical and Experimental Observations. Futura, Mount Kisco, NY: 1985.
6. Schaper W. The Collateral Circulation of the Heart. Elsevier, Amsterdam, Netherlands: 1971.
7. Schaper W, Schaper J. Collateral Circulation—Heart, Brain, Kidney, Limbs. Dordrecht: Kluwer Academic, 1993.
8. Folkman J, D'Amore A. Blood vessel formation: what is its molecular basis? Cell 1996;87:1153–1155.

9. Freedman SB, Isner JM. Therapeutic angiogenesis for coronary artery disease. Ann Intern Med 2002;136:54–71.

10. Unger EF. Experimental evaluation of coronary collateral development. Cardiovasc Res 2001;49:497–506.

11. Litvak J, Siderides LE, Vineberg AM. Experimental production of coronary artery insufficiency and occlusion. Am Heart J 1957;53:505–518.

12. Roth DM, Maruoka Y, Rogers J, et al. Development of collateral circulation in left circumflex ameroid-occluded swine myocardium. Am J Physiol 1987;253:H1279–H1288.

13. Roth DM, White FC, Nichols ML, et al. Effect of long-term exercise on regional myocardial function and coronary collateral development after gradual coronary artery occlusion in pigs. Circulation 1990;82:1778–1789.

14. Simons M. Myocardial ischemia and growth factor therapy. In: Dormandy JA, Dole WP, Rubanyi GM, eds. Therapeutic Angiogenesis. Springer, Berlin: 1999:125.

15. White FC, Carroll SM, Magnet A, et al. Coronary collateral development in swine after coronary artery occlusion. Circ Res 1992;71:1490–1500.

16. Radke PW, Heinl-Green A, Frass OM, et al. Evaluation of the porcine ameroid constrictor model of chronic myocardial ischemia for therapeutic angiogenesis studies. JACC 2003;41(6):331A.

17. Operschall C, Falivene L, Clozel JP, Roux S. A new model of chronic cardiac ischemia in rabbits. J Appl Physiol 2000;88:1438–1445.

18. Fujita M, Mikuniya A, Takayashi M, et al. Acceleration of coronary collateral development by heparin in conscious dogs. Jpn Circ J 1987;51:395–402.

19. Vineberg AM. The vineberg operation. 1. Revascularization of the heart. J Am Med Assoc 1966;195(Suppl):43–47c.

20. Kraitchman DL, Bluemke D, Chin BB, et al. A minimally invasive method for creating coronary stenosis in a swine model for MRI and SPECT imaging. Invest Radiol 2000;35:445–451.

21. Huwer H, Winning J, Vollmar B, et al. Microvascularization and ventricular function after local alginate-encapsulated angiogenic growth factor treatment in a rat cryothermia-induced myocardial infarction model. Microvasc Res 2001;62:211.

22. Huwer H, Rissland J, Vollmar B, et al. Angiogenesis and microvascularization after cryothermia-induced myocardial infarction: a quantitative fluorescence microscopic study in rats. Basic Res Cardiol 1999;94:85–93.

23. Chilian WM, Mass HJ, Williams SE, et al. Microvascular occlusions promote coronary collateral growth. Am J Physiol 1990;258:H1103–H1111.

24. Sabbah HN, Stein PD, Kono T, et al. A canine model of chronic heart failure produced by multiple sequential coronary microembolizations. Am J Physiol 1991;260:H1379–H1384.

25. Zimmermann R, Arras M, Ullmann C, et al. Time course of mitosis and collateral growth following coronary embolization in the porcine heart. Cell Tissue Res 1997;287:583–590.

26. Schaper W, Munoz-Chapuli R, Wolf C, et al. Collateral circulation of the heart. In: Ware JA, Simons M, eds. Angiogenesis and Cardiovascular Disease. Oxford University Press, Oxford, UK: 1999:159–198.

27. Li J, Brown LF, Hibberd MG, et al. VEGF, flk-1, and flt-1 expression in a rat myocardial model of angiogenesis. Am J Physiol 1996;270:H1803–H1811.

28. Takeshita S, Rossow S, Kearney M, et al. Time course of increased cellular proliferation in collateral arteries after administration of vascular endothelial growth factor in a rabbit model of lower limb vascular insufficiency. Am J Pathol 1995;147:1649–1660.

29. Ware JA, Simons M. Angiogenesis and Cardiovascular Disease. Oxford University Press, Oxford, UK: 1999.
30. Xie MH, Holcomb I, Deuel B, et al. FGF-19, a novel fibroblast growth factor with unique specificity for FGFR4. Cytokine 1999;11:729–735.
31. Battler A, Scheinowitz M, Bor A, et al. Intracoronary injection of basic growth factor enhances angiogenesis in infarcted swine myocardium. J Am Coll Cardiol 1993;22:2001–2006.
32. Yanagisawa-Miwa A, Uchida Y, Nakamura F, et al. Salvage of infarcted myocardium by angiogenic action of basic fibroblast growth factor. Science 1992;257:1401–1403.
33. Roth DM, Maruoka Y, Rogers J, et al. Development of coronary collateral circulation in left circumflex ameroid-occluded swine myocardium. Am J Physiol 1987;253:H1279–H1288.
34. Banai S, Jaklitsch MT, Shou M, et al. Angiogenic-induced enhancement of collateral blood flow to ischemic myocardium by vascular endothelial growth factor in dogs. Circulation 1994;89:2183–2189.
35. Takeshita S, Zheng LP, Brogi E, et al. Therapeutic angiogenesis: a single intraarterial bolus of vascular endothelial growth factor augments revascularization in a rabbit ischemic hind limb model. J Clin Invest 1994;93:662–670.
36. Baird A, Walicke P. Fibroblast growth factors. Br Med Bull 1989;45:438–452.
37. Mack CA, Patel SR, Schwartz EA, et al. Biologic bypass with the use of adenovirus-mediated gene transfer of the complementary deoxyribonucleic acid for vascular endothelial growth factor 121 improves myocardial perfusion and function in the ischemic porcine heart. J Cardiovasc Surg 1998;115:168–177.
38. Patel SR, Lee LY, Mack CA, et al. Safety of direct myocardial administration of an adenovirus vector encoding vascular endothelial growth factor 121. Hum Gene Ther 1999;10:1331–1348.
39. French BA, Mazur W, Bolli R. Direct in vivo gene transfer into porcine myocardium using replication-deficient adenoviral vectors. Circulation 1994;90:2414–2424.
40. Kornowski R, Leon MB, Fuchs S, et al. Electromagnetic guidance for catheter-based transendocardial injection: a platform for intramyocardial angiogenesis therapy. J Am Coll Cardiol 2000;35:1031–1039.
41. Tio RA, Tkebuchava T, Scheuerman TH, et al. Intramyocardial gene therapy with naked DNA encoding vascular endothelial growth factor improves collateral flow to ischemic myocardium. Hum Gene Ther 1999;10:2953–2960.
42. Aoki M, Morishita R, Taniyame Y, et al. Angiogenesis induced by hepatocyte growth factor in noninfarcted myocardium and infarcted myocardium: up-regulation of essential transcription factor for angiogenesis. Gene Ther 2000;7:417–427.
43. Taniyama Y, Morishita R, Hiraoka K, et al. Therapeutic angiogenesis induced by human hepatocyte growth factor gene in rat diabetic hind limb ischemia model: molecular mechanisms of delayed angiogenesis in diabetes. Circulation 2001;104:2344–2350.
44. Lazarous DF, Shou M, Stiber JA, et al. Adenoviral-mediated gene transfer induces sustained pericardial VEGF expression in dogs: effect on myocardial angiogenesis. Cardiovasc Res 1999;44:294–302.
45. Giordano F, Ping P, McKirnan MD, et al. Intracoronary gene transfer of fibroblast growth factor-5 increases blood flow and contractile function in an ischemic region of the heart. Nat Med 1996;2:534–539.
46. Asahara T, Murohara T, Sullivan A, et al. Isolation of putative progenitor endothelial cells for angiogenesis. Science 1997;275:964–967.
47. Tomita S, Li RK, Weisel RD, et al. Autologous transplantation of bone marrow cells improves damaged heart function. Circulation 1999;100(19 Suppl):II247–II256.

48. Kobayashi T, Hamano K, Li TS, et al. Enhancement of angiogenesis by the implantation of self bone marrow cells in a rat ischemic heart model. Surg Res 2000;89:189–195.
49. Schatteman GC, Hanlon HD, Jiao C, et al. Blood-derived angioblasts accelerate blood-flow restoration in diabetic mice. J Clin Invest 2000;106:571–578.
50. Shintani S, Murohara T, Ikeda H, et al. Augmentation of postnatal neovascularization with autologous bone marrow transplantation. Circulation 2001;103:897–903.
51. Orlic D, Kajstura J, Chimenti S, et al. Bone marrow cells regenerate infarcted myocardium. Nature 2001;410:701–705.
52. Fuchs S, Baffour R, Zhou YF, et al. Transendocardial delivery of autologous bone marrow enhances collateral perfusion and regional function in pigs with chronic experimental myocardial ischemia. J Am Coll Cardiol 2001;37:1726–1732.
53. Kim EJ, Li RK, Weisel RD, et al. Angiogenesis by endothelial cell transplantation. J Thorac Cardiovasc Surg 2001;122:963–971.
54. Kocher AA, Schuster MD, Szabolcs MJ, et al. Neovascularization of ischemic myocardium by human bone-marrow-derived angioblasts prevents cardiomyocyte apoptosis, reduces remodeling and improves cardiac function. Nat Med 2001;7:430–436.
55. Kobayashi T, Hamano K, Li TS, et al. Angiogenesis induced by the injection of peripheral leukocytes and platelets. J Surg Res 2002;103:279–286.
56. Hamano K, Li TS, Kobayashi T, et al. Therapeutic angiogenesis induced by local autologous bone marrow cell implantation. Ann Thorac Surg 2002;73:1210–1215.
57. Post MJ, Laham R, Sellke FW, Simons M. Therapeutic angiogenesis in cardiology using protein formulations. Cardiovasc Res 2001;49:522–531.
58. Simons M, Bonow RO, Chronos NA. Clinical trials in coronary angiogenesis: issues, problems, consensus: an expert panel summary. Circ 2000;102:E73–E86.
59. Pearlman JD, Laham RJ, Post M, et al. Medical imaging techniques in the evaluation of strategies for therapeutic angiogenesis. Curr Pharm Des 2002;8:1467–1496.
60. Wilke NM, Zenovich AG, Jerosch-Herold M, Henry TD. Cardiac magnetic resonance imaging for the assessment of myocardial angiogenesis. Curr Interv Cardiol Rep 2001;3:205–212.
61. Pearlman JD, Laham RJ, Simons M. Coronary angiogenesis: detection in vivo with MR imaging sensitive to collateral neocirculation—preliminary study in pigs. Radiology 2000;214:801–807.
62. Lederman RJ, Guttman MA, Peters DC. Catheter-based endomyocardial injection with real-time magnetic resonance imaging. Circulation 2002;105:1282–1284.
63. Li JJ, Ueno H, Pan Y, et al. Percutaneous transluminal gene transfer into canine myocardium in vivo by replication-defective adenovirus. Cardiovasc Res 1995;30:97–105.
64. Vale PR, Losordo DW, Tkebuchava T, et al. Catheter-based myocardial gene transfer utilizing nonfluoroscopic electromechanical left ventricular mapping. J Am Coll Cardiol 1999;34:246–254.
65. Goncalves LM, Epstein SE, Piek JJ. Controlling collateral development: the difficult task of mimicking mother nature. Cardiovasc Res 2001;49:495–496.
66. Reed MJ, Corsa A, Pendergrass W, et al. Neovascularization in aged mice: delayed angiogenesis is coincident with decreased levels of transforming growth factor beta1 and type I collagen. Am J Pathol 1998;152:113–123.
67. Swift ME, Kleinman HK, DiPietro LA. Impaired wound repair and delayed angiogenesis in aged mice. Lab Invest 1999;79:1479–1487.
68. Reed MJ, Corsa AC, Kudravi SA, et al. A deficit in collagenase activity contributes to impaired migration of aged microvascular endothelial cells. J Cell Biochem 2000;77:116–126.

69. Simons M. Therapeutic coronary angiogenesis: a fronte praecipitium a tergo lupi? Am J Physiol Heart Circ Physiol 2002;280:H1923–H1927.

70. Harada K, et al. Basic fibroblast growth factor improves myocardial function in chronically ischemic porcine hearts. J Clin Invest 1994;94:623–630.

71. Lopez JJ, Edelman ER, Stamler A, et al. Basic fibroblast growth factor in a porcine model of chronic myocardial ischemia: a comparison of angiographic, echocardiographic and coronary flow parameters. J Pharmacol Exp Ther 1997; 282:385–390.

72. Sato K, Laham RJ, Pearlman JD, et al. Efficacy of intracoronary versus intravenous FGF-2 in a pig model of chronic myocardial ischemia. Ann Thorac Surg 2000;70: 2113–2118.

73. Laham RJ, Rezaee M, Post M, et al. Delivery of fibroblast growth factor-2 induces neovascularization in a porcine model of chronic myocardial ischemia. J Pharmacol Exp Ther 2000;292:795–802.

74. Unger EF, Banai S, Shou M, et al. Basic fibroblast growth factor enhances myocardial collateral flow in a canine model. Am J Physiol Heart Circ Physiol 1994;266: H1588–H1595.

75. Lazarous DF, Scheinowitz M, Shou M, eta l. Effects of chronic systemic administration of basic fibroblast growth factor on collateral development in the canine heart. Circulation 1995;91:145–153.

76. Uchida Y, Yanagisawa-Miwa A, Nakamura F, et al. Angiogenic therapy of acute myocardial infarciton by intrapericardial injection of basic fibroblast growth factor and heparin sulfate: an experiment study. Am Heart J 1995;130:1182–1188.

77. Shou M, Thirumurti V, Rajanayagam S. Effect of basic fibroblast growth factor on myocardial angiogenesis in dogs with mature collateral vessels. J Am Coll Cardiol 1997;29:1102–1106.

78. Villanueva FS, Abraham JA, Schreiner GF, et al. Myocardial Contrast Echocardiography can be used to assess the microvascular response to vascular endothelial growth factor-121. Circulation 2002;105:759–765.

79. Baffour R, Berman J, Garb JL, Rhee SW, Kaufman J, Friedmann P. Enhanced angiogenesis and growth of collaterals by in vivo administration of recombinant basic fibroblast growth factor in a rabbit model of acute lower limb ischemia: dose-response effect of basic fibroblast growth facotr. J Vasc Surg 1992;16:181–191.

80. Takeshita S, Pu LQ, Stein LA, et al. Intramuscular administration of vascular endothelial growth factor induces dose-dependent collateral artery augmentation in a rabbit model of chronic limb ischemia. Circulation 1994;90:II228–II234.

81. Edelman ER, Nugent MA, Smith LT, Karnovsky MJ. Basic fibroblast growth factor enhances the coupling of intimal hyperplasia and proliferation of vasa vasorum in injured rat arteries. J Clin Invest 1992;89:465–473.

4 The Coronary Microcirculation and Angiogenesis

Pierre Voisine, Joanna J. Wykrzykowska,
Munir Boodhwani, David G. Harrison,
Roger J. Laham, and Frank W. Sellke

CONTENTS

INTRODUCTION

Resistance circulation of the heart is important in regulating the delivery of blood and nutrients to the myocardium. There has been a long-standing interest in studying its properties; however, prior to the mid-1980s, technical limitations made it difficult to directly study coro-

From: *Contemporary Cardiology: Angiogenesis and Direct Myocardial Revasularization*
Edited by: R. J. Laham and D. S. Baim © Humana Press Inc., Totowa, NJ

nary microvessels either *in situ* or in vitro. Traditionally, studies of the coronary microcirculation had been limited to indirect assessments using measurements of coronary flow and calculations of coronary resistance, which provided a great deal of insight into the properties of the intact coronary circulation. Significantly more has been learned in the last 15 yr as new in vivo and in vitro approaches have been developed for direct study of coronary microvessels *(1–4)*. Furthermore, development of microangiography methods allowed for visualization of the coronary microcirculation in mammals *(5,6)*. The most important finding of these studies was the inhomogeneity of the resistance vessels *(7)*.

As are other vascular beds, the coronary microcirculation is composed of resistance arterioles, capillaries, and small veins (venules). The unique features of the coronary microcirculation allow it to function in the setting of a contracting support structure, to interact with the surrounding tissue, and to respond to dynamic changes in requirements for nutrients. These features of the coronary microcirculation have been described previously in extensive review articles *(8–11)* and entire books *(12,13)*. Thorough re-analysis of all facets of coronary physiology is covered in these prior reviews. The following paragraphs will discuss and emphasize some of the critical aspects of coronary circulation physiology, particularly as they relate to the coronary microcirculation. We will focus on how the physiology and pharmacology of the coronary microcirculation pertains to angiogenesis.

DEFINITIONS: THE CORONARY RESISTANCE CIRCULATION AS DEFINED BY PRESSURE GRADIENTS

Resistance vessels are those over which pressure losses occur. Traditionally, resistance vessels were considered to be precapillary arterioles (25–50 μm). Vessels of larger dimensions were thought to have little role in the regulation of perfusion. For the coronary circulation, this concept was radically changed in the 1980s by Nellis et al. *(1)* and, subsequently, Chilian and co-workers *(2)*. Their experiments demonstrated that approx 50% of the total coronary vascular resistance is present in vessels larger than 100 μm in diameter, particularly under conditions of ischemia and hypoxia *(14)*. The pressure decreases could be observed in vessels as large as 300 μm. The distribution of vascular resistance is not static and the size of vessels regulating vascular resistance depends on the tone of the vasculature (Fig. 1) *(2,15)*. Under conditions of vasodilatation following intravenous administration of dipyridamole, a significant redistribution of microvascular resistance occurs. Similarly to what is seen in myocardial ischemia (>50% stenosis), a greater proportion of vascular resistance is then attributable to larger arteries and veins *(16)*. As much

Basal flow

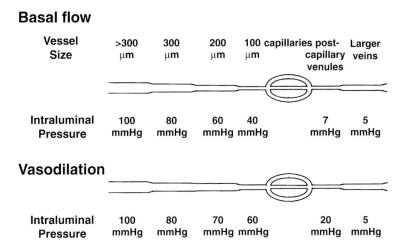

Vessel Size	>300 μm	300 μm	200 μm	100 μm	capillaries	post-capillary venules	Larger veins
Intraluminal Pressure	100 mmHg	80 mmHg	60 mmHg	40 mmHg		7 mmHg	5 mmHg

Vasodilation

Intraluminal Pressure	100 mmHg	80 mmHg	70 mmHg	60 mmHg		20 mmHg	5 mmHg

Fig. 1. Intravascular pressures in the coronary microcirculation under basal conditions and during vasodilation with dipyridamole. Dipyridamole infusion reduced pressures in small arteries <170 μm while increasing venular pressures resulting in redistribution of microvascular resistance. Adapted from refs. *15* and *16*.

as 30% of resistance may reside in the venous circulation under conditions of maximal vascular dilatation, in contrast with predictions derived from older traditional theories of vascular regulation. These observations have led to numerous studies, both in vivo and in vitro, examining the properties of these larger (100–300 μm) microvessels.

Another unique feature of the coronary circulation is that pressure losses are observed not only as vessel sizes decrease, but also as they penetrate from the epicardium to the endocardium *(17)*. The influence of extravascular forces is differentially distributed across the myocardium and becomes especially important at the subendocardial level *(15)*. During maximal vasodilatation, this pressure gradient increases from a few (8–10) to more than 20 mmHg, and can further increase in the setting of cardiac hypertrophy (Fig. 2) *(18)*. The net result is a reduction of perfusion pressure in the subendocardium, providing a potential explanation to the susceptibility of hypertrophied hearts to develop subendocardial ischemia.

REGULATION OF CORONARY VASOMOTOR TONE: ENDOGENOUS AND EXOGENOUS CONTROL

Vasomotor tone results from the complex interaction of circulating substances, properties intrinsic to the vessel wall, surrounding parenchymal tissue, neuronal influences, and extra-vascular factors. Proper-

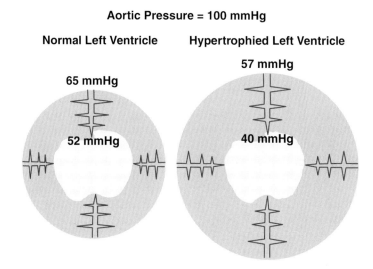

Fig. 2. Transmural losses of coronary perfusion pressure in normal and hyper-trophied hearts. Pressures were measured using micropuncture-servo null tech-niques in hearts perfused via the left main coronary artery at 100 mmHg. Adapted from ref. *18*.

ties intrinsic to the vessel wall and interactions with adjacent tissues may work together to promote metabolic regulation and autoregulation. In the coronary circulation, there is evidence that all of these are integrated to play a role in setting microvascular tone, and there are longitudinal gradients of metabolic, myogenic, and flow-dependent responses *(19)*. The major contributing factors are summarized in Fig. 3 *(15)*.

Myogenic Tone

Myogenic tone is a property of the vascular smooth muscle in most vessels, including coronary microvessels *(3)*. The myogenic response is an increase in wall tension, or a decrease in vessel diameter, in response to an increase in vascular transmural pressure according to Laplace's law. Vessels contract in response to an increased intraluminal pressure to normalize wall tension and prevent vascular injury *(20)*. Myogenic reactivity lends an important contribution to regulation of blood flow and maintenance of basal vascular tone. It has been postulated as one mechanism of autoregulation. We will discuss the molecular mecha-nisms that mediate myogenic response later.

Depolarization of the vascular smooth muscle cells (VSMCs) in response to increased intraluminal pressure or stretch causes influx of Ca^{2+} *(22–24)*. The 30-pS nonselective mechanosensitive cation chan-

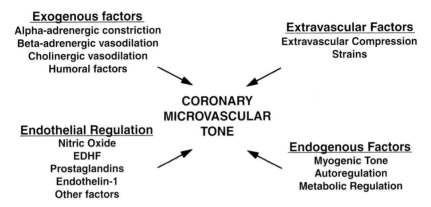

Fig. 3. Major factors contributing to regulation of coronary microvascular tone (**A**) mechanosensor induced calcium influx, the role of L-type calcium channels and the downstream mediators; (**B**) Diacylglycerol and 20-hydroxyeicosatrienoic acid pathways. Adapted from ref. *11*.

nel belonging to the transient receptor potential channels (TRPCs) family has recently been discovered as a potential effector of this initial calcium influx *(25)*. As calcium enters the vascular muscle cell and depolarizes it, this in turn activates L-type (voltage-gated) calcium channels, leading to increased intracellular calcium and vasoconstriction. Calcium-activated as well as voltage-dependent potassium channels, responsible for compensatory potassium efflux and hyperpolarization, provide a feedback mechanism for depolarization and vasoconstriction *(21,26)*. The density of L-type calcium channels is greatest in arteries with smallest diameters *(27)*. This mechanism plays a pivotal role in myogenic microvascular constriction *(24)*.

In addition to the stretch-activated calcium channels, activation of phospholipase C *(28,29)* also plays a role in vasomotor tone, resulting in the production of diacylglycerol and inositol 1,4,5-trisphosphate (IP_3). While IP_3 triggers the release of Ca^{2+} from the sarcoplasmic reticulum *(30)*, diacylglycerol activates protein kinase C (PKC) *(31,32)*. PKC positively feedbacks on calcium influx.

20-Hydroxyeicosatetraenoic acid (20-HETE) and epoxyeicosatrienoic acids (EETs), the metabolic products of arachidonic acid by cytochrome P-450 enzymes, also play critical roles in the regulation of vascular tone *(33)*. Whereas EETs are endothelium-derived vasodilators that hyperpolarize VSMCs through activation of K^+ channels, 20-HETE is a vasoconstrictor produced in VSMCs that reduces the open-state probability of Ca^{2+}-activated K^+ channels *(33)*. The involvement of 20-

HETE in the regulation of coronary vascular tones is suggested by recent data showing that it can induce contraction of small porcine coronary arteries by two mechanisms, one endothelium-dependent, involving the cyclooxygenase-dependent generation of vasoconstrictor prostanoids, and the other endothelium-independent, involving the activation of Rho-kinase, phosphorylation of myosin light chain MLC20, and sensitization of the contractile apparatus to Ca^{2+} (34).

Mitogen-activated protein (MAP) kinase pathways have also been investigated for their contributing role in myogenic tone. They are involved in the mechanotransduction of wall tension of rat skeletal muscle arterioles exposed to pressure (35). In a recent study, vasomotor dysfunction of the coronary microcirculation following cardiopulmonary bypass and cardioplegic arrest in humans was found to be mediated in part by alterations in the MAP/extracellular signal regulated kinase (ERK)1/2 pathway (36).

Myogenic tone in coronary vessels is independent of the endothelium (37); however, it varies among species and is influenced both by vessel size and ventricular transmural heterogeneity. Spontaneous tone and myogenic responses are often observed in porcine and primate coronary vessels. In contrast, they are uncommonly seen in canine coronary microvessels. The magnitude of the myogenic response of porcine arterioles has been shown to be less significant in microvessels larger than 150 μm (38), and of maximal importance in intermediate arterioles (50–80 μm) (39). Myogenic responses to increases in pressure are greater in coronary microvessels from the subepicardium than in vessels from the subendocardium (3). This increased dilatation capacity of subepicardial arterioles functions as a possible protective mechanism to ischemia. Interestingly, exercise training also seems to increase the capacity for coronary arterioles to generate myogenic tone (40). The physiological relevance of this remains unclear, but recent evidence suggests that exercise-induced alterations in PKC signaling underlie the enhanced myogenic contraction (32).

Metabolic Regulation and Autoregulation

The tone of the coronary microcirculation and, consequently, levels of myocardial perfusion, are tightly coupled to the state of myocardial oxygen consumption. When myocardial oxygen needs are increased, coronary flow rises accordingly. This is partly a result of myocardial oxygen extraction being near maximum even under resting conditions. Thus, myocardial ability to extract additional oxygen with increased demand is limited.

Autoregulation refers to the ability of a vascular bed to constrict and dilate, in order to maintain flow constant during changes in perfusion pressure. In the coronary circulation, autoregulation is most effective between pressures of 40 and 160 mmHg. The range of pressures over which autoregulation can be observed is different for the subendocardium, as compared with the subepicardium. Thus, flow will begin to decrease at pressures <70–75 mmHg in the subendocardium, as opposed to substantially lower pressures in the more superficial layers of the heart (41). Importantly, chronic hypertension shifts the range of pressures over which autoregulation occurs in the subendocardium such that flow will begin to decline at even higher pressures. This may be related to changes in subendocardial perfusion pressure (discussed earlier) and thus may also explain the propensity for the subendocardium to develop ischemia in the setting of myocardial hypertrophy. Of note, during both autoregulation and metabolic regulation, studies using direct observations of the coronary microcirculation indicate that the predominant changes in vasomotion occur in vessels <100 μm in diameter.

The signaling molecules linking flow to demand and participating in the autoregulation process have been the subject of extensive investigation, but remain poorly defined (42). Prostaglandins (43), nitric oxide (NO) (44), tissue levels of oxygen, carbon dioxide, hydrogen ions, and potassium have all been considered as candidates (45). Flow-induced dilation, in contrast with myogenic response, is endothelium-dependent and is dependent on as-yet unidentified mechanoreceptors. Extensive research spanning 40 yr has been devoted to understanding a potential role of adenosine as a mediator of either autoregulation or metabolic regulation. Adenosine was thought to be a likely candidate because it is a potent vasodilator, and accumulates as a result of increased cardiac work or ischemia. Several earlier studies showed adenosine levels in the heart and coronary sinus correlating with myocardial work and coronary perfusion (46). Despite this, antagonists of the adenosine receptor and degradation of adenosine with adenosine deaminase have only minor effects on myocardial perfusion at rest or during a variety of interventions. More recent studies in canine models of either pacing-induced metabolic stimulation under β-blockade and anesthesia (46) or exercise-induced stimulation in the steady state (47) showed that adenosine is not required for the local metabolic control of coronary flow. These results suggest that reactive hyperemia relies primarily on mediators other than adenosine.

A role for ATP-sensitive potassium channels in regulation of myocardial perfusion has also been described, and linked to adenosine-induced vasodilation. Studies in pig subepicardial coronary arterioles have led to the proposition that adenosine activates both endothelial and smooth muscle cell pathways via their respective K_{ATP} channels. The opening of K_{ATP} channels through activation of pertussis toxin-sensitive G proteins in the endothelium leads to the production and release of NO. Subsequently, NO activates smooth muscle guanylyl cyclase resulting in vasodilation. The activation of smooth muscle K_{ATP} channels, on the other hand, leads to vasodilation through hyperpolarization, independently of G proteins and cAMP/cGMP pathways *(48)*. Blockade of these channels with glibenclamide inhibits vasodilation of coronary microvessels less than 100 µm in diameter caused by reduction in perfusion pressure *(49)*. Blocking K_{ATP} channels also reduces basal coronary perfusion in vivo *(50,51)*. These two separate pathways of potassium channel opening and adenosine receptor activation interact to modulate myocardial flow during exercise and during changes in myocardial perfusion pressure *(51)*. The concept of redundancy in control of such an important process as coronary metabolic and autoregulation is extremely important. It may explain why previous studies examining these pathways in isolation were negative. More recently, the role of K_{ATP} channels in coronary vasodilation and modulation of coronary blood flow was also demonstrated in patients *(52)*. It was also demonstrated that K_{ATP} channel-mediated vasodilation is impaired in diabetics *(53)*. The role of endothelial function in autoregulation as well as coronary vascular tone as a whole is well recognized and considered in a further section. In contrast with the importance of vasodilatory substances produced by myocytes in relation to oxygen consumption, constrictors such as endothelin-1 seem to have decreased influence on vascular tone during increased metabolism *(54)*.

Extravascular Forces

The coronary circulation is exposed to a large number of extravascular forces produced by contraction of adjacent myocardium and intraventricular pressures. Extravascular influences may become more evident during ischemia or in the setting of other pathological processes leading to decreased tissue compliance or increased tissue edema. For example, collateral perfusion is particularly sensitive to changes in heart rate (more frequent extravascular compression) and ventricular diameter (stretch) *(13,55)*.

Extravascular pressure might collapse coronary vessels under certain circumstances. In 1978, Bellamy reported that flow through the epicardial coronary arteries halted when aortic pressure fell to values ranging from 25 to 50 mmHg *(56)*. This observation and others highlighted the possibility that extravascular forces might be sufficiently high to collapse vessels when intraluminal pressures declined to values below this "critical closing pressure." It soon became apparent, however, that flow in the coronary microcirculation continued even when the arterial driving pressure was minimally higher than coronary venous pressure. Modeling and various experimental interventions determined that this continued forward flow in microvessels despite decreases of antegrade blood flow in larger upstream arteries was explained by capacitance of the coronary circulation (57). Kanatsuka and colleagues used a floating microscope to visualize epicardial capillaries. They were able to show that red cells continued to flow, even after perfusion had stopped in the more proximal vessels. Using this approach, they showed that the "stop-flow" pressure in the epicardial coronary microvessels was only a few mmHg higher than right atrial pressure (58). They did not observe cessation of epicardial coronary microvessel flow at any pressure. Therefore, it seems likely that the concept of "critical closing pressure" is not applicable to all vessels in the coronary circulation. It is conceivable that vessels deeper in the subendocardium may collapse as a result of pressure transmitted from the ventricular chamber, particularly when left-ventricular diastolic pressure is very high. Myocardial contrast echocardiography studies in dogs show an increase in capillary resistance as coronary blood flow decreases. They provide an alternative explanation for the critical coronary closing pressure (59). Most recent data from Sun and co-workers (60) shows that cardiac contraction with consequent vessel deformation causes increase in endothelial nitric oxide synthase (eNOS) phosphorylation and increase in NO production and vasodilation. This NO release is greater in the subendocardium that in the subepicardium.

Neurohumoral Control of the Circulation

In the past three decades, there has been a significant amount of research on the role of the sympathetic and parasympathetic nervous systems in regulating coronary perfusion (61). In awake animals, α-adrenergic stimulation produces rather marked reductions in coronary flow, suggesting constriction of coronary resistance vessels (57). Administration of β-adrenergic stimuli results in marked coronary vasodilation, because of a direct effect on the β-adrenergic receptors in the coronary microvessels and indirectly by increasing myocardial metabolic demand. Sympathetic nerve stimulation results in coronary vasodilation. β-Adrenergic antagonists, on the other hand, cause transient vasoconstriction. In vitro, however, α-adrenergic stimulation has minimal contractile effects on coronary microvessels (62). Selective pharmacological α_2 adrenergic stimulation results in is rather potent vasodilation of all sized coronary microvessels, predominantly as a result of a release of endothelium-derived NO. β-Adrenergic stimulation produces a potent relaxation of all coronary arteries, but especially small resistance vessels *(62)*. In vitro, the β_2-adrenergic receptor-subtype predominates in vessels less than 100 microns in diameter *(62)*. In vivo, however, mixed β_1- or β_2-adrenergic receptor population controls vascular resistance. Larger coronary vessels are regulated by a mixed β_1- and β_2-adrenoceptor subtype population, or a predominant β_1-adrenergic mechanism.

Activation of cholinergic receptors by either vagal stimulation or the infusion of acetylcholine produces a uniform vasodilation of coronary vessels *(63)*. This vasodilation is predominantly mediated by endothelium-derived NO. The release of a hyperpolarizing factor (discussed later) *(64)* and prostaglandin substances *(65)* may also play a role in vessel response to vasoactive substances. The role of endothelium-derived factors, in regulation of coronary microvascular tone, is discussed more thoroughly later in this chapter.

Effects of Humoral Agents on the Coronary Microcirculation

The response of the coronary microcirculation to a variety of humoral agents is very heterogeneous. For example, serotonin *(66)* constricts vessels greater than 100 microns in diameter, but causes potent vasodilation of smaller arteries. In contrast, vasopressin produces greater constriction in microvessels less than 100 microns in diameter than in larger microvessels *(66,67)*. In the larger epicardial coronary arteries, vasopressin causes predominantly vasodilation. Endothelin-1 acts as a vasoconstrictor when administered to the adventitial surface of coronary microvessels. The degree of this constriction is inversely related to the size of the vessels. Paradoxically, when endothelin-1 is administered intra-arterially it acts as a vasodilator, presumably via release of NO *(68)*. After myocardial infarction, the effect of endothelin on coronary vasomotor tone appears to be attenuated *(69)*. Activation of other receptors, such as the thromboxane receptor *(65)*, results in uniform constriction of all coronary arterioles and veins.

Endothelial Regulation of the Coronary Microcirculation

In addition to direct influences on the vascular smooth muscle, numerous neurohumoral stimuli modulate coronary vascular tone via their effect on the endothelium. As in all other circulations, the coronary endothelium releases a variety of substances, which modulate tone of the resistance vessels. These substances include NO, prostaglandins, a hyperpolarizing factor, endothelin, and reactive oxygen species. Among these various factors, NO plays a predominant role. The enzyme responsible for production of NO is eNOS (or NOS-3), a 133-kDa protein constitutively expressed by endothelial cells. The biochemical mechanisms responsible for function of the NO synthases have recently been elucidated. For all isoforms, an electron donor (nicotinamide adenine dinucleotide phosphate, or NADPH) binds to a site at the carboxyl terminus of the protein. Electrons are then transferred from NADPH to the flavins flavin-adenine dinucleotide (FAD) and flavin mononucleotide (FMN) noncovalently bound within the reductase domain. For the neuronal NOS and eNOS, electrons are stored on the flavins until the enzyme is activated by calcium/calmodulin (Ca/CaM). When calmodulin binds to the enzyme, electrons are transferred to a prosthetic heme group in the oxygenase domain. Upon heme reduction, catalysis of arginine to citrulline and NO occurs. The NO thus formed diffuses to underlying vascular smooth muscle, where it stimulates soluble guanylate cyclase. This increases cyclic guanosine monophosphate (cGMP) and results in vasodilation via activation of cGMP-dependent protein kinase *(70)*. There is substantial evidence that NO may undergo reactions with other molecules, such as those containing compounds to form biologically active nitroso intermediates *(71)*. Calcium/calmodulin binding is a prerequisite for activity of eNOS. There is evidence, however, that phosphorylation *(72)*, membrane binding *(73)*, and association with the integral membrane protein caveolin *(74)*, can also modulate eNOS activity. eNOS is constitutively expressed in the endothelium, but its expression is subject to regulation. Factors such as shear stress *(75)*, the state of endothelial cell growth *(76)*, hypoxia *(77)*, exposure to oxidized low density lipoprotein, and exposure to cytokines all affect expression of eNOS. eNOS expression is regulated by changes in mRNA half-life rather than changes in the rate of its transcription. Moreover, the bioavailability of NO can also be decreased by a lack of substrate or cofactors for eNOS *(78)*, alterations of cellular signaling resulting in inappropriate activation of eNOS *(79)*, and accelerated degradation of NO by reactive oxygen species *(80)*. An endogenous competitor of L-arginine for eNOS, called asymmetric dimethylarginine, can also decrease NO availability. Dimethylarginine level is elevated in conditions such as hypercholesterolemia associated with both endothelial dysfunction and impaired angiogenic response *(81)*. In the coronary circulation, the release of NO confers a state of basal vasodilation, and administration of NO synthase antagonists produce an increase in resting coronary resistance *(82)*. When substances such as acetylcholine and bradykinin are administered, coronary microvessels of all sizes dilate.

In smaller vessels of both the coronary and peripheral circulations, factors other than NO can modulate endothelium-dependent vascular relaxation. One such factor is the endothelium-derived hyperpolarizing factor (EDHF). Even before the endothelium was found to be critical in modulating vascular tone, it was known that certain relaxing substances would hyperpolarize vascular smooth muscle. It was subsequently shown that this phenomenon was endothelium-dependent *(83)*. This hyperpolarizing effect occurs via opening of vascular smooth muscle potassium channels, and the channel type involved has been the subject of substantial interest. These have largely been characterized using pharmacological means. In cerebral vessels, a voltage-regulated potassium channel has been implicated in endothelium-dependent hyperpolarization *(84)*, whereas others have suggested that the EDHF acts on large conductance potassium channels. When the vascular smooth muscle is hyperpolarized, voltage-sensitive calcium channels are closed, leading to a reduction in intracellular calcium. There is debate as to the nature of the hyperpolarizing factor, and some investigators have suggested that it is simply NO acting in a fashion independent of guanylate cyclase. Recent data supports the concept that the hyperpolarizing factor is a cytochrome P_{450} fatty acid metabolite *(85)*, although this remains controversial *(86)*. Endothelium-derived potassium *(87)*, electrical communications through gap junctions between endothelial cells and VSMCs *(88)*, L-S-nitrosothiols *(89)*, and hydrogen peroxide *(90)* have also been suggested. In the coronary circulation, the importance of the hyperpolarizing factor in modulating endothelium-dependent vascular relaxation seems to increase as vessel size decreases *(91)*.

Prostaglandin synthesis by the endothelium also contributes to modulation of tone in the coronary microcirculation. Interestingly, the production of prostaglandins seems to inhibit production of NO during hypoxia *(92)*, although the mechanism for this has not been clarified.

CONSIDERATIONS REGARDING THE CORONARY VENULES IN MODULATION OF OVERALL CORONARY VASCULAR RESPONSIVENESS

The arterial microcirculation is considered to be the predominant regulator of coronary blood flow. However, venules may have a considerable importance under conditions of vascular dilation, as noted previously *(16)*, such as exercise, metabolic stress, or reperfusion after myocardial ischemia. The venous circulation may also influence myocardial stiffness and diastolic properties of the heart. Veins can respond differently to agonists and neuronal stimulation compared with arteries in the same vascular bed *(65,93)*. Thus, a consideration of the venous circulation apart from the arterial circulation may be warranted under certain physiologic and clinical conditions.

Not only is vasomotor regulation differentially controlled between the venous and arterial microcirculations, but certain reactions to pathologic stimuli occur preferentially on one side of the capillary bed. For example, postcapillary venules are the initiating site of neutrophil adherence and transmigration *(94)*, whereas arterioles seldom manifest these initial changes in the inflammatory response. In addition, complement fragment C5a causes neutophil adherence in venules but not in arterioles, suggesting that different mechanisms mediate neutrophil–endothelial adherence in the two vessel types. The mechanism of C5a-induced neutrophil adherence has recently been shown to involve the activation of Src kinase, Src/β-catenin association, and β-catenin phosphorylation *(95)*. Neutrophil adherence, in turn, causes dysfunction of the endothelial cell barrier leading to hyperpermeability which is seen in ischemia and other inflammatory disease states *(96)*. While ischemia-reperfusion has been determined to cause endothelial dysfunction in veins *(97)*, under similar conditions arterioles appear to be more susceptible to a reduction in endothelium-dependent relaxation than coronary venules *(98)*.

ROLE OF ENDOTHELIAL FACTORS IN VASCULAR GROWTH, DEVELOPMENT, AND RESPONSE TO INJURY

The role of endothelial mediators, in particular the role of NO and NO-related factors on the growth of vascular cells and blood vessels, has been a subject of recent interest. This research was largely spurred by observations made in 1989 by Garg and Hassid that nitrovasodilators and NO-donors, such as sodium nitroprusside and *S*-nitrosopenacillamine, reduced growth of VSMCs and fibroblasts in culture *(99)*. In these initial studies, very large concentrations of the nitrovasodilators seemed to be necessary to produce this effect, and there was initially some skepticism regarding the physiological importance of this finding. Subsequent studies have largely supported their premise, implicating NO as an inhibitor of smooth muscle growth. Treatment of rabbits with L-nitroarginine methyl ester (L-NAME, which inhibits NO formation) markedly increases the neointimal development following vascular balloon injury *(100)*. Likewise, local transfection of the rat carotid artery with the eNOS cDNA reduces the intimal proliferation that follows balloon injury *(101)*. The vascular response to injury is enhanced in mice deficient in eNOS *(102)*. This effect of NO on vascular smooth muscle growth is mediated by cGMP and can be mimicked by cGMP analogs

(103). Interestingly, atrial natriuretic factor (which increases cGMP via activation of a particulate guanylate cyclase) shares this property of nitric oxide *(104)*. Similarly, C-type natriuretic peptide (CNP), produced by endothelial cells, can also inhibit smooth muscle growth *(103)*. There is some debate whether the antigrowth effects of NO or the natriuretic peptide are mediated by cAMP or cGMP dependent protein kinases *(103,105)*. Protein kinase A, with its effects on the protein levels of p21 and p53, has also been implicated as a possible mechanism of growth inhibition of VSMCs by eNOS *(106)*. NO exerts its effects on vascular smooth muscle not only through growth inhibition, but also through promotion of apoptosis *(107)*.

Studies evaluating the effects of NO on the progression of atherosclerosis have shown that it can have both protective and atherogenic effects. Studies in eNOS deficient mice fed an atherogenic diet showed reduced fatty streaks compared to controls *(108)*, and it has also been demonstrated that eNOS over-expression leads to accelerated atherosclerosis in apoE-deficient mice *(109)*. On the other hand, Kuhlencordt et al. demonstrated distal coronary arteriosclerosis with myocardial ischemia and left-ventricular failure in apoE and eNOS double knockout mice, suggesting a protective effect of NO *(110)*. These potentially conflicting results may be related to different cellular and molecular mechanisms through which NO exerts its effects as well as the differing spatio-temporal profile of NO within the vasculature. A particular cGMP dependent protein kinase (cGKI) has been implicated in the proatherogenic effects of nitric oxide on VSMCs *(111)*. Further elucidation of NO signaling pathways may reveal novel molecular targets for the treatment of atherosclerosis.

These effects of NO on VSMCs have obvious implications for neointimal formation following vessel injury as well as atherosclerosis. Consequently, there has been substantial interest in using NO donors, or organic nitrates, as approachs to modify the atherosclerotic process or to prevent restenosis following angioplasty. Studies to date using these drugs have not shown any obvious benefit. However, the potential use of these agents as modulators of mitogenesis and proliferation may not yet be realized.

Although NO and cGMP-elevating agents inhibit the growth of fibroblasts and vascular smooth muscle, they do not alter the rate of growth of endothelial cells as assessed by cell number or [^{3}H]-thymidine incorporation *(76)*. This is important because, as discussed previously, one of the most potent stimuli for increasing expression of the eNOS is proliferation. Proliferating cells express about sixfold as much eNOS mRNA as confluent cells *(76)*. This is associated with a threefold increase in eNOS protein and NO production by the proliferating cells as compared with nongrowing cells. If one considers this in terms of the ability of the vessel to respond to injury, it makes teleological sense. Following endothelial denudation, the proliferating endothelial cells compensate by producing large amounts of NO as they grow back to recover the exposed intima. This increased NO production would tend to minimize platelet adhesion and vascular smooth muscle proliferation in the area. Because endothelial cell proliferation is relatively insensitive to the growth inhibitory effects of NO, this permits rapid re-endothelialization of a denuded region, even in the presence of large quantities of NO. In addition to the effects of eNOS, recent studies have also demonstrated a role for reactive oxygen species and the NADPH oxidase system in the regulation of endothelial cell growth (112). Rat coronary endothelial cell growth seems to involve cross-talk between reactive oxygen species and NO and their respective signaling pathways.

ROLE OF NITRIC OXIDE IN THE ANGIOGENIC PROCESS

NO not only influences the rate of vascular smooth muscle growth and the vascular response to injury, but also has tremendous effects on new vessel growth. The process of blood vessel formation involves several distinct steps, including (1) increased vascular permeability and dissolution of the bond between the endothelium and basement membrane; (2) migration; (3) reattachment of endothelial cells; (4) proliferation and migration; and (5) the formation of a tubule which is the rudimentary vascular structure (113). The cellular and molecular changes required for the angiogenic and vasculogenic processes, and the exact roles of growth factors and NO, are as yet poorly understood. Almost universally, pathological conditions that may lead to angiogenesis, such as tissue hypoxia and inflammation, are associated with the production and release of growth factors. Indeed, increased expression of fibroblast growth factor (FGF) receptor-1 and the vascular endothelial growth factor (VEGF) receptors flt-1 and flk-1 is known to occur in both acute (114) and chronic (115) myocardial ischemia (Fig. 4). This would suggest that these substances are critical to the formation of new blood vessels. However, the process of angiogenesis in vivo is a complex one which is regulated by a variety of proangiogenic and anti-angiogenic factors.

There is also a strong relation between the release of NO with subsequent activation of guanylate cyclase and the regulation of blood vessel growth and development. But again, the relationship is not well defined and at times seems contradictory. For example, substance P and growth factors such as VEGF and FGF, all of which stimulate release of NO

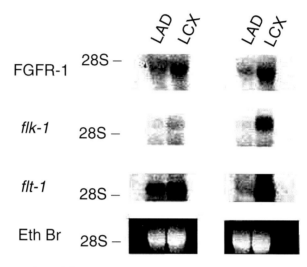

Fig. 4. Expression of fibroblast growth factor (FGF)-2 (FGFR1) and vascular endothelial growth factor (VEGF) (flt-1,flk-1) receptors in chronically ischemic myocardium *(115)*.

(115–117), induce new vessel formation in vivo. This is in addition to increasing the permeability, migration, and proliferation of postcapillary endothelial cells in tissue culture *(116,118)*. Moreover, VEGF enhances the expression of eNOS in native and cultured endothelial cells, an effect that may be important in the process of VEGF-induced angiogenesis *(119)*. Inhibitors of NOS suppress angiogenesis and the proliferative effect of VEGF. Uhlmann et al. *(120)* measured the proliferation and migration of choroidal endothelial cells after VEGF stimulation in the presence or absence of L-NAME, a NO inhibitor. They found that pretreatment with L-NAME attenuated the VEGF-induced angiogenic response, in direct correlation with a reduction in basal NO release. In addition, mice deficient in eNOS have decreased VEGF expression and decreased myocardial angiogenesis and capillary development *(121)*.

It was recently reported that VEGF-stimulated NO release is inhibited by the blockade of VEGF receptor 1 (VEGFR-1). VEGFR-1, via NO-dependent mechanisms, negatively regulates VEGFR-2-mediated endothelial cell proliferation and promotes formation of capillary networks in human umbilical vein endothelial cells *(122)*. It was suggested that VEGFR-1 may be a signaling receptor that promotes endothelial cell differentiation into vascular tubes, in part by limiting VEGFR-2-mediated endothelial cell proliferation via NO, which seems to be a molecular switch for endothelial cell differentiation. NO may also play a crucial role in the VEGF-mediated angiogenic response of VSMCs. The effect of exogenous and endogenous NO on the synthesis of VEGF by rat and human VSMCs was recently examined by exposing cells to exogenous NO donors, or to the genetic augmentation of eNOS or inducible NOS (iNOS) *(123)*. NO-donors potentiated by twofold the generation of VEGF protein by rat or human VSMCs. Similarly, rat or human VSMCs transiently transfected with plasmid cDNA encoding eNOS or iNOS synthesized up to threefold more VEGF than those transfected with control plasmid cDNA, an effect which was reversed after treatment with L-NAME.

In comparison with VEGF, a lesser number of studies have tied the angiogenic effects of FGF-2 to local NO availability. Still, NO likely acts as an important signal in the angiogenic response to FGF-2 as well. Presumably NO terminates the proliferative actions of FGF-2 and promotes the differentiation of endothelial cells into vascular tubes *(124)*. This role is supported by another study that showed that the inhibition of endothelial NOS by L-NAME attenuated endothelial cell migration, but not proliferation, in vitro *(125)*. These authors also demonstrated that endogenous endothelium-derived NO maintains the functional expression of integrin $\alpha_v\beta_3$, which is a mediator for endothelial migration, survival, and angiogenesis. This would suggest that endothelium-derived NO plays a crucial role in mediating angiogenesis by supporting endothelial cell migration, at least partly via an integrin-dependent mechanism.

It has also been demonstrated that tube development by growing endothelial cells in three-dimensional gels in response to transforming growth factor-β is dependent on NO and inhibited by antagonists of NOS *(126)*. Moreover, the stimulated synthesis and release of endothelium-derived NO by VEGF and FGF-2 has been shown to be largely regulated by tyrosine kinases *(115)*. further implicating the role of NO in blood vessel formation mediated by these two proteins. Interestingly, activity of the tyrosine kinase Src was also found to protect endothelial cells from apoptosis during VEGF-mediated angiogenesis in chick embryos and mice *(127)*.

Convincing in vivo evidence that endothelial factors play a major role in mediating the angiogenic response was found in murine studies of apoE-hypercholesterolemic mice. These mice exhibit attenuated collateral vessel formation in response to a FGF-2 disk angiogenesis system in a hind-limb ischemia model *(81,128)*. This inhibition was fully reversed by the oral administration of L-arginine, which is the substrate for endothelial NO production. In a porcine model of chronic myocardial ischemia, evidence was recently produced that hypercholesterolemia-induced endothelial dysfunction blocked the angiogenic response to both FGF *(129)* and VEGF *(130)*. Overall, the bulk of evidence suggests that NO production and perhaps other yet-unidentified endothelial factors play a significant role in mediating the endogenous as well as the exogenous angiogenic responses. This likely accounts for the attenuated effects of angiogenic therapy observed in humans with end-stage, inoperable coronary artery disease (CAD) who display significant endothelial dysfunction

To summarize, the ultimate effect of NO on vascular cellularity and growth is complex. Experimentally, NO clearly suppresses vascular thickening and intimal proliferation following balloon injury, and inhibits growth of VSMCs in culture. The ultimate effect on vessel growth of NO and related molecules seems to depend on the model employed and whether a separate stimulus for angiogenesis is applied. The therapeutic benefit of NO donors on microcirculatory development in a clinical setting (for example, to stimulate new vessel growth in the heart) remains questionable. A major problem with the use of the currently available NO-generating compounds in humans is that they cannot be used for prolonged periods of time because of the development of tolerance (in the case of the organic nitrates), toxicity (in the case of sodium nitroprusside), or generation of reactive oxygen species (in the case of molsidimine-like drugs).

THE CORONARY MICROCIRCULATION IN DISEASE STATES

A variety of systemic and cardiac diseases affect the coronary microcirculation. These may be considered functional alterations involving changes in responsiveness of the coronary microvessels, and structural effects such as alterations of the number and diameter of the coronary microvessels.

Pathophysiological Alterations of Functional Properties of the Coronary Microcirculation

A particularly important aspect of endothelial regulation of vasomotion is that endothelial-mediated vasodilation is abnormal in a variety of pathological conditions. These include atherosclerosis, hypercholesterolemia, diabetes, hypertension, cigarette smoking, and aging. The mechanisms underlying these abnormal endothelium-dependent responses have been the subject of substantial debate. Deficiencies of the substrate for eNOS, L-arginine, and the co-factor tetrahydrobiopterin have all been implicated, as well as the endogenous competitor of L-arginine for eNOS, asymmetric dimethylarginine. Abnormalities of G protein signaling, resulting in reduced activation of eNOS in response to endothelial cell receptor activation, have also been shown to occur. A substantial body of data suggests that in some of these conditions (hypercholesterolemia, hypertension, and diabetes), increased production of vascular superoxide ($\cdot O_2^-$) occurs. Superoxide reacts very rapidly with NO$\cdot$, leading to the formation of the toxic peroxynitrite anion. Although peroxynitrite can produce vasodilation, it is a very weak vasodilator, and as a result this reaction significantly reduces the amount of bioavailable NO.

The initial studies demonstrating abnormal endothelium-dependent vascular relaxation in various disease models were performed in larger vessels. Subsequent experiments have shown that most, if not all, of these disease processes also affect the coronary microcirculation in a similar fashion. This is of particular interest in the case of hypercholesterolemia and atherosclerosis. One of the first examples of an alteration in coronary microvessels in atherosclerosis was made in vessels from monkeys fed a high-cholesterol diet for 18 mo *(131)*. These animals developed advanced atherosclerotic lesions in larger vessels, and had abnormal vasodilation in response to acetylcholine, the calcium ionophore A23187, and thrombin in those vessels. On the other hand, coronary microvessels from the same animals had dramatically impaired relaxations to the same acetylcholine, bradykinin, and the calcium ionophore A23187, and in some cases, these agents produced paradoxical constrictions (Fig. 5). Similar findings have been made in other animal models of diet-induced atherosclerosis. Subsequent studies performed using in vivo techniques showed that vasoconstriction caused by serotonin and ergonovine (both known to be modulated by the endothelium) was markedly enhanced in the coronary microcirculation of hypercholesterolemic monkeys *(132)*. These findings are striking because the coronary microcirculation is spared from the development of overt atherosclerosis. Thus, vessels that have been exposed to a high cholesterol milieu, even in the absence of atherosclerosis, develop abnormal vasomotion. Although it is difficult to perform such studies in human vessels, investigators have used Doppler techniques to measure coronary flow in humans. Diminished flow responses to acetylcholine have been demonstrated in humans with hypercholesterolemia *(133)*. Importantly, this abnormality of vascular function has been corrected by reduction of serum cholesterol *(133)*, or through anti-oxidant therapy. Similar observations have been made in either humans or experimental models of hypertension *(134)*, ischemia followed by reperfusion *(98,135)*, and diabetes *(136)*. Indeed, altered endothelial regulation of vasomotion has

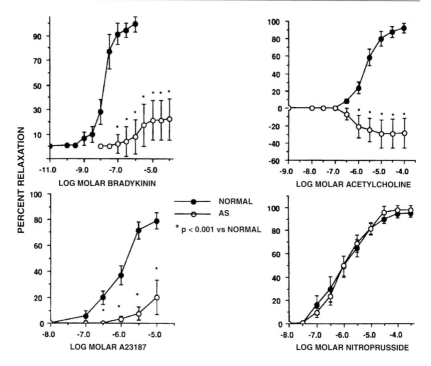

Fig. 5. Effect of atherosclerosis on endothelium-dependent and endothelium-independent vasodilation. Cynomolgus monkeys were made atherosclerotic by feeding a high cholesterol diet for 18 mo. Coronary microvessels ranging from 70 to 140 μm in diameter were studied in a pressurized state using video microscopy. Following preconstriction, the various vasoactive agents were added in a cumulative fashion. Relaxations were expressed as a percent of preconstricted tension. Data are from ref. *68.*

been found in the coronary arteries of patients with chest pain and normal coronary arteries, and it is thought that, at least in some instances, this might contribute to their clinical symptoms. In addition, abnormalities in microvascular relaxation resulting from endothelial dysfunction have been linked to poorer prognosis in patients with atherosclerotic disease.

A particularly important clinical setting in which endothelial function is altered in the coronary microcirculation is following cardioplegic arrest and extracorporeal circulation *(137)*. This abnormality persists for some time after cardiopulmonary bypass, and normalizes thereafter. Obviously, such a deficit in endothelial function may have important clinical implications because of the frequency in which cardioplegia is used in cardiovascular surgery. It is not uncommon for patients undergoing coronary artery bypass grafting, with seemingly complete coronary revascularlization, to exhibit signs of myocardial ischemia during the hours following surgery. It is conceivable that alterations of endothelial function may contribute to this alteration in cardiac function. In addition, it is likely that the arteriopathy often observed after cardiac transplantation is in part related to endothelial injury as a result of inadequate vascular preservation.

A condition that rather strikingly alters coronary vascular reactivity is the development of collateral vessels. When a coronary artery is gradually occluded, flow to the subtended myocardium does not cease, but persists via perfusion through collateral vessels. When these vessels fully develop, they are capable of providing normal resting perfusion to the region previously served by the occluded vessel, albeit at a lower perfusion pressure. Because collateral vessels represent "new" vessels, and because of their obvious pathophysiological importance, there has been interest in factors that might modulate their reactivity. To perform such studies, investigators have used ameroid constrictors to produce gradual occlusion of coronary arteries in dogs and pigs, and removed mature collateral vessels subsequently. For the most part, these vessels have demonstrated normal endothelium-dependent vascular relaxation and normal responses to most agents studied in vivo. In mature canine collateral vessels, however, constrictions to vasopressin are markedly enhanced when compared to the effect of vasopressin on similar sized native coronary arteries *(138)*. In vivo, vasopressin has been shown to markedly reduce perfusion to collateral-dependent myocardium in doses that have no effect on normally perfused myocardium *(139)*. This effect may be limited to pharmacologic properties of vasopressin. Studies of pigs with developed collaterals have failed to demonstrate an effect of a vasopressin antagonist on collateral perfusion during exercise *(140)*. Interestingly, the coronary arterioles nourished by collaterals develop markedly abnormal vascular reactivity characterized by impaired endothelium-dependent vascular relaxations and enhanced constrictions to vasopressin (Fig. 6) *(138)*. These observations were originally made in vitro in microvessels from a canine model of collateral development, but have since been reproduced in a porcine model of chronic ischemia *(141,142)*.

The mechanism of the impaired microvascular endothelium-dependent relaxation in the collateral-dependent region has not been determined. It may, however, be related to increased local levels in NO as a result of increased expression of iNOS leading to reduced activity of eNOS *(143)*. Recent studies have demonstrated a marked increase in iNOS expression in chronically ischemic myocardium *(144)*. Alternatively, changes in shear stress or pulsatile flow in the collateral dependent microvasculature may contribute to the altered vascular reactivity *(145)*. In a recent study *(130)*, the inhibition of the angiogenic response

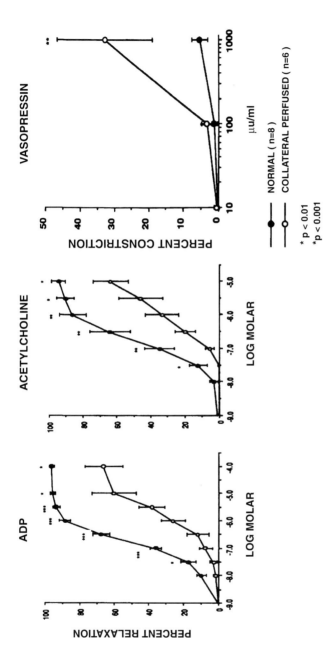

Fig. 6. Alterations of vascular reactivity in microvessels from collateral-perfused myocardium. Collaterals were produced by placement of an ameroid constrictor on the circumflex coronary artery of dogs for 3–6 mo. Following this, coronary microvessels ranging from 100 to 220 were studied in vitro. Of note, vasodilation in response to the calcium ionophore A23187 and nitroglycerin were not altered in these vessels. Data are from ref. 138.

86

to exogenous VEGF in a porcine model of chronic myocardial ischemia, hypercholesterolemia-induced endothelial dysfunction was associated with a decrease in expression of eNOS and VEGF in the ischemic area. In addition, chronic treatment of hypercholesterolemic animals with L-arginine reversed the hypercholesterolemia-induced endothelial dysfunction (Fig. 7) and restored the angiogenic response to VEGF, normalizing collateral dependent perfusion in the ischemic territory *(146)* (Fig. 8). Finally, changes in intracellular calcium mobilization have been observed in collateral vessels *(147)*, which may be responsible for changes in vascular tone and responses.

Studies have addressed the possibility that collateral growth and coronary microvessel function might be altered by the direct perivascular application or infusion of angiogenic growth factors such FGF-1 or FGF-2, or VEGF. Indeed, such studies have shown that these therapeutic interventions are not only associated with improved myocardial function and improved perfusion in chonic ischemic models, but also with normalization of endothelium-dependent relaxation in the collateral-dependent vasculature *(141,142,148)*. The cause of this enhancement of endothelium-dependent relaxation is not fully understood, but several mechanisms may be involved. Both FGF-2 and VEGF release NO *(115)*, which may improve collateral perfusion and decrease tissue ischemia. As stated earlier, expression of receptors for both FGF-2 and VEGF is selectively increased in chronically ischemic myocardium *(115)*, suggesting that these growth factors are functionally upregulated. This may also explain why enhanced endothelium-dependent relaxation only occurs in the collateral-dependent region and not in the normally perfused myocardium after the perivascular exogenous administration of VEGF or FGF-2. Alternatively, FGF-2 and VEGF may counteract the effects of substances detrimental to vascular function or stabilize NO or NOS. Another possibility is that the growth factors induce enough collateral formation to prevent a reduction in myocardial blood flow or in pulsatile perfusion. In summary, treatment of collateral-dependent vessels with angiogenic growth factors may enhance endothelium-dependent relaxation, in addition to improving other aspects of cardiac performance. This may, at least in theory, be the basis for a clinical improvement in patients after therapeutic angiogenesis suffering inoperative myocardial ischemia.

ACUTE MICROVASCULAR EFFECTS OF GROWTH FACTORS

One potential problem associated with the intravascular administration of VEGF, FGF-2, and other angiogenic growth factors is the periph-

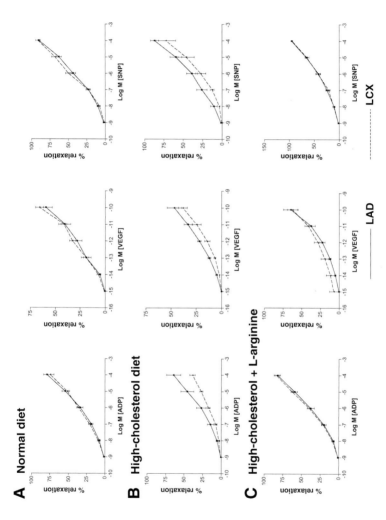

Fig. 7. Microvascular reactivity studies after 4 wk of vascular endothelial growth factor (VEGF) treatment in a porcine model of myocardial ischemia with (**B,C**) or without (**A**) hypercholesterolemia-induced endothelial dysfunction. Graphs show percent relaxation to increasing concentrations of vasodilating agents following preconstriction with U46619. SNP, sodium nitroprusside; ADP, adenosine diphosphate. From ref. *146.*

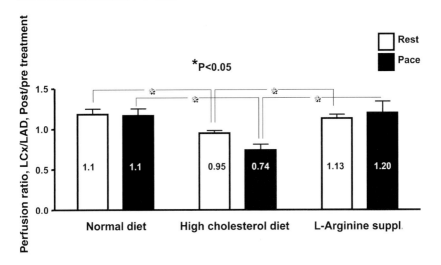

Fig. 8. Post- vs prevascular endothelial growth factor (VEGF) treatment ratios of ischemic (left circumflex artery [LCX]) vs nonischemic (left anterior descending artery [LAD]) blood flows in a porcine model of myocardial ischemia with hypercholesterolemia-induced endothelial dysfunction (high-cholesterol diet) compared to controls (normal diet), and the effect of L-arginine supplementation (high-cholesterol + L-arginine). From ref. *146*.

eral vasodilation. The angiogenic potential of FGF-2 is largely independent of the release of NO, whereas VEGF-induced vessel formation is potently coupled to the release of NO. The intravascular infusions of FGF-2 and VEGF are poorly tolerated, owing to their vasodilatory effects *(115,149)* and resulting systemic hypotension. Profound hypotension is obviously not well tolerated by patients with severe and inoperable coronary artery disease. VEGF-induced relaxation may be inhibited by the concomitant administration of L-NAME, suggesting a possible method to counter the vasodilatory effect of acute administration of VEGF. Interestingly, VEGF produces a rapid tachyphylaxis to subsequent bolus injections of the growth factor, and also to the injection of other endothelium-dependent vasoactive agents such as serotonin. The relaxations to sodium nitroprusside and adenosine are not affected, suggesting a selectively acquired defect in the endothelial vasodilatory mechanism *(149)*. Examples of these vascular effects are shown in Fig. 9.

   Although the predominant effect of VEGF may lie in the NO-guanylate pathway, other pathways may also be important. Relaxation of vessels by VEGF is not affected to the same degree by the tyrosine kinase inhibitor genistein as it is by an inhibitor of NOS, nor is VEGF-

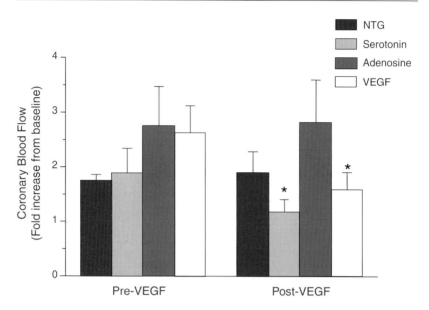

Fig. 9. Normalization of hypercholesterolemia induced endothelial dysfunction, as measured by endothelial dependent microvascular relaxation, in pigs
supplemented chronically with L-arginine. From ref. *145*.

induced relaxation totally inhibited by L-NAME *(115)*. This suggests
that VEGF-induced relaxation may have an endothelial component independent of NO, or that it may release NO through a mechanism unrelated to its two different tyrosine kinase receptors *(149)*. The VEGF-
induced release of platelet-activating factor (PAF), which may cause
vasodilation in low concentrations, increases vascular permeability in intact
vessels and cultured aortic endothelial cells *(150)*. The cyclooxygenase-2
(COX-2) pathway has also been shown to be upregulated in response to
hypoxia as well as exogenous VEGF administration, eventually leading
to the synthesis and release of vasodilatory prostanoids *(151)*. An
understanding of the acute vascular effects of growth factors may increase our understanding of the initial steps in blood vessel development
and growth, and also help clinicians deal with hypotension associated
with the intravascular administration of VEGF and other growth factors.

Structural Changes in the Coronary Microcirculation

For years, it has been observed that patients with cardiac hypertrophy
resulting from a variety of causes have chest pain suggestive of myocardial ischemia. This has led to an extensive body of research examining

potential alterations of structure of the coronary microcirculation in a variety of conditions associated with cardiac hypertrophy. In both experimental animals and humans with cardiac hypertrophy, there is a reduction in the maximal capacity of the coronary circulation to dilate in response to either reactive hyperemia or pharmacological stimuli *(12,152)*. Two hypotheses have been proposed to explain this defect in vasodilator function. One is that as the myocardium hypertrophies, the coronary resistance circulation does not increase to keep pace with the larger myocardial mass. Thus, peak flow normalized to myocardial mass is reduced because of this relative paucity of coronary arterioles. A second structural alteration of the microcirculation, which occurs in hypertension, is actual loss of coronary resistance vessels.

It has been assumed that these studies examining a loss of maximal vasodilator reserve reflect a structural alteration of the coronary microcirculation because they are observed during maximal pharmacological stimulation. Thus, the resultant flow must reflect the driving pressure for perfusion and the cross-sectional area of the coronary resistance circulation. The pharmacological agents employed in these studies have included adenosine, dipyridamole, or papaverine. Many of these observations were made prior to understanding the importance of the endothelium in modulation of vasodilation, but in fairness, it is likely that most of these changes in maximal vasodilation were not due to altered release of vasodilator substances from the endothelium. The vasodilation caused by adenosine and papaverine is not greatly influenced by the endothelium. In addition, loss of endothelial function is not always associated with an impaired maximal vasodilation to adenosine. Nevertheless, it is possible that some of impaired vasodilator responses, attributed to losses of vascular cross-sectional area, were in fact the result of changes in endothelial function.

There are structural changes in the coronary microcirculation that occur with hypertension and myocardial hypertrophy which alter autoregulation and the perfusion pressure in the subendocardium, as discussed previously.

PHARMACOLOGY OF THE CORONARY MICROCIRCULATION

The response of the coronary microcirculation to a variety of neurohumoral stimuli is heterogeneous. Similarly, a variety of pharmacologic agents such as organic nitrates, adenosine, dipyridamole, and certain inhalation anesthetics exert heterogeneous effects on the coronary microcirculation.

The organic nitrates represent a diverse group of compounds, which contain a nitrate ester moiety. Unlike many other nitrovasodilators, the organic nitrates do not spontaneously release NO, but must undergo a three-electron reduction of the nitrogen atom, which is eventually released as NO *(153)*. Both enzymatic and nonenzymatic mechanisms for this "biotransformation" have been implicated. Enzymatic processes predominate in vivo. The enzyme systems involved have only been partially characterized, and it appears that only certain tissues, such as coronary circulation, are capable of this enzymatic process. It was noted as early as the 1960s *(154,155)* that the organic nitrates produced prolonged vasodilation of the larger epicardial coronary arteries but produced only minimal and short-lived increases in coronary flow. More recent in vitro and in vivo studies confirm that coronary microvessels >200 μm in diameter are potently dilated in response to nitroglycerin, whereas vessels <100 μm in diameter are dilated only minimally by suprapharm- acological concentrations (>1 μmol/L) of the drug *(138,156)*. This property of nitroglycerin is shared by other organic nitrates, and is likely related to the common requirement for biotransformation of the nitrate ester. Nitrovasodilators, such as *S*-nitrosocysteine (a nitrosothiol) and sodium nitroprusside either yield NO spontaneously or upon a one-electron reduction. They potently dilate all size coronary microvessels. The smaller coronary microvessels (<100 μm in diameter) can respond to NO, but are simply incapable of biotransforming nitroglycerin to the free NO gas. Subsequent studies have shown that this biotransformation process likely requires glutathione. The ability of large, but not small, coronary microvessels to respond to nitroglycerin may be related to variations in intracellular glutathione levels in different sized microvessels *(157)*. Figure 10 illustrates the responses of coronary microvessels to various nitrovasodilators.

This pharmacological property of the organic nitrates to dilate larger coronary arteries preferentially over the smaller coronary microvessels likely confers their anti-anginal properties. Drugs that dilate the smaller (<100 μm) coronary microvessels have been implicated in producing the coronary steal phenomenon. By sparing coronary microvessels <100 μm in diameter, the organic nitrates avoid this untoward effect. They still posses the beneficial effects of dilating venous capacitance vessels (reducing cardiac preload), epicardial coronary arteries (sites of coronary stenoses), and coronary collateral vessels. This profile of differential vascular activity may explain the tremendously beneficial effects these drugs and other agents with similar heterogeneous vasomotor effects *(158)* have in the treatment of myocardial ischemia.

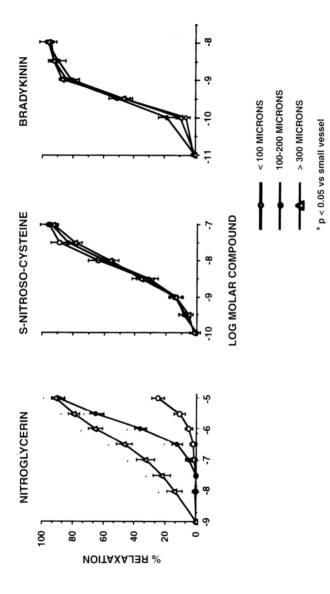

Fig. 10. The effect of nitroglycerin, a nitric oxide donor, and endogenously released nitric oxide on various sized coronary microvessels. Vessels less then 100 μm in diameter are much less responsive to nitroglycerin than larger classes of vessels. A simple nitric oxide donor, such as S-nitrosocysteine, produces similar degrees of vasodilation in all sized coronary microvessels, as does endogenously reduced nitric oxide. From ref. 67.

93

Adenosine has an effect on the coronary microvessels that is precisely the opposite of that caused by organic nitrates. Although adenosine is not generally considered a pharmacological agent, it is worth mentioning here because it is used therapeutically for treatment of arrhythmias, and diagnostically to induce myocardial ischemia. Dipyridamole is also often used for this latter purpose, and its effect is mediated by its ability to both enhance adenosine's release and inhibit its degradation. Adenosine produces potent vasodilation of coronary microvessels <100 μm in diameter and only modest dilation of larger vessels.

The dyhydropyridine type calcium channel antagonists produce uniform vasodilation of all classes of coronary microvessels via their effect on L-type voltage gated channels. The greatest effect is observed in smallest vessels due to the density of L-type channels being inversely proportional to the vessel diameter. There has not been a reported comparison of the effect of the other subtypes of calcium channel antagonists. More recently, calcium channel blockers have been used to prevent no-reflow phenomenon after myocardial infarction *(159)*.

As indicated in the section entitled "Metabolic Regulation and Autoregulation" in this chapter, there is a great deal of interest in the role of potassium channels in modulating coronary flow. A variety of potassium channel opening agents, principally those that affect the K_{ATP} channel, have been studied in terms of their ability to alter coronary hemodynamics. These agents, which include drugs such as cromakalim, lemakalim, and bemikalim, are potent vasodilators of all vessels, and markedly increase coronary flow when administered in vivo. The exact profile of coronary microvessels dilated by these agents has not been examined, but they are capable of hyperpolarizing smooth muscle of very small coronary arterioles. A potentially useful therapeutic agent is nicorandil, an organic nitrate with potassium channel opening properties. Not surprisingly, nicorandil dilates all sized coronary microvessels under normal conditions; however, it becomes selective for vessels larger than 100 μm in diameter when K_{ATP} channels are blocked by glibenclamide *(160)*.

Angiotensin-converting enzyme (ACE) inhibitors do not have a direct vasodilatory effect on large epicardial arteries but do dilate microvessels. Indirectly they potentiate endothelium-dependent vasodilatory action of NO and EDHF. ACE is present in the coronary vessel wall. It converts angiotensin I to angiotensin II with concomitant breakdown of bradykinins. ACE inhibitors decrease the level of angiotensin II and increase bradykinins, which in turn increase NO *(161,162)*, prostaglandins and EDHF. In dog experiments, ACE inhibitors increased the coronary blood flow in ischemic myocardium and normalized endocardial to epicardial flow ratio (163). They also appear to have antioxidant properties (164) and exert an antiproliferative/microvascular remodeling effect (165).

The inhibitory effect of angiotensin II on angiogenesis has long been known, and the pro-angiogenic properties of ACE inhibitors were thought to be mediated through angiotension II withdrawal (166,167), and to involve the bradykinin and eNOS pathway (168). Recent evidence suggests that angiotensin II is a humoral regulator if peripheral angiogenesis involving two receptor subtypes with opposing actions, the activation of AT1 and AT2 leading respectively to inhibition and stimulation of the angiogenic response (169).

3-Hydroxy-3methylglutaryl (HMG)-coenzyme A reductase inhibitors (or statins) also exert direct beneficial effects on the endothelium, in part through an increase in NO production (170). They can promote angiogenesis independently of direct changes in eNOS expression, but rather by stabilization of eNOS mRNA (171), and modulation of hsp90 and caveolin abundance, contributing to eNOS availability and functionality to potentiate the NO-dependent, protein kinase AKT-activated angiogenic process (172,173). Although these pro-angiogenic properties can be observed at low doses, statins could paradoxically exert antiangiogenic effects at high dose (174), in association with decreased endothelial release of VEGF, increased endothelial apoptosis (175), and of Rho A geranylgeranylation and membrane localization (176).

SUMMARY

In this review, we have summarized some of the newer concepts regarding physiological, pathophysiological, and pharmacological control of the coronary microcirculation. Whenever possible, we have focused on studies that have directly examined the coronary microvessels using some of the newer technology (in vitro preparations or *in situ* observations). It is not possible, however, to understand these studies without consideration of some of the more classical studies of the intact coronary circulation performed in intact animals or isolated hearts. Although these older approaches, in general, employed indirect techniques, they provided a wealth of insight and understanding of coronary blood flow regulation. In reviewing this literature, it is clear that many of the methods used in the last three decades for study of the coronary circulation and microcirculation have largely been abandoned, or are being used in relatively few laboratories. In part, this is a result of the fact that the research questions that have arisen regarding vascular function have necessitated the use of more basic techniques, including cell culture and molecular biological approaches. Another reason for this is the difficulty of these studies and the expense of larger animals used in many of the physiological experiments. A relatively recent development has been the ability to make many in vivo measurements of coronary hemodynamics in human subjects in the catheterization laboratory, bypassing the absolute need for large animal studies of flow. Nevertheless, as vascular biology research examines more fundamental questions, it will be important not to lose sight of the need to take basic observations back to the intact circulation. As emphasized in this chapter, properties of peripheral vessels cannot be extrapolated to the coronary circulation, and properties of one size or class of coronary microvessel may not be present in another size or class of coronary microvessel. Future studies will be most successful when fundamental observations can be tested in intact vessels and circulations, including the coronary circulation.

REFERENCES

1. Nellis SH, Liedtke AJ, Whitesell L. Small coronary vessel pressure and diameter in an intact beating rabbit heart using fixed-position and free-motion techniques. Circ Res 1981;49:342–353.
2. Chilian WM, Eastham CL, Marcus ML. Microvascular distribution of coronary vascular resistance in beating left ventricle. Am J Physiol 1986;251:H779–H788.
3. Kuo L, et al. Myogenic activity in isolated subepicardial and subendocardial coronary arterioles. Am J Physiol 1988;255(6Pt2):H1558–H1562
4. Ashikawa K, et al. A new microscopic system for the continuous observation of the coronary microcirculation in the beating canine left ventricle. Microvasc Res 1984;28:387–394.
5. Yada T, et al. In vivo observation of subendocardial microvessels of the beating porcine heart using a needle probe videomicroscope with a CCD camera. Circ Res 1993;72:939–946.
6. Mori H, et al. Visualization of penetrating transmural arteries in situ by monochromatic synchroton radiation. Circulation 1994;89:863–871.
7. Jones CJH, et al. Regulation of coronary blood flow: coordianation of heterogenous control mechanisms in vascular microdomains. Cardiovasc Res 1995;29:585–596.
8. Feigl EO. Coronary physiology. Physiol Rev 1983;63:1–205.
9. Hoffman JI. Transmural myocardial perfusion. Prog Cardiovasc Dis 1987;29:429–464.
10. Duncker DJ, Bache RJ. Regulation of coronary vasomotor tone under normal conditions and during acute myocardial hypoperfusion. Pharmacol Ther 2000;86:87–110.
11. Komaru T, Knatsika H, Shirato K. Coronary microcirculation. Physiology and Pharmacology. Pharmacol Ther 2000;86:217–261.
12. Marcus M. The coronary circulation in health and disease. First ed. McGraw-Hill, New York, NY: 1983.
13. Schaper W. The pathophysiology of myocardial perfusion. 1 ed. Elsevier/North Holland Biomedical, Amsterdam, The Netherlands: 1979.
14. Kanatsuka H, et al. Heterogenous changes in epimyocardial microvascular size during graded coronary stenosis. Evidence of the microvascular site fro autorogulation. Circ Res 1990;66:389–396.
15. Muller JM, et al. Intergrated regulation of pressure and flow in the coronary microcirculation. Cardiovasc Res 1996;32:668–678.

16. Chilian WM, Layne SM, Klausner EC, Eastham CL, Marcus ML. Redistribution of coronary microvascular resistance produced by dipyridamole. Am J Physiol 1989;256:H383–H390.
17. Chilian WM. Microvascular pressures and resistances in the left ventricular subepicardium and subendocardium. Circ Res 1991;69:561–570.
18. Fujii M, Nuno DW, Lamping KG, Dellsperger KC, Eastham CL, Harrison DG. Effect of hypertension and hypertrophy on coronary microvascular pressure. Circ Res 1992;71:120–126.
19. Kuo L, et al. Longitudinal gradients for endothelium-dependent and independent vascular responses in the coronary microcirculation. Circulation 1995;92:518–525.
20. Miller FJ Jr, Dellsperger KC, Gutterman DD. Myogenic constriction of human coronary arterioles. Am J Physiol 1997;273:H257–H264.
21. Brayden JE, Nelson MT. Regulation of arterial tone by activation of calcium-dependent potassium channels. Science 1992;256:532–535.
22. Nelson MT, et al. Calcium channels, potassium channels, and voltage-dependence of arterial smooth muscle. Am J Physiol 1990;259(1 Pt 1):C3–C18.
23. Meininger GA, et al. Calcium measurement in isolated arterioles during myogenic and agonist stimulation. Am J Physiol 1991;261(3 Pt 2):H950–H959
24. Hill MA, Meininger GA. Calcium entry and myogenic phenomena in skeletal muscle arterioles. Am J Physiol 1994;267:H1088–H1092.
25. Park KW, Dai H-B, Lowenstein E, Darvish E, Sellke FW. Heterogeneous vasomotor responses of rabbit microvessels to isoflurane. Anesthesiology 1994;81:1190–1197.
26. Knot HJ, Nelson MT. Regulation of membrane potential and diameter by voltage-dependent K^+ channels in rabbit myogenic cerebral arteries. Am J Physiol 1995;269:H348–H355.
27. Bowles DK, et al. Heterogeneity of L-type calcium current density in coronary smooth muscle. Am J Physiol 1997;273(4 Pt 2):H2083–H2089
28. Osol G, Laher I, Cipolla M. Protein kinase C modulates basal myogenic tone in resistance arteries from the cerebral circulation. Circ Res 1991;68:359–367.
29. Narayanan J, Imig M, Roman RJ, Harder DR. Pressurization of isolated renal arteries increases inositol trisphosphate and diacylglycerol. Am J Physiol 1994;266:H1840–H1845.
30. Large WA. Receptor-operated Ca^{2+}-permeable nonselective cation channels in vascular smooth muscle: a physiologic perspective. J Cardiovasc Electrophysiol 2002;13:493–501.
31. Slish DF, Welsh DG, Brayden JE. Diacylglycerol and protein kinase C activate cation channels involved in myogenic tone. Am J Physiol 2002;283:H2196–H2201.
32. Korzick DH, Laughlin MH, Bowles DK. Alterations in PKC signaling underlie enhanced myogenic tone in exercise-trained porcine coronary resistance arteries. J Appl Physiol 2004;96:1425–1432.
33. Roman RJ. P-450 metabolites of arachidonic acid in the control of cardiovascular function. Physiol Rev 2002;82:131–185.
34. Randriamboavonjy V, Busse R, Fleming I. 20-HETE-induced contraction of small coronary arteries depends on the activation of Rho-kinase. Hypertension 2003;41:801–806.
35. Massett MP, Zoltan U, Csiszar A, Kaley G, Koller A. Different roles of PKC and MAP kinases in arteriolar constrictions to pressure and agonists. Am J Physiol 2002;283:H2282–H2287.
36. Khan TA, Bianchi C, Ruel M, Voisine P, Li J, Liddicoat JR, Sellke FW. Mitogen-activated protein kinase inhibition and cardioplegia-cardiopulmonary bypass reduce coronary myogenic tone. Circulation 2003;108(Suppl 1):II348–II353.

37. Kuo L, Chilian WM, Davis MJ. Coronary arteriolar myogenic response is independent of endothelium. Circ Res 1990;66:860–866.

38. Nakayama K, Osol G, Halpern W. Reactivity of isolated porcine coronary resistance arteries to cholinergic and adrenergic drugs and transmural pressure changes. Circ Res 1988;62:741–748.

39. Liao JC, Kuo L. Interaction between adenosine and flow-induced dilation in coronary microvascular network. Am J Physiol 1997;272:H1571–H1581.

40. Muller JM, Myers PR, Laughlin MH. Exercise training alters myogenic responses in porcine coronary resistance arteries. J Appl Physiol 1993;75:2677–2682.

41. Boatwright RB, Downey HF, Bashour FA, Crystal GJ. Transmural variation in autoregulation of coronary blood flow in hyperperfused canine myocardium. Circ Res 1980;47:599–609.

42. Davis PF. Flow-mediated endothelial mechanotransduction. Physiol Rev 1995;75: 519–560.

43. Jimenez AH, et al. Effects of oxygen tension on flow-induced vasodilation in porcine coronary arterioles. Microvasc Res 1996;51:365–377.

44. Kuo L, et al. Interaction of pressure- and flow-induced responses in porcine coronary resistance vessels. Am J Physiol 1991;261(6 Pt 2):H1706–H1715

45. Olsson RA, Bunger R. Metabolic control of coronary blood flow. Prog Cardiovasc Dis 1987;29:369–387.

46. Yada T, Richmond KN, Van Bibber R, Kroll K, Feigl EO. Role of adenosine in local metabolic coronary vasodilation. Am J Physiol 1999;276:H1425–H1433.

47. Duncker DJ, Stubenitsky R, Verdouw PD. Role of adenosine in the regulation of coronary blood flow in swine at rest and during treadmill exercise. Am J Physiol 1998;275:H1663–H1672.

48. Hein TW, Kuo L. cAMP-independent dilation of coronary arterioles to adenosisne: role of nitric oxide, G proteins, and K_{ATP} channels. Circ Res 1999;85:634–642.

49. Komaru T, Kanatsuka H, Dellsperger K, Takishima T. The role of ATP-sensitive potassium channels in regulating coronary microcirculation. Biorheology 1993;30:371–380.

50. Duncker DJ, Van Zon NS, Altman JD, Pavek TJ, Bache RJ. Role of K+ ATP channels in coronary vasodilation during exercise. Circulation 1993;88:1245–1253.

51. Duncker DJ, van Zon NS, Ishibashi Y, Bache RJ. Role of K+ ATP channels and adenosine in the regulation of coronary blood flow during exercise with normal and restricted coronary blood flow. J Clin Invest 1996;97:996–1009.

52. Farouque HM, et al. Effect of ATP-sensitive channel inhibition on coronary netabolic vasodilation in humans. Arterioscler Thromb Vasc Biol 2004;24(5):905–910.

53. Miura H, et al. Diabetes mellitus impairs vasodilation to hypoxia in human coronary arterioles: reduced activity of ATP-sensitive potassium channels. Circ Res 2003;92(2):151–158.

54. Merkus D, Duncker DJ, Chilian WM. Metabolic regulation of vascular tone: role of endothelin-1. Am J Physiol 2002;283:H1915–H1921.

55. Conway RS, Kirk ES, Eng C. Ventricular preload alters intravascular and extravascular resistances of coronary collaterals. Am J Physiol 1988;254:H532–H541.

56. Bellamy RF. Diastolic coronary artery pressure-flow relations in the dog. Circ Res 1978;43:92–101.

57. Eng C, Jentzer JH, Kirk ES. The effects of the coronary capacitance on the interpretation of diastolic pressure-flow relationships. Circ Res 1982;50:334–341.

58. Kanatsuka H, Ashikawa K, Komaru T, Suzuki T, Takishima T. Diameter change and pressure-red blood cell velocity relations in coronary microvessels during long diastoles in the canine left ventricle. Circ Res 1990;66:503–510.

59. Jayaweera AR, Wei K, Coggins M, Bin JP, Goodman C, Kaul S. Role of capillaries in determining CBF reserve: new insights using myocardial contrast echocardiography. Am J Physiol 1999;277:H2363–H2372.
60. Sun, et al. Mechanical compression elicits NO-dependent increases in coronary flow. Am J Physiol Heart Circ Physiol 2004;287:H2454–H2460.
61. Young MA, Knight DR, Vatner SF. Autonomic control of large coronary arteries and resistance vessels. Prog Cardiovasc Dis 1987;30:211–234.
62. Wang SY, Friedman M, Johnson RG, Weintraub RM, Sellke FW. Adrenergic regulation of coronary microcirculation after extracorporeal circulation and crystalloid cardioplegia. Am J Physiol 1994;267:H2462–H2470.
63. Lamping KG, Chilian WM, Eastham CL, Marcus ML. Coronary microvascular response to exogenously administered and endogenously released acetylcholine. Microvasc Res 1992;43:294–307.
64. Hammarstrom AK, Parkington HC, Coleman HA. Release of endothelium-derived hyperpolarizing factor (EDHF) by M3 receptor stimulation in guinea-pig coronary artery. Br J Pharmacol 1995;115:717–722.
65. Sellke FW, Dai HB. Responses of porcine epicardial venules to neurohumoral substances. Cardiovasc Res 1993;27:1326–1332.
66. Lamping KG, Kanatsuka H, Eastham CL, Chilian WM, Marcus ML. Nonuniform vasomotor responses of the coronary microcirculation to serotonin and vasopressin. Circ Res 1989;65:343–351.
67. Sellke FW, Myers PR, Bates JN, Harrison DG. Influence of vessel size on the sensitivity of porcine microvessels to nitroglycerin. Am J Physiol 1990;258:H515–H520.
68. Lamping KG, Clothier JL, Eastham CL, Marcus ML. Coronary microvascular response to endothelin is dependent on vessel diameter and route of administration. Am J Physiol 1992;263:H703–H709.
69. Merkus D. Contribution of endothelium to coronary vasomotor tone. Am J Physiol Heart Circ Physiol 2005;28:H871–H880.
70. Murad F. Cyclic guanosine monophosphate as a mediator of vasodilation. J Clin Invest 1986;78:1–5.
71. Myers PR, Minor RL Jr, Guerra R Jr, Bates JN, Harrison DG. The vasorelaxant properties of the endothelium-derived relaxing factor more closely resemble S-nitrosocysteine than nitric oxide. Nature 1990;345:161–163.
72. Corson M, James N, Latta S, Nerem R, Berk B, Harrison D. Phosphorylation of endothelial nitric oxide synthse in response to fluid shear stress. Circ Res 1996;79:984–991.
73. Venema RC, Sayegh HS, Arnal J-F, Harrison DG. Role of the enzyme calmodulin-binding domain in membrane association and phospholipid inhibition of endothelial nitric oxide synthase. J Biol Chem 1995;270:14705–14711.
74. Michel J, Feron O, Sacks D, Michel T. Reciprocal regulation of endothelial nitric-oxide synthase by Ca^{2+}-calmodulin and caveolin. J Biol Chem 1997;272:15583–15586.
75. Uemetsu M, Ohara Y, Navas JP, et al. Regulation of endothelial cell nitric oxide synthase mRNA expresiion by shear stress. Am J Physiol 1995;269:C1371–C1378.
76. Arnal J-F, Yamin J, Dockery S, Harrison DG. Regulation of endothelial nitric oxide synthase mRNA, protein and activity during cell growth. Am J Physiol (Cell Physiol) 1994;267:C1381–C1388.
77. McQuillan LP, Leung GK, Marsden PA, Kostyk SK, Kourembanas S. Hypoxia inhibits expression of eNOS via transcriptional and posttranscriptional mechanisms. Am J Physiol 1994;267:H1921–H1927.
78. Pou S, Pou WS, Bredt DS, Snyder SH, Rosen GM. Generation of superoxide by purified brain nitric oxide synthase. J Biol Chem 1992;267:24173–24176.

79. Shimokawa H, Flavahan NA, Vanhoutte PM. Loss of endothelial pertussis toxin-sensitive G protein function in atherosclerotic porcine coronary arteries. Circulation 1991;83:652–660.
80. Harrison DG. Endothelial function and oxidant stress. Clin Cardiol 1997;20:II-11–II-17.
81. Jang JJ, Ho HKV, Kwan HH, Fajardo LF, Cooke JP. Angiogenesis is impaired by hypercholesterolemia—role of asymmetric dimethylarginine. Circulation 2000;102:1414–1419.
82. Amezcua JL, Palmer RM, de Souza BM, Moncada S. Nitric oxide synthesized from L-arginine regulates vascular tone in the coronary circulation of the rabbit. Br J Pharmacol 1989;97:1119–1124.
83. Taylor SG, Weston AH. Endothelium-derived hyperpolarizing factor: a new endogenous inhibitor from the vascular endothelium. Trends Pharmacol Sci 1988;9:272–274.
84. Petersson J, Zygmunt PM, Hogestatt ED. Characterization of the potassium channels involved in EDHF-mediated relaxation in cerebral arteries. Br J Pharmacol 1997;120:1344–1350.
85. Campbell WB, Gebremedhin D, Pratt PF, Harder DR. Identification of epoxyeicosatrienoic acids as endothelium-derived hyperpolarizing factors. Circ Res 1996;78:415–423.
86. Fulton D, McGiff JC, Wolin MS, Kaminski P, Quilley J. Evidence against a cytochrome P_{450}-derived reactive oxygen species as the mediator of the nitric oxide-independent vasodilator effect of bradykinin in the perfused heart of the rat. J Pharmacol Exp Ther 1997;280:702–709.
87. Edwards G, Dora KA, Gardener MJ, Garland CJ, Weston AH. K^+ is an endothelium-derived hyperpolarizinf factor in rat arteries. Nature 1998;396:269–272.
88. Taylor HJ, Chaytor AT, Evance WH, Griffith TM. Inhibition of the gap junctional component of endothelium-dependent relaxations in rabbit iliac artery by 18-alpha glycyrrhetinic acid. Br J Pharmacol 1998;125:1–3.
89. Batenburg WW, et al. L-S nitrosothiols: endothelium-derived hyperpolarizing factors in porcine coronary arteries? J Hypertens 2004;22:1927–1936.
90. Yada T, Shimokawa H, Hiramatsu O, Kajita T, Shigeto F, Goto M, Ogasawara Y, Kajiya F. Hydrogen peroxide, an endogenous endothelium-derived hyperpolarizing factor, plays an important role in coronary autoregulation in vivo. Circulation 2003;107:1040–1045.
91. Shimokawa H, Yasutake H, Fujii K, et al. The importance of the hyperpolarizing mechanism increases as the vessel size decreases in endothelium-dependent relaxations in rat mesenteric circulation. J Cardiovasc Pharmacol 1996;28:703–711.
92. Xu XP, Tanner MA, Myers PR. Prostaglandin-mediated inhibition of nitric oxide production by bovine aortic endothelium during hypoxia. Cardiovasc Res 1995;30:345–350.
93. Klassen G, Armour J. Epicardial coronary venous pressure measurements: autonomic responses. Can J Physiol Pharmacol 1982;60:698–706.
94. Yuan Y, Mier R, Chilian W, Zawieja D, Granger H. Interaction of neutrophils and endothelium in isolated coronary venules and arterioles. Am J Physiol 1995;268:H490–H498.
95. Tinsey JH, Ustinova EE, Xu W, Yuan SY. Src-dependent, neutrophil-mediated vascular hyperpermeability and beta-catenin modification. Am J Physiol Cell Physiol 2002;283(6):C1745–C1751.
96. Yuan SY, Wu MH, Ustinova EE, et al. Myosin light chain phosphorylation in neutrophil-stimulated coronary microvascular leakage. Circ Res 2002;90(11):1214–1221.

97. Lefer D, Nakanishi K, Vinten-Johansen J, Ma X, Lefer A. Cardiac venous endothelial dysfunction after myocardial ischemia and reperfusion in dogs. Am J Physiol 1992;263:H850–H856.

98. Piana RN, Wang SY, Friedman M, Sellke FW. Angiotensin-converting enzyme inhibition preserves endothelium-dependent coronary microvascular responses during short-term ischemia-reperfusion. Circulation 1996;93:544–551.

99. Garg UC, Hassid A. Nitric oxide-generating vasodilators and 8-bromo-cyclic guanosine monophosphate inhibit mitogenesis and proliferation of cultured rat vascular smooth muscle cells. J Clin Invest 1989;83:1774–1777.

100. Cayatte AJ, Palacino JJ, Horten K, Cohen RA. Chronic inhibition of nitric oxide production accelerates neointima formation and impairs endothelial function in hypercholesterolemic rabbits. Arterioscler Thromb 1994;14:753–759.

101. von der Leyen HE, Gibbons GH, Morishita R, et al. Gene therapy inhibiting neointimal vascular lesion: in vivo transfer of endothelial cell nitric oxide synthase gene. Proc Natl Acad Sci USA 1995;92:1137–1141.

102. Moroi M, Zhang L, Yasuda T, Virmani R, Gold HK, Fisman MC, Huang PL. Interaction of genetic deficiency of endothelial nitric oxide, gender and pregnancy in vascular response to injury in mice. J Clin Invest 1998;101:1225–1232.

103. Yu SM, Hung LM, Lin CC. cGMP-elevating agents suppress proliferation of vascular smooth muscle cells by inhibiting the activation of epidermal growth factor signaling pathway. Circulation 1997;95:1269–1277.

104. Itoh H, Pratt RE, Ohno M, Dzau VJ. Atrial natriuretic polypeptide as a novel antigrowth factor of endothelial cells. Hypertension 1992;19:758–761.

105. Cornwell TL, Arnold E, Boerth NJ, Lincoln TM. Inhibition of smooth muscle cell growth by nitric oxide and activation of cAMP-dependent protein kinase by cGMP. Am J Physiol 1994;267:C1405–C1413.

106. D'Souza FM, Sparks RL, Chen H, Kadowitz PJ, Jeter JR Jr. Mechanis of eNOS gene transfer inhibition of vascular smooth muscle cell proliferation. Am J Physiol Cell Physiol 2003;284(1):C191–C199

107. Pollman MJ, Yamada T, Horiuchi M, Gibbons GH. Vasoactive substances regulate vascular smooth muscle cell apoptosis. Countervailing influences of nitric oxide and angiotensin II. Circ Res 1996;79:748–756.

108. Shi W, Wang X, Shih DM, Laubach VE, Vavab M, Lusis AJ. Paradoxical reduction of fatty streak formation in mice lacking endothelial nitric oxide synthase. Circulation 2002;105:2078.

109. Ozaki M, Kawashima S, Yamashita T, et al. Overexpression of endothelial nitric oxide synthase accelerates atherosclerotic lesion formation in apoE-deficient mice. J Clin Invest 2002;110:331–340.

110. Kuhlencordt PJ, Gyurko R, Han F, et al. Accelerated atherosclerosis, aortic aneurysm formation, and ischemic heat disease in apolipoprotein E/endothelial nitric oxide synthase double-knockout mice. Circulation 2001;104:448.

111. Wolfsgruber W, Feil S, Brummer S, Kuppinger O, Hofmann F, Feil R. A proatherogenic role for cGMP-dependant protein kinase in vascular smooth muscle cells. PNAS 2003;100(23):13519–13524.

112. Bayraktutan U. Nitric oxide synthase and NAD(P)H oxidase modulate coronary endothelial cell growth. J Mol Cell Cardiol 2004;36(2):277–286.

113. Ware J, Simons M. Angiogenesis in ischemic heart disease. Nat Med 1997;3:158–164.

114. Li J, Brown L, Hibberd M, Grossman J, Morgan J, Simons M. VEGF, flk-1, flt-1 expression in a rat myocardial infarction model of angiogenesis. Am J Physiol 1996;270:H1803–H1811.

115. Sellke FW, Wang SY, Stamler A, et al. Enhanced microvascular relaxations to VEGF and bFGF in chronically ischemic porcine myocardium. Am J Physiol 1996;271:H713–H720.

116. Wu H, Yuan Y, McCarthy M, Granger H. Acidic and basic FGF's dilate arterioles of skeletal muscle through a NO-dependent mechanism. Am J Physiol 1996;271:H1087–H1093.

117. Ziche M, Morbidelli L, Masini E, et al. Nitric oxide mediates angiogenesis in vivo and endothelial cell growth and migration in vitro promoted by substance P. J Clin Invest 1994;94:2036–2044.

118. Morbidelli L, Chang CH, Douglas JG, Granger HJ, Ledda F, Ziche M. Nitric oxide mediates mitogenic effect of VEGF on coronary venular endothelium. Am J Physiol 1996;270:H411–H415.

119. Bouloumie A, Schini-Kerth VB, Busse R. Vascular endothelial growth factor up-regulates nitric oxide synthase expression in endothelial cells. Cardiovasc Res 1999;41:773–780.

120. Uhlmann S, Friedrichs U, Eichler W, Hoffmann S, Wiedemann P. Direct measurement of VEGF-induced nitric oxide production by choroidal endothelial cells. Microvasc Res 2001;62:179–189.

121. Zhao X, Lu X, Feng Q. Deficiency in endothelial nitric oxide synthase impairs myocardial angiogenesis. Am J Physiol Heart Circ Physiol 2002;283(6):H2371–H2378.

122. Bussolati B, Dunk C, Grohman M, Kontos CD, Mason J, Ahmed A. Vascular endothelial growth factor receptor-1 modulates vascular endothelial growth factor-mediated angiogenesis via nitric oxide. Am J Pathol 2001;159:993–1008.

123. Jozkowicz A, Cooke JP, Guevara I, et al. Genetic augmentation of nitric oxide synthase increases the vascular generation of VEGF. Cardiovasc Res 2001;51:773–783.

124. Babaei S, Teichert-Kuliszewska K, Monge JC, Mohamed F, Bendeck MP, Stewart DJ. Role of nitric oxide in the angiogenic response in vitro to basic fibroblast growth factor. Circ Res 1998;82:1007–1015.

125. Murohara T, Witzenbichler B, Spyridopoulos I, et al. Role of endothelial nitric oxide synthase in endothelial cell migration. Arterioscler Thromb Vasc Biol 1999;19:1156–1161.

126. Papapetropoulos A, Desai KM, Rudic RD, et al. Nitric oxide synthase inhibitors attenuate transforming-growth-factor-beta 1-stimulated capillary organization in vitro. Am J Pathol 1997;150:1835–1844.

127. Eliceiri BP, Paul R, Schwartzberg PL, Hood JD, Leng J, Cheresh DA. Selective requirement for Src kinases during VEGF-induced angiogenesis and vascular permeability. Mol Cell 1999;4:915–924.

128. Duan J, Murohara T, Ikeda H, et al. Hypercholesterolemia inhibits angiogenesis in response to hindlimb ischemia: nitric oxide-dependent mechanism. Circulation 2000;102:III370–III376.

129. Ruel M, Wu GF, Khan TA, et al. Inhibition of the cardiac angiogenic response to surgical FGF-2 therapy in a swine endothelial dysfunction model. Circulation 2003;108(Suppl 1):II335–II340.

130. Voisine P, Bianchi C, Ruel M, et al. Inhibition of the cardiac angiogenic response to exogenous vascular endothelial growth factor (VEGF) therapy in a porcine model of endothelial dysfunction. Surgery 2004;136:407–415.

131. Sellke FW, Armstrong ML, Harrison DG. Endothelium-dependent vascular relaxation is abnormal in the coronary microcirculation of atherosclerotic primates. Circulation 1990;81:1586–1593.

132. Chilian WM, Dellsperger KC, Layne SM, et al. Effects of atherosclerosis on the coronary microcirculation. Am J Physiol 1990;258:H529–H539.

133. Drexler H, Zeiher AM, Meinzer K, Just H. Correction of endothelial dysfunction in coronary microcirculation of hypercholesterolaemic patients by L-arginine. Lancet 1991;338:1546–1550.
134. Treasure CB, Klein JL, Vita JA, et al. Hypertension and left ventricular hypertrophy are associated with impaired endothelium-mediated relaxation in human coronary resistance vessels. Circulation 1993;87:86–93.
135. Quillen JE, Sellke FW, Brooks LA, Harrison DG. Ischemia-reperfusion impairs endothelium-dependent relaxation of coronary microvessels but does not affect large arteries. Circulation 1990;82:586–594.
136. Matsunaga T, Okumura K, Ishizaka H, Tsunoda R, Tayama S, Yasue H. Impairment of coronary blood flow regulation by endothelium-derived nitric oxide in dogs with alloxan-induced diabetes. J Cardiovasc Pharmacol 1996;28:60–67.
137. Sellke FW, Shafique T, Schoen FJ, Weintraub RM. Impaired endothelium-dependent coronary microvascular relaxation after cold potassium cardioplegia and reperfusion. J Thorac Cardiovasc Surg 1993;105:52–58.
138. Sellke FW, Quillen JE, Brooks LA, Harrison DG. Endothelial modulation of the coronary vasculature in vessels perfused via mature collaterals. Circulation 1990;81:1938–1947.
139. Peters KG, Marcus ML, Harrison DG. Vasopressin and the mature coronary collateral circulation. Circulation 1989;79:1324–1331.
140. Symons JD, Longhurst JC, Stebbins CL. Response of collateral-dependent myocardium to vasopressin release during prolonged intense exercise. Am J Physiol 1993;264:H1644–H1652.
141. Harada K, Friedman M, Lopez J, et al. Vascular endothelial growth factor administration in chronic myocardial ischemia. Am J Physiol 1996;270:H1791–H1802.
142. Sellke FW, Wang SY, Friedman M, et al. Basic FGF enhances endothelium-dependent relaxation of the collateral-perfused coronary microcirculation. Am J Physiol 1994;267:H1303–H1311.
143. Ravichandran L, Johns R, Rengasamy A. Direct and reversible inhibition of endothelial nitric oxide synthase by nitric oxide. Am J Physiol 1995;268:H2216–H2223.
144. Laham RJ, Simons M, Tokufuji M, Hung D, Sellke FW. Modulation of myocardial perfusion and vascular reactivity by pericardial basic fibroblast growth factor: insight into ischemia-induced reduction in endothelium-dependent vasodilation. J Thorac Cardiovasc Surg 1998;116:1022–1028.
145. Uematsu M, Ohara Y, Navas JP, et al. Regulation of endothelial cell nitric oxide synthase mRNA expression by shear stress. Am J Physiol 1995;269:C1371–C1378.
146. Voisine P, Bianchi C, Khan TA, et al. Normalization of coronary microvascular reactivity and improvement in myocardial perfusion by surgical VEGF therapy combined with oral supplementation of L-arginine in a porcine model of endothelial dysfunction. J Thorac Cardiovasc Surg 2005; in press.
147. Rapps J, Jones A, Sturek M, Magliola L, Parker J. Mechanisms of altered contractile responses to vasopressin and endothelin in canine collateral arteries. Circulation 1997;95:231–239.
148. Bauters C, Asahara T, Zheng L, et al. Recovery of disturbed endothelium-dependent flow in the collateral-perfused rabbit ischemic hindlimb after administration of vascular endothelial growth factor. Circulation 1995;91:2802–2809.
149. Lopez J, Laham R, Carrozza J, et al. Hemodynamic effects of intracoronary VEGF delivery-Evidence of tachyphylaxis and NO dependence of response. Am J Physiol 1997;273:H1317–H1323.
150. Sirois M, Edelman E. VEGF effect on vascular permeability is mediated by synthesis of platelet-activating factor. Am J Physiol 1997;272:H2746–H2756.

151. Wu G, Mannam AP, Wu J, et al. Hypoxia induces myocyte-dependent COX-2 regulation in endothelial cells: role of VEGF. Am J Physiol Heart Circ Physiol 2003;285(6):H2420–H2429

152. Marcus ML, Harrison DG, Chilian WM, e tal. Alterations in the coronary circulation in hypertrophied ventricles. Circulation 1987;75:I 19–I 25.

153. Thatcher GRJ, et al. Nitrates and NO release: contemporary aspects in biological and medicinal chemistry. Free Radic Biol Med 2004;37(8):1122–1143.

154. Winbury MM, Howe BB, Weiss HR. Effect of nitrates and other coronary dilators on large and small coronary vessels; an hypothesis for the mechanism of action of nitrates. J Pharmacol Exp Ther 1969;168:70–95.

155. Fam WM, McGregor M. Effect of nitroglycerin and dipyridamole on regional coronary resistance. Circ Res 1968;22:649–659.

156. Kurz MA, Lamping KG, Bates JN, Eastham CL, Marcus ML, Harrison DG. Mechanisms responsible for the heterogeneous coronary microvascular response to nitroglycerin. Circ Res 1991;68:847–855.

157. Wheatley RM, Dockery SP, Kurz MA, Sayegh HS, Harrison DG. Interactions of nitroglycerin and sulfhydryl-donating compounds in coronary microvessels. Am J Physiol 1994;266:H291–H297.

158. Park KS, Kim Y, Lee YH, Earm YE, Ho WK. Mechanosensitive cation channels in arterial smooth muscle cells are activated by diacylglycerol and inhibited by phospholipase C inhibitor. Circ Res 2003;93:557–564.

159. Werner GS, et al. Intracoronary verapamil for reversal of no-reflow during coronary angioplasty for acute myocardial infarction. Catheter Cardiovasc Interv 2002;57(4):444–451.

160. Akai K, Wang Y, Sato K, et al. Vasodilatory effect of nicorandil on coronary arterial microvessels: its dependency on vessel size and the involvement of the ATP-sensitive potassium channels. J Cardiovasc Pharmacol 1995;26:541–547.

161. Kichuk MR, et al. Regulation of nitric oxide production in human coronary microvessels and the contribution of local kinin formation. Circulation 1996;94: 44–51.

162. Chen R, et al. important role of nitric oxide in the effect of angiotensin converting enzyme inhibitor imipaprine on vascular injury. Hypertension 2003;42(4):542–547.

163. Kitakaze M, et al. Beneficial effects of inhibition of angiotensin converting enzyme on ischemic myocardium during coronary hypoperfusion in dogs. Circulation 1995;92:950–961.

164. Piana RN, et al. Angiotensin converting enzyme inhibition preserves endothelium-dependent coronary microvascular responses during short-term ischemia-reperfusion. Circulation 1996;93:544–551.

165. Dzau VJ, et al. The relevance of tissue angiotensin converting enzyme: manifestations in mechanistic and endpoint data. Am J Cardiol 2001;88(9A):1L–20L.

166. Unger T, Mattfeldt T, Lamberty V, et al. Effect of early onset angiotensin enzyme inhibition on myocardial capillaries. Hypertension 1992;20:478–482.

167. Fabre JE, Rivard A, Magner M, Silver M, Isner JM. Tissue inhibition of angiotensin-converting enzyme activity stimulates angiogenesis in vivo. Circulation 1999;99:3043–3049.

168. Silvestre JS, Bergaya S, Tamarat R, Duriez M, Boulanger CM, Levy BI. Proangiogenic effect of angiotensin-converting enzyme inhibition is mediated by the bradykinin B(2) receptor pathway. Circ Res 2001;89:678–683.

169. Walther T, Menrad A, Orzechowski HD, Siemeister G, Paul M, Schirner M. Differntial regulation of in vivo angiogenesis by angiotensin II receptors. FASEB J 2003;17:2061–2067.

170. Corsini A, Bellosta S, Baetta R, Funagalli R, Paoletti R, Bernini F. New insights into the pharmacodynamic and pharmacokinetic properties of statins. Pharmacol Ther 1999;84:413–428.
171. Laufs U, Liao JK. Direct vascular effects of HMG-CoA reductase inhibitors. Trends Cardiovasc Med 2000;10:143–148.
172. Brouet A, Sonveauzx P, Dessy C, Moniotte S, Balligand JL, Feron O. Hsp90 and caveolin are key targets for the proangiogenic nitric oxidemediated effects of statins. Circ Res 2001;89:866–873.
173. Kureishi Y, Luo Z, Shiojima I, et al. The HMG-CoA reductase inhibitor simvastatin activates the protein kinase Akt and promotes angiogenesis in normocholesterolemic animals. Nat Med 2000;6:1004–1010.
174. Urbich C, Dernbach E, Zeiher AM, Dimmeler S. Double-edged role of statins in angiogenesis signaling. Circ Res 2002;90:737–744.
175. Weis M, Heeschen C, Glassford AJ, Cooke JP. Statins have biphasic effects on angiogenesis. Circulation 2002;105:739–745.
176. Park HJ, Kong D, Iruela-Arispe L, Begley U, Tang D, Galper JB. 3-hydroxy-3-methylglutaryl coenzyme A reductase inhibitors interfere with angiogenesis by inhibiting the geranylgeranylation fo RhoA. Circ Res 2002;91:143–150.

5

Local and Regional Vascular Delivery Strategies for Therapeutic Angiogenesis and Myogenesis

Erik T. Price, MD, Alan C. Yeung, MD, and Mehrdad Rezaee, MD, PhD

CONTENTS

INTRODUCTION

An estimated 15% of patients with ischemic heart disease are not amenable to conventional methods of revascularization *(1–3)*, and an additional 12–22% may be limited to incomplete percutaneous coronary intervention (PCI) or surgical procedures *(1,4–7)*. These so-called no-option patients often progress to end-stage ischemic cardiomyopathy with an annual mortality in excess of 30% *(8)*. Treatment options for this

From: *Contemporary Cardiology: Angiogenesis and Direct Myocardial Revasularization*
Edited by: R. J. Laham and D. S. Baim © Humana Press Inc., Totowa, NJ

group remain limited to multidrug medical management, myocardial reduction surgery, left-ventricular (LV) assist device placement, or cardiac transplantation. The current estimation is that 100,000 patients per year in this group would potentially benefit from alternative therapies *(2,3,9)*. Over the past decade, cardiac angiogenesis and myogenesis have emerged as such alternatives.

The efforts to develop alternative treatments have been mostly directed toward understanding cardiac vascular and muscle regeneration and the various protein, gene, and cellular mediators of these biological processes. Semantic differences between neovascularization, angiogenesis, arteriogenesis, and vasculogenesis are important and are further discussed in recent reviews *(4,10,11)*. For the purposes of this chapter, these processes will be collectively referred to as angiogenesis. Myogenesis and cellular myoplasty refer to mammalian cellular transplantation into the myocardium *(12–17)*. A comparative analysis of the many agents that may facilitate cardiac angiogenesis or myogenesis is beyond the scope of this chapter and is deferred to expert reviews *(4,10–29)*.

The potential availability of myogenic and angiogenic factors has created an unusual situation in medicine where potent reagents are at hand, but the optimal delivery modalities to target these to the cardiac tissue are not yet established *(30–33)*. This chapter will provide an overview of the delivery modalities that may facilitate the anticipated efficacy of therapeutic cardiac angiogenesis and cellular cardiomyoplasty. Conceptualized criteria of an ideal delivery system are presented in Table 1. Safety issues are most pertinent for application in patients with severe cardiac disease and multiple co-morbidities *(4,33–35)*. Safety issues addressed, delivery modalities should be applicable to the broadest patient population. If these treatments are to become routine, this modality should be practical for both the patient and practitioner and reproducible across a wide spectrum of operator skills. The ideal method of cardiac delivery must efficiently deliver the desired product to clinically relevant regions of targeted myocardium and also promote product retention for sustained biological activity. These parameters may serve as guidelines for future development as well as useful tools for comparison of currently available modalities.

SYSTEMIC CARDIAC DELIVERY

Systemic delivery is well established with respect to cardiac pharmaceuticals. Theoretical advantages are evident, with noninvasive procedural practicality, cost efficiency, and broad patient applicability. For these reasons, the systemic route for protein growth factor and gene

Table 1
Proposed Parameters for an Ideal Myocardial Delivery System

Safety
  Minimal procedure-related complications
    (corporal invasiveness, local invasiveness, myocardial damage, coronary
    vascular damage, ventricular perforation, pericardial tamponade,
    arrhythmia)
Applicability
  Broad spectrum of patients
  Useful across a broad range of disease types
    (acute ischemia, sub-acute infarction, chronic infarction, ischemic
    cardiomyopathy, nonischemic cardiomyopathy)
Practicality
  For the patient
    (minimally invasive, limited procedural discomfort, limited procedural time,
    outpatient vs inpatient, single administration)
  For the practitioner
    (standard equipment, standard skill set, procedural efficiency, independence)
Efficiency
  Procedural efficiency
    (high delivery success rate, reproducible, time efficient)
  Product delivery efficiency
Precision
  Maximal delivery to targeted areas
    (regionality within the myocardium)
  Minimal delivery to nontargeted areas
    (diffusion, wash-out)
Retained Activity
  Location of delivery allowing prolonged retention for maximal beneficial
    biological effect

product delivery has been actively investigated. In early investigations of fibroblast growth factor (FGF) and vascular endothelial growth factor (VEGF), systemic intravenous delivery produced consistently poor acute and chronic myocardial protein uptake with widely variable clinical effects *(36–39)*. Follow-up studies have primarily used the systemic route to establish comparative superiority of alternative methods *(32,40–43)*. In composite, these studies demonstrated acute myocardial retention that was consistently <1% after systemic delivery, with significant first-pass product uptake in both liver and lungs and no significant improvement in collateral development, angiogenesis, myocardial perfusion, or function.

Clinical application in 59 no-option patients treated with either systemic ($n = 14$) or intracoronary ($n = 35$) FGF at variable doses claimed overall clinical effectiveness with attenuation of regional stress-induced ischemia *(44)*. However, systemic and intracoronary subsets were grouped together for final analysis, preventing interpretation of independent effects of systemic delivery. In a larger (VEGF in Ischemia for Vascular Angiogenesis;VIVA) clinical trial of protein growth factor delivery, 178 patients received VEGF by both intravenous and intracoronary routes of administration *(45)*. Although the individual effects of each route were again not separable, the composite underwhelming results of this study may further attest to inadequacies of the peripheral intravenous delivery of protein growth factor formulations.

The small amount of protein or gene product reaching the myocardium may be physiologically predicted, with only 3% of the cardiac output per minute perfusing the myocardium *(47)*, and effective filtering (35–50% of total acute delivery) by combined pulmonary, hepatic, renal, and reticuloendothelial systems *(38,40)*. Product loss through the pulmonary circulation has been seen to be most prominent for protein growth factors. As noted above, the average efficiency of myocardial delivery using the systemic route is <1% acutely, with myocardial retention falling appreciably within 24 h *(32,40,41)*.

Procedural modifications have not provided significant improvement. Atrial, ventricular cavity, and even pulmonary artery infusion distal to Swan Ganz balloon occlusion demonstrate similarly poor myocardial uptake *(32)*. Higher dosing and repetitive or continuous administration improve total myocardial uptake *(41,43)* but are not easily translated into the clinical setting. Furthermore, these modifications do not appreciably alter tissue specificity, with potentially serious clinical consequences of product delivery to unintended organs and potent systemic side effects. An example of this is the dose-dependent hypotension seen with intravenous VEGF (and to a lesser extent FGF) *(43,48–50)*. The potential risks in combination with relative delivery inefficiency continue to challenge intravenous introduction of protein and genetic agents.

Systemic methods of cellular transplant were examined by delivery of human mesenchymal stem cells (hMSCs) into the left ventricular cavity of immunodeficient mice *(51)*. At 4 d the majority of transplanted cells were identified in the spleen, liver, and lungs, with cells identifiable in the hearts of 75% of the animals. In the remaining animals, rare transplanted cells were identified with estimated myocardial delivery of 0.44%. Additional studies using radiolabeled MSCs delivered by the same systemic method resulted in similar <1% total cardiac activity at 4 h *(52)*. Independent systemic delivery of endothelial precursor cells

(EPCs) demonstrated superiority of ventricular cavity over peripheral vein delivery, with 1-h myocardial retention of up to 4.7 ± 1.55% of transplanted cells *(53)*. Although the efficiency afforded by the systemic method varies between protein, gene, and cellular products, the generally poor myocardial retention and lack of tissue specificity make it unlikely that this approach will find broad utility in future.

DIRECT INTRAMYOCARDIAL INJECTION

Transepicardial needle injection into the myocardium is the most straightforward and extensively studied of the delivery methods. Direct muscular injection of protein growth factors for the treatment of peripheral ischemia is well established *(54–56)*, and direct intramyocardial delivery of these same angiogenic agents has been addressed in a number of studies demonstrating higher efficiency and preclinical efficacy *(42,57–59)*. Direct intramyocardial injection (DIMI) may provide acute delivery efficiencies of 5–30%, depending upon the product delivered *(21,60)*. Chronic retention has been less well documented, with suggestions of significant tissue efflux over a relatively short period of time *(60)* and unchanged safety concerns related to nontargeted tissue uptake. Unlike systemic or other vascular delivery, direct injection may minimize dose-dependent toxicity (e.g., VEGF- and FGF-mediated hypotension) through focal product concentration and depot tissue release *(60)*. Most studies have not quantitatively examined delivery efficiency, but the lower than expected retention of protein products by standard injection is thought to be due to active and passive egress through the needle tract, incomplete penetration of injection needle, and interstitial pathways during each cardiac cycle *(19,33)*.

In an attempt to enhance sustained biological effects, several unique gene transfer approaches have been combined with DIMI *(18,61–73)*. Transepicardial injection of plasmids encoding VEGF (ph.VEGF) in murine and porcine models demonstrated dose-dependent gene expression, with peak VEGF protein levels between 1 and 5 d, and variable transgene duration from 3 d to 3 wk *(61,62)*. Whereas some studies have reported beneficial effects related to angiogenesis and enhanced myocardial blood flow, others have demonstrated no clinical effects *(63,64)*.

In a recent comparison with viral vectors (adenovirus, adeno-associated virus, and herpes simplex virus), uncomplexed and complexed naked DNA proved inefficient for direct intramyocardial delivery (less than one positive cell per heart), whereas all viral vectors produced significant transgene expression up to 21 d *(66)*. DIMI of Ad.VEGF to rat myocardium produced peak gene expression at 24–72 h that remained detectable for up to 3 wk *(67)*. Similar transepicardial delivery of

Ad.VEGF to ischemic pigs improved regional stress perfusion and function for up to 4 wk *(68)*. Examining myocardial protective effects, Ad.FGF injected into rabbit myocardium that was infarcted 12 d later showed evidence of angiogenesis in the pretreated areas with 50% reduction in the myocardial area at risk *(69)*. This study broadens the potential application of angiogenic gene transfer from chronic ischemia and infarct to acute injury and even prophylactic treatment.

Delivery of adeno-associated vectors by DIMI methods has proven equally efficacious in preclinical studies, with documented myocardial transgene expression lasting for up to 8 wk *(70)*. Also documented was improved segmental wall motion concurrent with a greater than threefold increase in total arteriolar wall area in animals treated with AAV.FGF compared to controls *(71)*. Others have effectively delivered HJV.HGF gene product to the myocardium with resultant improvements in neovascularization, regional function, and perfusion *(72,73)*. In these studies the effect of endogenous upregulation of HGF expression was not determined.

Successful cellular cardiomyoplasty, by DIMI and other methods, has recently undergone comprehensive review *(12)*. These authors examined myocardial delivery of cardiomyocytes (fetal, neonatal, or adult), skeletal myoblasts, and various stem cells (embryonic stem cells, mesenchymal or bone marrow stem cells, endothelial progenitor cells, and uncharacterized progenitor cell mixtures). No significant differences were seen in cell engraftment capabilities among various cell types, although quantitative analyses of acute and chronic transplant efficiency and cellular distribution were not independently examined. It remains unclear if cellular transplant facilitates functional improvement through differentiation into physiologically active cardiomyocyte cell types, through angiogenesis, or potentially through physical effects on remodeling with alteration in the mechanical properties of scar or ischemic tissues. The degree to which targeted delivery by transepicardial injection may affect these variables is under exploration, and this modality remains a viable investigational and treatment approach.

Because of the relative invasiveness of DIMI, clinical experience has been predictably more complex. In a phase I trial in five patients with symptomatic myocardial ischemia, naked plasma DNA encoding for VEGF was directly injected into myocardial areas of injury via mini-thoracotomy *(74)*. Injections were safe, and at 30 and 60 d postdelivery there were significant reductions in angina, improvement in regional perfusion, and angiographic evidence of enhanced collateral flow in treated patients. In a follow-up study, 20 patients received similar treatment with improved perfusion and collateral formation again documented up to 60 d, and anginal improvement out to 3 mo *(75)*. DIMI was also used to deliver Ad.VEGF to 21 coronary artery disease (CAD) patients, either concurrent with bypass surgery (*n* = 15) or as stand-alone therapy via mini-thoracotomy (*n* = 6) *(76)*. Delivery using both methods was performed without procedurally related adverse events, demonstrating improvement in angina class and regional ventricular function at 30 d, but no significant change in perfusion or exercise performance. Direct injection of FGF in 20 patients undergoing coronary bypass surgery (in the area of left internal mammary artery [LIMA] to left anterior descending artery [LAD] anastamosis) resulted in augmented neovascularization in the anastomotic region at 1 yr *(77)*. Skeletal myoblast transplant by DIMI methods concurrent with surgical revascularization has likewise proven safe and feasible in a small number of patients *(17)*.

DIMI claims superiority with respect to targeted myocardial distribution. However, although a large amount of product may be introduced into focal myocardial areas, this process depends on limited epicardial visualization to identify site(s) of interest. Direct delivery is at best focal and not regional without numerous injections, and limited with respect to septal and deep myocardial access *(19)*. Preclinical and clinical studies support the angiogenic and myogenic potential of DIMI, and this modality remains an attractive delivery option, especially as part of a hybrid procedure with mechanical revascularization.

PERCUTANEOUS INTRAMYOCARDIAL DELIVERY

Percutaneous intramyocardial delivery (PIMD) has evolved based on the focal efficiency of intramyocardial injection and the potential to optimize safety, practicality, and patient applicability. Competitive device development has produced a variety of technologies, each combining catheter-based transendocardial needle injection with unique properties to facilitate intramyocardial localization, delivery, and retention. Integrated electromechanical myocardial mapping, standard fluoroscopic, ultrasound, or even magnetic resonance imaging (MRI) are being applied to target myocardial delivery of angiogenic factors or mammalian cells.

The NOGA™ Biosense system combines three-dimensional (3D) electromechanical ventricular mapping with a catheter-based needle injection system (Biosense-Webster). Early NOGA-guided PIMD of tracer dye in pigs confirmed procedural safety *(78)*. PIMD of Ad.luciferase or Ad.VEGF with this system was successful in 91% of attempts, providing focal transgene expression in 97% of successful injections (rapid fall-off beyond 1-cm delivery point radius) and similar VEGF protein levels using percutaneous endocardial or transepicardial needle delivery

(79). Using similar methods, autologous bone marrow cells have been delivered to areas of porcine myocardial ischemia, with evidence of improved collateral flow and regional myocardial function in areas corresponding to cellular transplant *(80)*.

Intracardiac echocardiography (ICE) was combined with fluoroscopy as an alternative to NOGA guidance for directed PIMD of gene products in pigs *(81)*. ICE/fluoroscopy successfully directed intramyocardial injection in 88–100% of attempts, with enhanced appreciation for injectate leakage. Focal transgene expression was identified in 95.2% of injection sites, but cardiomyocyte transfection efficiency was <1% after plasmid-LacZ delivery. Guided PIMD has also proven feasible for the introduction of myoblasts and endothelial progenitor cells in swine, with efficient acute cellular engraftment and significant improvement in regional collateral development, capillary density, and LV-ejection fraction (EF) *(82,83)*.

Clinical experience includes a phase I study in six no-option patients receiving plasmid DNA encoding for VEGF delivered to ischemic regions by NOGA-Biosense *(84)*. Treated patients had significantly reduced angina for up to 1 yr. In a follow-up phase I and II, placebo-controlled, double-blind study, 19 similar patients *(85)* were treated with ph.VEGF, resulting in a significant improvement in anginal class. Delivery of autologous bone marrow (ABM) cells with the NOGA-Biosense system was performed, targeting areas of myocardial ischemia in 10 patients *(86)*. Successful cellular delivery resulted in improvement of angina score and regional ischemia in injection territories at 3 mo. PIMD of ABM cells was similarly performed in 14 separate patients with end-stage ischemic heart disease using preprocedural SPECT imaging combined with real-time NOGA mapping and a NOGA Myostar™ injection catheter (Cordis Corporation, Miami Lakes, FL) *(87)*. At 4 mo, treated patients had improved EF as compared to pretreatment baseline. Larger phase I and II studies are currently underway, with anticipated efficacy studies using this PIMD method to follow.

The Stiletto™ endomyocardial injection system (Boston Scientific, Natick, MA) has also been tested for adenoviral delivery in a pig model with successful injection in 80% of attempted sites and efficient local transfection (30.1 ± 6.8 β-Gal cells/HPF) *(88)*. Separate quantitative distribution analysis of Stiletto™ endomyocardial injection of neutron-activated microspheres revealed $43 \pm 15\%$ acute myocardial retention, with delivery efficiency inversely related to injectate volume *(60)*. This device has recently been modified to incorporate an MR receiver coil within the delivery catheter for successful MR-guided focal myocardial injection *(89)*. This combined technology has been applied for the first-

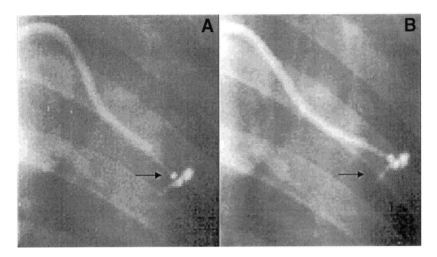

Fig. 1. Contrast media is injected into the myocardium to illustrate attachment of helical needle, the injection site, lack of backleak, and the stability of engagement during cardiac cycle. The anchoring of the infusion catheter into the myocardium maintains the delivery position with cardiac motion: (**A**) during relaxation; (**B**) during systolic contraction. The arrow demonstrates the stability of the anchoring tip with cardiac motion. This ability to maintain position allows for slow infusion of the contrast dye into the myocardium. From ref. *91.*

ever temporal noninvasive tracking of PIMD cell transplant *(90)*. Porcine mesenchymal stem cells labeled with iron fluorophores were delivered under real-time 3D MR guidance to normal and infarcted pig hearts. Serial MR imaging for up to 21 d was able to identify MR signals down to a minimum dose of 10^5 cells, with histological evaluation confirming intact MSCs retaining fluorophores. This novel PIMD modification provides the unique opportunity for combined MR myocardial functional assessment, rtMRI-guided cellular transplantation, and temporal noninvasive cellular tracking.

Another PIMD platform, the BioCardia™ catheter delivery system (BioCardia, South San Francisco, CA) uses a deflectable guiding catheter to direct endomyocardial approximation of a needle delivery catheter to targeted sites of injection (Fig. 1). The delivery catheter contains a helical needle infusion tip for effective anchoring and defined delivery depth. The feasibility and safety of this delivery system for introduction of biomaterial and gene products have been demonstrated in porcine models as well as in patients *(91–93)*. Effective applications for cell delivery have also been documented using this platform to deliver mesenchymal stem cells to areas of infarcted porcine myocardium *(94)*. Results demonstrated successful engraftment for up to 8 wk, with MSCs located in areas of neovascularization and transplant cell expression of markers suggesting myogenic differentiation. A separate feasibility study in a porcine model of LAD infarct demonstrated accurate myocardial cell transplant using the BioCardia system *(95)*. Three weeks after PIMD, a large number of viable transplanted cells were histologically identifiable, with 98.4% of these cells localized to the anteroseptal walls, 95.8% localized to the endocardial half, and 96.8% within infarct or 5-mm border zone (Fig. 2).

The overall delivery efficiencies of PIMD methods are likely equivalent if not superior to those of direct transepicardial injection *(4,60,79)*. Moreover, although temporal retention of protein and gene products has not been completely addressed, chronic cellular viability has been documented after PIMD transplant *(60,90,95)*. NOGA mapping provides a large amount of information for precise electromechanical myocardial targeting, but it remains a complicated system requiring special equipment and operator skill and significant procedural time. Furthermore, it is not clear that extensive precision for delivery is required, as small areas of infarct or ischemia are not indications for these alternative treatments. MR-guided Stiletto delivery is attractive but not yet widely available and again requires a high level of technical imaging and percutaneous proficiency. Methods utilizing standard fluoroscopic or ultrasound guidance may optimize procedural practicality.

As needle injection systems, each of these PIMD platforms induces myocardial damage associated with both needle insertion and tissue disruption. The acceptable amount of myocardial damage and the degree to which this mechanical disruption is harmful or potentially beneficial have not been determined. Furthermore, spring-loaded systems lack both depth control and myocardial anchoring, with potential for under- or overpenetration of the intended myocardial area. Between 3 and 20% of intended injections miss with these systems. While transmyocardial extension has not been prominent, most practitioners avoid injections into tissue less than 4 mm thick, often delivering to border-zone areas in preference over thinned myocardial scar. For the purpose of angiogenesis, border-zone injection may be inconsequential or even beneficial, but for intended myogenesis in areas of chronic infarct this may limit the efficacy. The BioCardia system may have advantages with fixed endocardial engagement and a helical injection tract improving acute delivery success, retention, and delivery depth.

Issues related to myocardial penetration, arrhythmia, product retention, and catheter compatibility will need further clarification as the

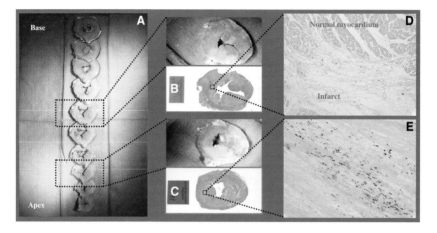

Color Plate 1, Fig. 2 (*see* discussion in Chapter 5, and full caption on p. 117). Percutaneous intramyocardial delivery (Biocardia™) cellular delivery. From ref. *95*.

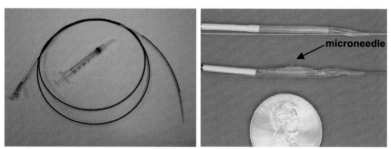

EndoBionics MicroSyringe™

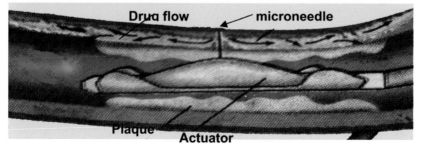

Color Plate 2, Fig. 3 (*see* discussion in Chapter 5, and full caption on p. 120). Catheter-based adventitial drug-delivery system.

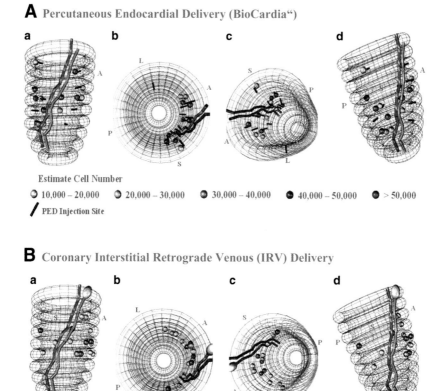

A Percutaneous Endocardial Delivery (BioCardia")

a   b   c   d

Estimate Cell Number

◯ 10,000 – 20,000   ◓ 20,000 – 30,000   ● 30,000 – 40,000   ● 40,000 – 50,000   ● > 50,000

╱ PED Injection Site

B Coronary Interstitial Retrograde Venous (IRV) Delivery

a   b   c   d

Estimate Cell Number

◯ 20,000 – 40,000   ◓ 40,000 – 60,000   ● 60,000 – 80,000   ● 80,000 – 100,000   ● > 100,000

⬭ AIV Balloon Occlusion Site

Color Plate 3, Fig. 5 (*see* discussion in Chapter 5, and full caption on p. 128). (Top) Percutaneous endocardial delivery (BioCardia™). (Bottom) Coronary interstitial retrograde venous (IRV) delivery. From ref. *95*.

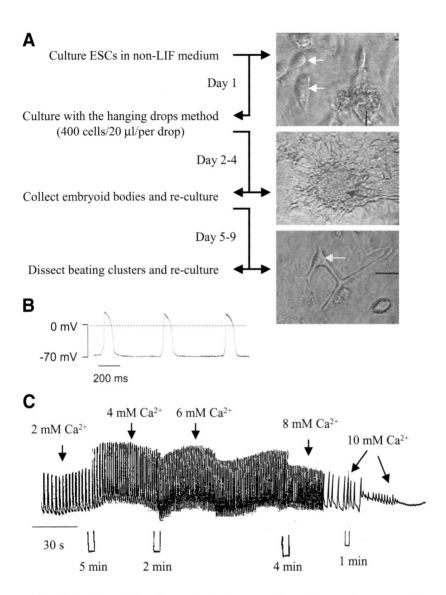

A

Culture ESCs in non-LIF medium

Day 1

Culture with the hanging drops method
(400 cells/20 µl/per drop)

Day 2-4

Collect embryoid bodies and re-culture

Day 5-9

Dissect beating clusters and re-culture

B

0 mV

-70 mV

200 ms

C

2 mM Ca^{2+} 4 mM Ca^{2+} 6 mM Ca^{2+} 8 mM Ca^{2+} 10 mM Ca^{2+}

30 s

5 min   2 min   4 min   1 min

Color Plate 4, Fig. 1 (*see* discussion in Chapter 11, and full caption on p. 287).
Action potentials and cell contractions of cardiomyocytes differentiated from
mouse embryonic stem cells (ESCs).

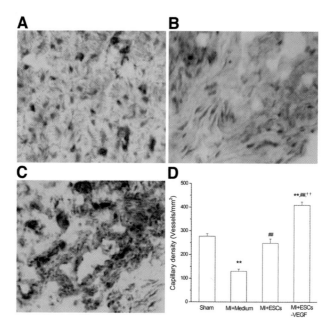

Color Plate 5, Fig. 2 (*see* discussion in Chapter 11, and full caption on p. 297). Immunostaining for blood vessel endothelial cells by the anti-von Willebrand Factor (vWF) antibody in mouse myocardial sections.

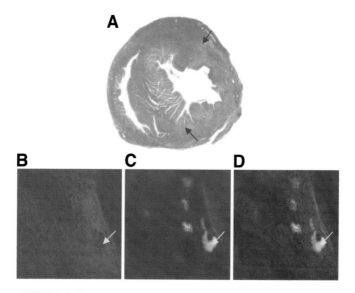

Color Plate 6, Fig. 3 (*see* discussion in Chapter 11, and full caption on p. 299). Antibody immunostaining against tumor necrosis factor (TNF)-α (red) and green fluorescent protein (GFP) (green) in infarcted myocardium.

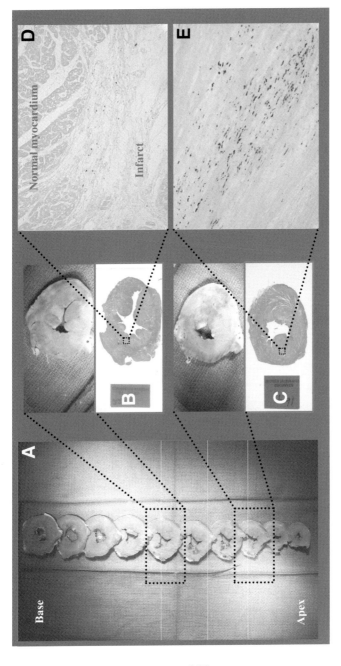

Fig. 2. Percutaneous intramyocardial delivery (Biocardia™) cellular delivery. Left ventricles were sectioned from base to apex in 1-cm rings (**A**). Specially prepared slides preserved anatomical ring orientation (**B,C**). Native cardiac tissue and infarct (H&E) were delineated from labeled fibroblasts (blue iron cyanate reaction) (**D**: ×10; **E**: ×20). From ref. 95.

percutaneous intramyocardial delivery techniques play a larger role in clinical practice *(4,60)*. However, the many advantages of the PIMD system make it extremely attractive for future applications in cardiac angiogenesis and cellular cardiomyoplasty.

INTRAPERICARDIAL AND PERIVASCULAR DELIVERY

The pericardial space and adjacent tissues may serve as a reservoir for sustained release to the myocardium, a property that has been exploited for various pharmaceutical deliveries *(96–99)*. Access to this space and adjacent epicardial perivascular tissue may be accomplished in a less invasive and procedurally practical manner, avoiding intramyocardial penetration, intravascular or ventricular lumen manipulation, and associated mechanical, inflammatory, and immunological consequences. Without direct myocardial introduction, this method remains less applicable to cellular delivery but retains the potential for facilitated angiogenesis using both surgical and percutaneous techniques.

The surgical approach has focused primarily on delivery of growth factors complexed to sustained-release particles placed under direct visualization in the perivascular tissue of visceral pericardium and underlying epicardium. In a pig left circumflex artery (LCX) ameroid constrictor model, FGF in ethylene vinyl acetate polymer was delivered to perivascular (pv) areas immediately adjacent to the LCX *(100)*. After 7–9 wk, coronary blood flow was significantly increased in the ischemic territory, with associated improvement in both regional and global ventricular function in FGF-treated animals. In a similar model, FGF heparin-alginate beads were delivered to epicardial perivascular areas at the time of LCX ameroid constrictor placement *(101)*. After 5–8 wk, FGF-bead-treated animals had a fourfold reduction in infarct size and improved coronary blood flow and regional mechanical function during rapid pacing. Early clinical application involved injection of free FGF to epicardial areas adjacent to diseased LAD arteries in 20 patients receiving LIMA grafts *(77,102)*. Follow-up angiography at 3 mo and 3 yr showed persistent local increase in collateral vessels within the LAD territory. In a randomized, double-blind, placebo-controlled trial in 24 patients, heparin-alginate FGF beads ($n = 16$) or placebo ($n = 8$) were implanted at the time of coronary artery bypass grafting (CABG) in perivascular epicardial locations corresponding to ungraftable myocardial territories *(103,104)*. Patients who received pv-delivered FGF had significantly improved angina scores compared to controls at 6 mo and improved nuclear perfusion in the ungraftable treated territories. As with gene-delivery systems, temporal product levels and distribution have been difficult to quantify using sustained-release pv methods.

Bolus infusion of radiolabeled basic fibroblast growth factor (bFGF) through a silastic catheter placed within the pericardial space of dogs resulted in "cardiac" recovery of 19% of product 150 min after injection *(32)*. The majority of the label was located in "epimyocardial" tissue, with an order of magnitude drop in epicardial to endocardial distribution. Unlike intravenous (iv) and intracoronary (ic) routes, intrapericardial (ip) administration prevented significant hepatic uptake. Despite these encouraging feasibility results, the same group demonstrated that continuous pericardial infusion of large amounts of FGF over 1 wk failed to enhance collateral perfusion *(41)*. The distribution and pharmacokinetics of ip delivery of FGF has recently been re-examined, with 30.9% "cardiac" uptake at 1 h and 23.9% at 24 h *(106)*. However, "cardiac" measurements included both pericardium and myocardium, with diminished FGF recovery in targeted LAD and LCX intramyocardial territories. Intrapericardial delivery of VEGF through an osmotic pump positioned over the epicardial LCX artery in a porcine ameroid constrictor model improved left-to-left collateral index and myocardial perfusion *(107)*. Similar delivery of Ad.VEGF through a catheter in the pericardial space of dogs resulted in extensive transgene expression in the pericardium and epicardial surface (peak 3 d, lasting 8–14 d), but not within the mid-myocardial or endocardial tissue *(108)*. Serum VEGF levels did not increase, and there was no significant difference in collateral perfusion between VEGF and control groups.

Percutaneous coronary adventitial delivery has resurfaced as an alternative route for perivascular therapy. Recently a microsyringe system (MicroSyringe™) (Fig. 3) was developed for regulated drug injection into the adventitial space of coronary arteries *(109)*. The feasibility, safety, and distribution pattern of vascular treatment with this modality was tested by delivering Oregon green-labeled Paclitaxel (OGP), tacrolimus, microspheres, and mononuclear cells. A single injection of drugs or microspheres resulted in complete arterial wall coverage (longitudinal and circumferential), and injecting autologous mononuclear cells (MNCs) resulted in ectopic cell clusters (noncardiomyocyte) within the underlying myocardium. Perivascular depot delivery of angiogenic factors and pleuripotent cells using this MicroSyringe™ system may provide yet another means of facilitating angiogenesis and/or myogenesis within targeted myocardial areas.

Although the perivascular and intrapericardial methods may be less locally invasive, they are not without potential risks. Perivascular depot delivery has traditionally required open procedures similar to those for DIMI methods, and therefore are subject to the same procedural hazards and limitations. Complications with percutaneous intrapericardial de-

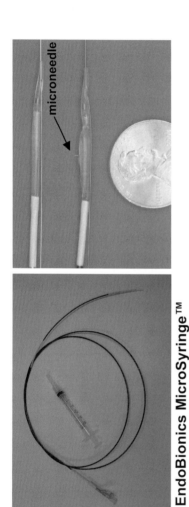

EndoBionics MicroSyringe™

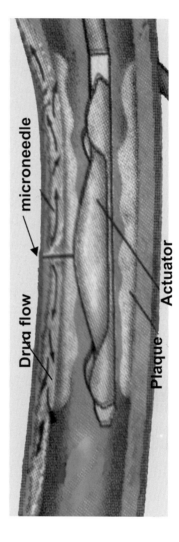

Fig. 3. Catheter-based adventitial drug-delivery system. The catheter system is designed for routine percutaneous application by a single operator (**A**). (**B**) 5 Fr intravascular devices that can deploy and retract a 150 μm × 1.0 mm needle mounted within an inflated semi-rigid polymer actuator. Upon actuator inflation (at 2 atm), the needle is designed to penetrate the external elastic lamina, facilitating direct drug delivery into the vessel wall (**C**).

livery have been minimal, but hemorrhagic and transudative effusions leading to tamponade have been noted *(108)*. Also, percutaneous intrapericardial delivery may exclude patients with prior coronary by-pass or pericardial surgery *(30)*. At first glance, the "cardiac" delivery efficiency of these methods appears on a par with other delivery modalities (12–19%), but as emphasized above, transmyocardial penetration may be severely limited. With product primarily confined to pericardial or epicardial surface tissues, the angiogenic efficacy of pv and ip delivery remains in question. Modifications affecting procedural access and myocardial penetration may enhance future applications.

INTRACORONARY DELIVERY

Intracoronary delivery of reagents for the treatment of coronary artery or myocardial disease may be performed through routine cardiac catheterization procedures. However, the efficiency of this route remains uncertain due to significant anterograde "wash-out," potentially effecting both safety and efficacy in applications for angiogenesis and myogenesis. Although early studies of FGF delivered by the ic route demonstrated proof of concept *(110–112)*, subsequent results have been more variable. Radiolabeled FGF delivered through the dog LAD resulted in acute tissue uptake and an elimination half-life of approx 50 min *(32)*. Intraluminal delivery through the left main coronary artery in a canine LCX ameroid model produced significant improvement in collateral perfusion when delivered by repeat bolus injection, but no improvement using single ic delivery *(41)*. Single ic infusion of radio-labeled FGF in normal and ischemic pigs resulted in a majority of acute protein uptake within the liver and a total cardiac activity of only 0.88 ± 0.89% at 1 h and 0.05 ± 0.04% at 24 h *(40)*, although FGF localized to ischemic tissue to a greater extent than normal myocardium.

Feasibility and efficacy of intracoronary administration of VEGF protein in ischemic pigs have also been examined *(43,48,107,113)*. VEGF administration by both intraluminal single-bolus ic delivery and local intravascular delivery through a balloon infusion catheter (InfusaSleeve, Local Med, Palo Alto, CA) produced significant improvement in collateral formation and myocardial flow, with corresponding improvement in regional function compared to controls *(107)*. This was complicated by hypotension, which was shown in follow-up studies to be ameliorated by nitric oxide sythetase inhibition *(43)*.

Successful angiogenic gene transfer by the ic route has also been documented in several preclinical investigations *(66,69,114–121)*. In ischemic swine receiving intracoronary Ad.FGF, successful transfection and myocardial transgene expression was evident for up to 2 wk with minimal gene product in noncardiac tissues (>95% first-pass myo-cardial retention) *(118)*. This highly efficient delivery correlated with significant improvements in regional ventricular function and blood flow and significantly increased capillary density. These noteworthy results have not been reproduced to the same degree in other ic gene transfer studies *(66,119)*. Bolus ic injection of Ad.VEGF in a porcine model demonstrated 33% less targeted transgene expression than comparative DIMI delivery *(66)*. Increase in intracoronary delivery pressure produced by intraluminal arterial occlusion and higher delivery flow rates improved ic gene transfer success *(120)*. Pressurized retrograde venous infusion of saline distal to coronary sinus occlusion also enhanced the effectiveness of ic gene transfer, supporting the concept of modality combination for delivery optimization *(121)*.

Despite only modest preclinical results for intracoronary administration of angiogenic mediators, several clinical studies have followed. In an uncontrolled, open-label, phase I study, 59 patients with coronary artery disease not amenable to revascularization received FGF by either ic ($n = 45$) or IV ($n = 14$) routes *(44)*. Combining ic and iv treatment groups at all doses, no significant improvement in global perfusion or inducible ischemia was seen. In the follow-up randomized, double blind, placebo-controlled clinical (FIRST) trial, 337 CAD patients received ic FGF *(122)*. At 90 d there were trends toward symptomatic improvement, but at 180 d there were no significant differences in any efficacy endpoint between the placebo and FGF groups. In the AGENT trial, replication-deficient adenovirus encoding for FGF ($n = 60$) or placebo ($n = 19$) was introduced through the coronary arteries of "no-option" patients *(123)*. Single ic injection produced no immediate adverse events. Although there were trends toward improvement in exercise testing with a treadmill (ETT) times at 4 wk, these results were insignificant across the study population. Subset analysis of patients with a baseline ETT of <10 min showed significant improvement in exercise tolerance. The second phase of this trial is currently underway.

Intracoronary delivery of VEGF to patients with CAD has met with similarly varied results. In an open-label phase I study, 14 patients received VEGF by selective coronary injection *(124)*. Stress single photon emission computed tomography (SPECT) imaging before and after treatment demonstrated dose-dependent segmental improvement in perfusion. In a larger, double-blind, placebo-controlled clinical trial, 178 patients received either placebo or VEGF by ic infusion, followed by iv VEGF administration (the VIVA trial) *(45)*. Myocardial perfusion and ETT performance at 60 d showed no significant benefit, and only marginal benefit in anginal class was present at 120 d in the high-dose group.

Local ic delivery of placebo, plasmid/liposome encoding VEGF, or Ad.VEGF was performed using a balloon perfusion-infusion catheter (Dispatch catheter, Boston Scientific) in 103 CAD patients undergoing percutaneous transluminal coronary angioplasty (PTCA) in Finland *(125)*. Myocardial perfusion at 6 mo was significantly improved in the Ad.VEGF-treated group.

Effective transplant of ic-delivered cells has also been demonstrated *(126,127)*. Although the acute myocardial retention of viable cells was limited, cellular migration to areas of injury and improvement in myocardial function were demonstrated. Intracoronary delivery of autologous bone marrow cells distal to PTCA balloon occlusion in 10 patients with acute myocardial infarction significantly decreased infarct size and improved regional myocardial function and perfusion at 3 mo *(128)*. In a different study, 20 patients with percutaneously reperfused acute myocardial infarction (AMI) were treated with intracoronary infusion of either bone marrow-derived ($n = 9$) or circulating ($n = 11$) progenitor cells (CD34/CD45+) *(129)*. At 4-mo follow-up, transplantation of progenitor cells was associated with significant improvement in global LV-EF, reduced end-systolic LV volume, improved coronary blood flow reserve in the infarct artery, and increased positron emission tomography (PET) viability within the infarct territory.

In the current era, cardiac catheterization and ic delivery are practical, procedurally safe, minimally invasive, and applicable to a wide cardiac patient population. However, given that myocardial ischemia is a function of partially or totally occluded coronary arteries, the intended ic route may not be available or may be limited to patients who have undergone prior revascularization or demonstrate adequate collateral circulation. Furthermore, product that is not picked up by the myocardium is rapidly cleared by anterograde blood flow. Although delivery distal to balloon occlusion may diminish this "wash-out," the arterial system precludes prolonged occlusion and repetitive or sustained intraluminal administration. The low efficiency of delivery, especially with protein and cells, requires technique modification, incorporation of molecular homing agents, and/or induction of transient local increase in product diffusion. Despite the limitation of ic delivery, the efficacy results in preliminary studies are encouraging and require corroboration in larger randomized trials.

RETROGRADE CORONARY VENOUS DELIVERY

The coronary venous system is also being exploited as a percutaneous vascular route to targeted myocardial areas. The coronary veins have been used by cardiac surgeons for over a century to establish retrograde

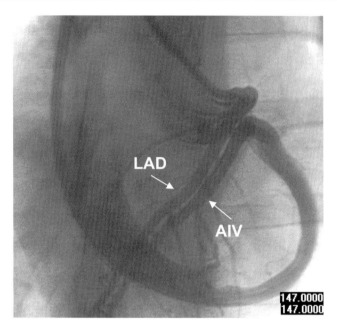

Fig. 4. Conserved proximity of the anterior interventricular vein (AIV) and left anterior descending artery (LAD) provides for regional intramyocardial delivery. In this antero-posterior view, co-injection of contrast into the AIV and LAD demonstrates the proximity of the vein and the artery.

flow of blood or cardioplegia solutions *(130–135)*, and coronary venous lead placement has now assumed a primary role in the treatment of both arrhythmia and heart failure *(136–140)*. Delivery of a wide range of pharmaceutical and biological agents has likewise been studied using various retrograde coronary venous (RCV) techniques *(141–146)*. In composite, these applications identify many unique characteristics of the coronary venous route, which may position it as a preferred method to achieve therapeutic angiogenesis or myogenesis.

Retrograde intravascular delivery requires only venous and right heart access, avoiding the potential complications and constraints of the left heart and arterial systems. Uninvolved in the process of atherogenesis, the coronary veins provide an unobstructed route to the myocardium and a compliant, low-pressure system amenable to safe catheter manipulation (Fig. 4). Furthermore, subselect coronary veins drain regional areas of myocardium that overlap arterial distributions in a highly conserved fashion *(147)*. These properties have recently been capitalized upon for delivery of protein growth factors, transgenes, and mammalian cells.

Intraluminal injection of materials through the coronary sinus or great cardiac vein results in minimal myocardial uptake, with product loss through anterograde venous drainage, veno-venous anastamoses, and alternative Thebesian systems *(148,149)*. Applying selective venous occlusion and intraluminal retrograde pressures that exceed that of venous drainage dramatically augments myocardial uptake *(150,151)*. These principles have been directed toward ongoing development of interstitial retrograde venous (IRV) delivery through the coronary veins *(95,152–155)*. The coronary IRV method incorporates single high-pressure retrograde infusion into selective branches of the coronary sinus and great cardiac veins. Infusion is performed distal to proximal venous balloon occlusion or in the subselected venous space between proximal and distal balloons. Intraluminal infusion pressures between 150 and 250 mmHg induce vascular disruption at the small venule and capillary level for myocardial extrusion without large epicardial vessel or persistent myocardial damage *(152)*.

In a porcine infarct model, IRV delivery of bFGF through anterior interventricular vein (AIV) resulted in an acute delivery efficiency of 13.4%, with >80% of detected bFGF localized to the ischemic myocardium and 21% improvement in flow within the ischemic LAD territory as compared to a placebo-treated group *(154)*. Furthermore, delivery of plasmid encoding the angiogenic factor Del-1 to the left ventricular myocardium using IRV techniques resulted in regional transgene expression in targeted (AIV/LAD) myocardial territories at levels similar to those shown to elicit capillary regrowth in hindlimb muscles of mice *(155)*. Nontargeted myocardial regions and noncardiac organs showed minimal transgene expression. Most recently, IRV techniques were used to successfully deliver porcine fibroblasts prelabeled with iron oxide nanoparticles to targeted areas of LV infarct *(95)* by single AIV infusion (150–250 mmHg). Labeled cells were preferentially localized to areas of LAD infarct and targeted anteroseptal regions (97.6%) as detected by Prussian blue (iron) staining. Cellular delivery efficiency 3 wk after IRV delivery was estimated to be $15.7 \pm 11.6\%$ with subset immunohistochemical analysis confirming viability and label retention of transplanted fibroblasts.

An electrocardiogram synchronized, gas-actuated infusion has been described to augment retrograde venous delivery during diastole and coronary venous drainage in systole *(156–160)*. This system has been applied for reporter gene delivery through the AIV of pigs. Combined with brief (10 min) LAD occlusion, this method significantly increased transgene expression in the targeted LAD territory, compared to ic delivery of the same gene products *(117)*. However, in the absence of concurrent arterial occlusion there was no further improvement over standard ic delivery. Cellular delivery using this automated pressure-regulated RCV technique for the purpose of cardiac angiogenesis and myogenesis is currently being investigated.

Myocardial delivery of autologous bone marrow cells through subselect branches of the coronary veins has also been performed using the TransVascular™ catheter system, which incorporates a phased-array ultrasound imaging system mounted next to an extendable nitinol needle (TransVascular Inc., Menlo Park, CA) *(161–163)*. In preliminary studies delivering autologous bone marrow cells in a collagen hydrogel to porcine myocardium, transplanted cells were microscopically identifiable up to 28 d postdelivery; however, cellular quantification by green fluorescent protein (GFP) expression was highly variable (2–51% at all time points) *(164)*. The feasibility of this platform in humans is currently being examined in Europe.

The anatomical complexity of the coronary venous system needs to be considered prior to developing effective delivery strategies *(165,166)*. Standard retrograde venous delivery efficiency is limited by product loss through alternative veno-venous anastamoses or Thebesian circuits. Although the presence of the coronary sinus, great cardiac vein, and their major tributaries (lateral cardiac vein, marginal cardiac vein, and AIV) is highly preserved in animal and human systems *(167)*, the intraluminal diameter of these vessels and degree of subbranching is widely variable. These differences may limit effective balloon occlusion and dramatically alter regional venous capacitance that determines retrograde infusion pressure. Further investigations are currently underway to optimize the delivery parameters and devices for all of the retrograde methods described above.

DIRECT COMPARISONS OF CARDIAC DELIVERY MODALITIES

Comparison of the current systems is required to determine the optimal method of cardiac delivery for therapeutic angiogenesis and/or myogenesis. Several studies have undertaken this task for a given protein, gene, or cellular product. For FGF delivery, various systemic, ic, and ip methods were examined in the same animal model *(32)*. This study demonstrated minimal acute myocardial retention after iv bolus injection or Swan Ganz delivery distal to pulmonary arterial occlusion (0.5% of total) or by left atrial infusion (1.3%) as compared with 3–5% by ic infusion and 19% after ip administration (with an order of magnitude drop in epicardial-to-endocardial distribution with ip delivery). The majority of labeled FGF was identified within the liver for all but the ip method. Independent comparisons of systemic and ic routes of FGF delivery in pigs revealed similar hepatic predominance, with total 1-h cardiac activities of $0.26 \pm 0.08\%$ (iv route), and $0.88 \pm 0.89\%$ (ic route), and 24-h values falling to $0.04 \pm 0.01\%$, and $0.05 \pm 0.04\%$, respectively *(40)*. Follow-up analysis of ip delivery revealed 30.9% cardiac uptake (pericardial and myocardial) at 1 h and 23.9% at 24 h *(106)*.

VEGF protein delivery comparisons are limited to studies of therapeutic effect. VEGF administration by ic delivery (luminal bolus injection and local balloon infusion) compared to ip delivery (osmotic pump infusion) demonstrated similar increases in collateral development, regional blood flow, and regional ventricular function for all delivery modalities *(107)*. However, separate comparisons of iv and ic methods of VEGF delivery in pigs showed that collateral vessel growth, myocardial blood flow, and microvascular function improved significantly in ic groups, but not in iv groups *(43)*.

In a rat model, ic and direct transepicardial injection of adenoviral vector coding for VEGF demonstrated superiority of DIMI gene transfer methods over the ic route, with peak gene expression 24–72 h after direct injection *(66)*. Separate investigations of adeno-associated vectors in mice comparing ic and DIMI methods resulted in transgene expression of less than 1% at 2 wk using ic delivery, but substantial myocardial expression at 8 wk that was comparable to direct injection *(69)*. Coronary venous delivery of an adenoviral vector in swine with transient LAD occlusion increased transgene expression in the targeted LAD area compared to ic delivery *(117)*. Comparisons of ic and RCV methods of adenoviral gene transfer in rabbits similarly found that transgene expression by RCV methods occurred only in the setting of simultaneous arterial occlusion *(121)*.

Despite the similarity of surgical and percutaneous methods of intramyocardial injection, few direct comparisons of these modalities have been performed. Using a pig model, percutaneous intramyocardial injection of labeled microspheres resulted in acute retention of $43 \pm 15\%$ of delivery product, whereas transepicardial injection demonstrated only $15 \pm 21\%$ retention *(60)*. Equivalent myocardial transgene expression using PIMD or DIMI methods has been reported *(4)*. Even fewer studies have directly compared separate modalities for cellular delivery. In a small feasibility study in pigs, fibroblasts were transplanted using the BioCardia PIMD and coronary venous IRV methods (Fig. 5). There was similar cellular recovery at 21 d, with PIMD resulting in cellular distribution to focal areas of injection and coronary venous IRV resulting in

A Percutaneous Endocardial Delivery (BioCardia")

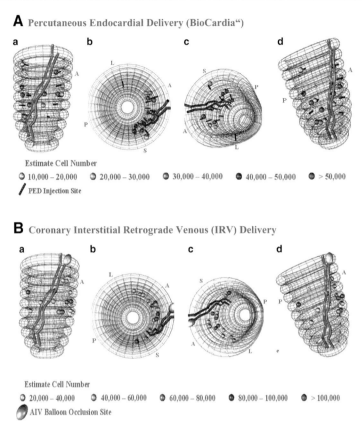

Estimate Cell Number

○ 10,000 – 20,000   ○ 20,000 – 30,000   ● 30,000 – 40,000   ● 40,000 – 50,000   ● > 50,000

/ PED Injection Site

B Coronary Interstitial Retrograde Venous (IRV) Delivery

Estimate Cell Number

○ 20,000 – 40,000   ○ 40,000 – 60,000   ● 60,000 – 80,000   ● 80,000 – 100,000   ● > 100,000

AIV Balloon Occlusion Site

Fig. 5. (top) Percutaneous endocardial delivery (BioCardia™). Composite distribution for percutaneous endocardial delivery in infarcted hearts at 21 d. 98.4% of cells were identified in anteroseptal walls, and 94.8% within a 4-cm longitudinal span of the mid left anterior descending artery (LAD) (**A,D**). The average depth of penetration was 3.4 ± 3.9 mm, with 95.8% localized to the endocardial half (**B,C**), and 96.8 within the infarct zone. (bottom) Coronary interstitial retrograde venous (IRV) delivery. Composite distribution for coronary IRV in infarcted hearts at 21 d. 97.6% of cells were identified in anteroseptal walls, and 92.5% within a 4-cm longitudinal span of the mid-LAD (**A,D**). These cells were an average 21.8 ± 7.9 mm from anterior ventricular vein, with 60.1% localized to the endocardial half (**B,C**), and 100% identified within the infarct zone. From ref. 95.

distribution consistent with regional venous drainage and both methods demonstrating preferential cellular recovery in areas of infarct (95).

Although results from these comparisons are based on different delivery techniques, biological agents, doses, and varying methods of analysis, they allow for a subjective assessment of how well each method

Table 2
Assessment of Delivery Methods

Delivery modality	Procedural safety	Procedural applicability	Procedural practicality	Delivery efficiency	Precision/ Regionality	Retained activity
Systemic	+ + + + +	+ + + + +	+ + + + +	+	+	+
DIMI	+ +	+ +	+	+ + + +	+ + + +	+ + +
PIMD	+ + + +	+ + + +	+ + + +	+ + + + +	+ + + +	++ +
pv	+ +	+ +	+ +	+ +	+ + +	+ +
ip	+ + +	+ + +	+ + +	+	+	+
ic	+ + + +	+ + + +	+ + + +	+ +	+ +	+
RCV	+ + + +	+ + + +	+ + + +	+ + ++	+ + + + +	+ + +
Alternatives	+ + +	+ + +	+ + +	+ + +	+ + +	+ +

DIMI, direct intramyocardial injection; PIMD, percutaneous intramyocardial delivery; pv, perivascular; ip, intrapericardial; ic, intracoronary; RCV, retrograde coronary venous.

meets ideal delivery parameters (Table 1) as well as objective review of method-dependent efficiency and distribution characteristics (Table 2).

ALTERNATIVE DELIVERY MODALITIES

Several additional delivery methods currently being developed and investigated deserve separate consideration. Some of the more intriguing alternatives involve application of therapeutic ultrasound, combined laser revascularization and DIMI techniques, electroporation conjugated delivery, tissue engineering, and autologous cellular mobilization.

External ultrasound focused on areas of vascular tissue in the presence of microbubble contrast agent and naked DNA has been shown to increase transgene expression by threefold *(168)*. Several variations of this method have recently been applied for enhanced myocardial delivery of viral vector and plasmid gene products by coronary arterial and venous routes *(169–172)*. Disappointing as stand-alone therapies for myocardial ischemia, double micro-ring (DMR) and other laser and radiofrequency technologies may have renewed applications when combined with direct angiogenic product delivery. Although percutaneous growth factor and transgene delivery does not appear to be augmented by radiofrequency injury *(173,174)*, transepicardial injection of these same products into surgical laser channels produces significant improvement in neovascularization and myocardial function *(175,176)*. In a separate combination of electrical and PIMD technologies, feasibility and safety have been demonstrated using a modified BioCardia catheter system (incorporating electrical pacing and electroporation capabilities) for augmented delivery to electrically stimulated tissue *(177)*.

Tissue engineering has also emerged as a feasible method for facilitated angiogenesis and/or myogenesis, with myocardial transplant of myoblast-derived bioartifical muscles (BAMs) or three-dimensional fibroblast scaffolds as "epicardial patches," increasing vascular growth up to threefold *(178–180)*. Finally, angiogenic and myogenic processes may be augmented through mobilization of endogenous cells that may have intrinsic tropism for and biological activity within areas of cardiac injury. Toward this end, recent studies have examined ischemic injury alone, granulocyte colony stimulating factor (G-CSF) and granulocyte-macrophage colony stimulating factor (GM-CSF), VEGF, statins, and many other biological products for progenitor cell mobilization *(15,181–185)*. The efficacy of these methods in promoting cardiac angiogenesis and/or myogenesis has yet to be fully established.

CONCLUSIONS

The ability to utilize potent biological mediators of both angiogenesis and myogenesis requires effective means for local and regional cardiovascular delivery. All of the modalities and strategies discussed above necessitate procedural optimization and further comparative investigation. A single technique will most likely not be sufficient to address every clinical situation, and delivery methods may differ in their ability to provide effective angiogenesis or cellular cardiomyoplasty. In addition to the established modalities described above, alternative delivery methods need to be more fully explored. Together these may define optimal strategies for cardiac delivery for upcoming generations of biological intervention agents.

REFERENCES

1. Jones EL, Craver JM, Guyton RA, Bone DK, Hatcher CR Jr, Riechwald N. Importance of complete revascularization in performance of the coronary bypass operation. Am J Cardiol 1983;51:7–12.
2. Mukherjee D, Bhatt DL, Roe MT, Patel V, Ellis SG. Direct myocardial revascularization and angiogenesis—how many patients might be eligible? Am J Cardiol 1999;84:598–600,A8.
3. Koransky ML, Robbins RC, Blau HM. VEGF gene delivery for treatment of ischemic cardiovascular disease. Trends Cardiovasc Med 2002;12(3):108–114.
4. Laham RJ, Simons M, Sellke F. Gene transfer for angiogenesis in coronary artery disease. Annu Rev Med 2001;52:485–502.
5. Folkman J. Angiogenic therapy of the human heart. Circulation 1998;97:628–629.
6. Bauters C. Growth factors as potential new treatment for ischemic heart disease. Clin Cardiol 1997;20(II):52–57.
7. McNeer JF, Conley MJ, Starmer CF, et al. Complete and incomplete revascularization at aortocoronary bypass surgery; experience with 392 consecutive patients. Am Heart J 1974;88:176–182.

8. Lucchese FA, Frota Filho JD, Blacher C, Pereira W, Lucio E, Beck L, Leonetti LA, Leaes PE. Partial left ventriculectomy: overall and late results in 44 class IV patients with 4-year follow-up. J Card Surg 2000;15:179–185.

9. Lowe HC, Burkoff D, Khachigian LM, MacNeill BD, Hayase M, Oesterle SN. Beyond angioplasty: novel developments in interventional cardiology. Intern Med J 2002;32:470–474.

10. Emanueli C, Madeddu P. Angiogenesis gene therapy to rescue ischemic tissues: achievements and future directions. Br J Pharmacol 2001;133(7):951–958.

11. Ware JA, Simons M. Angiogenesis in ischemic heart disease. Nat Med 1997;3(7): 158–164.

12. Dowell JD, Rubart M, Pasumarthi KBS, Soonpaa MH, Field LJ. Myocyte and myogenic stem cell transplantation in the heart. Cardiovasc Res 2003;58:336–350.

13. Perin EC, Geng YJ, Willerson JT. Adult stem cell therapy in perspective. Circulation 2003;107:935–938.

14. Orlic D, Hill JM, Arai AE. Stem cells for myocardial regeneration. Circ Res 2002;91:1092–1102.

15. Szmitko PE, Fedak PWM, Weisel RD, Stewart DJ, Kutryk MJB, Verma S. Endothelial progenitor cells: new hope for a broken heart. Circulation 2003;107:3093–3100.

16. Reffelmann T, Kloner RA. Cellular cardiomyoplasty—cardiomyocytes, skeletal myoblasts, or stem cells for regenerating myocardium and treatment of heart failure? Cardiovasc Res 2003;58(2):358–368.

17. Menasche P. Skeletal muscle satellite cell transplantation. Cardiovasc Res 2003;58:351–357.

18. Hammond HK, McKirnan MD. Angiogenic gene therapy for heart disease: a review of animal studies and clinical trials. Cardiovasc Res 2001;49:561–567.

19. Simons M, Bonow RO, Chronos NA, et al. Clinical trials in coronary angiogenesis: issues, problems, consensus: an expert panel summary. Circulation 2000;102(11):E73–E86.

20. Reinlib L, Field L. Cell transplantation as a future therapy for cardiovascular disease? A workshop of the National Heart, Lung, and Blood Institute. Circulation 2000;101:E182–E187.

21. Post MJ, Laham RJ, Sellke FW, Simons M. Therapeutic angiogenesis in cardiology using protein formulations. Cardiovasc Res 2001;49:522–531.

22. Sinnaeve P, Varenne O, Collen D, Janssens S. Gene therapy in the cardiovascular system: an update. Cardiovasc Res 1999;44(3):498–506.

23. Allen MD. Myocardial protection: is there a role for gene therapy? Ann Thorac Surg 1999;68(5):1924–1928.

24. Leor J, Prentice H, Sartorelli V, Quinones MJ, Patterson M, Kedes LK, Kloner RA. Gene transfer and cell transplant: an experimental approach to repair a 'broken heart.' Cardiovasc Res 1997;35:431–441.

25. Schwartz LB, Moawad J. Gene therapy for vascular disease. Ann Vasc Surg 1997;11(2):189–99.

26. Peppel K, Koch WJ, Lefkowitz RJ. Gene transfer studies for augmenting cardiac function. Trends Cardiovasc Med 1997;7:145–150.

27. Folkman J. Clinical applications of research on angiogenesis. NEJM 1995;333(26): 1757–1763.

28. Rowland RT, Cleveland JC, Meng X, Harken AH, Brown JM. Potential gene therapy strategies in the treatment of cardiovascular disease. Ann Thorac Surg 1995;60:721–728.

29. Losordo DW, Kawamoto A. Biological revascularization and the interventional molecular cardiologist: bypass for the next generation. Circulation 2002;106:3002–3005.

30. Kornowski R, Fuchs S, Leon MB, Epstein SE. Delivery strategies to achieve therapeutic myocardial angiogenesis. Circulation 2000;101(4):454–458.

31. Sellke FW, Ruel M. Vascular growth factors and angiogenesis in cardiac surgery. Ann Thorac Surg 2003;75(2):S685–S690.

32. Lazarous DF, Shou M, Stiber JA, Dadhania DM, Thirumurti V, Hodge E, et al. Pharmacodynamics of basic fibroblast growth factor: route of administration determines myocardial and systemic distribution. Cardiovasc Res 1997;36(1):78–85.

33. Epstein SE, Fuchs S, Zhou YF, Baffour R, Kornowski R. Therapeutic interventions for enhancing collateral development by administration of growth factors: basic principles, early results and potential hazards. Cardiovasc Res 2001;49(3):532–542.

34. Epstein SE, Kornowski R, Fuchs S, Dvorak HF. Angiogenesis therapy: amidst the hype, the neglected potential for serious side effects. Circulation 2001;104:115–119.

35. Isner JM, Vale PR, Symes JF, Losordo DW. Assessment of risks associated with cardiovascular gene therapy in human subjects. Circ Res 2001;89:389–400.

36. Unger EF, Banai S, Shou M, et al. Basic fibroblast growth factor enhances myocardial collateral flow in a canine model. Am J Physiol 1994;266:H1588–H1595.

37. Lazarous DF, Shou M, Scheinowitz M. Comparative effects of basic fibroblast growth factor and vascular endothelial growth factor on coronary collateral development and the arterial response to injury. Circulation 1996;94:1074–1082.

38. Lazarous DF, Scheinowitz M, Shou M, et al. Effects of chronic systemic administration of basic fibroblast growth factor on collateral development in the canine heart. Circulation 1995;91:145–153.

39. Thirumurti V, Shou M, Hodge E, Goncalves L, Epstein SE, Lazarous DF, Unger EF. Lack of efficacy of intravenous basic fibroblast growth factor in promoting myocardial angiogenesis, J Am Coll Cardiol 1998;31(Suppl 1):54.

40. Laham RJ, Rezaee M, Post M, Sellke FW, Braeckman RA, Hung D, et al. Intracoronary and intravenous administration of basic fibroblast growth factor: myocardial and tissue distribution. Drug Metab Dispos 1999;27(7):821–826.

41. Rajanayagam MA, Shou M, Thirumurti V, et al. Intracoronary basic fibroblast growth factor enhances myocardial collateral perfusion in dogs. J Am Coll Cardiol 2000;35(2):519–526.

42. Sakakibara Y, Tambara K, Sakaguchi G, et al. Toward surgical angiogenesis using slow-released basic fibroblast growth factor. Eur J Cardiothorac Surg 2003;24(1):105–112.

43. Sato K, Wu T, Laham RJ, et al. Efficacy of intracoronary or intravenous VEGF165 in a pig model of chronic myocardial ischemia. J Am Coll Cardiol 2001;37(2):616–623.

44. Udelson JE, Dilsizian V, Laham RJ, et al. Therapeutic angiogenesis with recombinant fibroblast growth factor-2 improves stress and rest myocardial perfusion abnormalities in patients with severe symptomatic chronic coronary artery disease. Circulation 2000;102:1605–1610.

45. Henry TD, Annex BH, McKendall GR, et al. (for the VIVA Investigators). Vascular endothelial growth factor in ischemia for vascular angiogenesis (the VIVA trial). Circulation 2003;107:1359–1365.

46. Li Y, Takemura G, Kosai KI, et al. Postinfarction treatment with an adenoviral vector expressing hepatocyte growth factor relieves chronic left ventricular remodeling and dysfunction in mice. Circulation 2003;107:2499–2506.

47. Strauer BE, Kornowski R. Stem cell therapies in perspective. Circulation 2003;107:929–934.

48. Hariawala MD, Horowitz JJ, Esakof D, et al. VEGF improves myocardial blood flow but produces EDRF-mediated hypotension in porcine hearts. J Surg Res 1996;63:77–82.

49. Lopez J, Laham RJ, Carrozza JC, et al. Hemodynamic effects of intracoronary VEGF delivery: evidence of tachyphylaxis and NO dependence of response. Am J Physiol 1997;273:H1317–H1323.

50. Yang R, Thomas GR, Bunting S, et al. Effects of vascular endothelial growth factor on hemodynamics and cardiac performance. J Cardiovasc Pharmacol 1996;27:838–844.

51. Toma C, Pittenger MF, Cahill KS, Byrne BJ, Kessler PD. Human mesenchymal stem cells differentiate to a cardiomyocytes phenotype in the adult murine heart. Circulation 2002;105:93–98.

52. Barbash IM, Chouraqui P, Baron J, et al. Systemic delivery of bone marrow-derived mesenchymal stem cells to the infarcted myocardium: feasibility, cell migration, and body distribution. Circulation 2003;108(7):863–868.

53. Aicher A, Brenner W, Zuhayra M, et al. Assessment of the tissue distribution of transplanted human endothelial progenitor cells by radioactive labeling. Circulation 2003;107:2134–2139.

54. Chleboun JO, Martins RN, Mitchell CA, Chirila TV. bFGF enhances the development of the collateral circulation after acute arterial occlusion. Biochem Biophys Res Comm 1992;185:510–516.

55. Walder CE, Errett CJ, Bunting S, et al. Vascular endothelial growth factor augments muscle blood flow and function in a rabbit model of hindlimb ischemia. J Cardiovasc Pharmacol 1996;27:91–98.

56. Takeshita S, Rossow ST, Kearney M, et al. Time course of increased cellular proliferation in collateral arteries after administration of vascular endothelial growth factor in a rabbit model of lower limb vascular insufficiency. Am J Pathol 1995;147:1649–1660.

57. Watanabe E, Smith DM, Sun J, Smart FW, Delcarpio JB, Roberts TB, et al. Effect of basic fibroblast growth factor on angiogenesis in the infarcted porcine heart. Basic Res Cardiol 1998;93(1):30–37.

58. Jiang ZS, Padua RR, Ju H, Doble BW, Jin Y, Hao J, et al. Acute protection of ischemic heart by FGF-2: involvement of FGF-2 receptors and protein kinase C. Am J Physiol Heart Circ Physiol 2002;282(3):H1071–H1080.

59. Edelberg JM, Lee SH, Kaur M, Tang L, Feirt NM, McCabe S, et al. Platelet-derived growth factor-AB limits the extent of myocardial infarction in a rat model: feasibility of restoring impaired angiogenic capacity in the aging heart. Circulation 2002;105(5):608–613.

60. Grossman PM, Han Z, Palasis M, Barry JJ, Lederman RJ. Incomplete retention after direct myocardial injection. Catheter Cardiovasc Interv 2002;55(3):392–397.

61. Sarkar N, Blomberg P, Wardell E, Eskandarpour M, Sylven C, Drvota V, et al. Nonsurgical direct delivery of plasmid DNA into rat heart: time course, dose response, and the influence of different promoters on gene expression. J Cardiovasc Pharmacol 2002;39(2):215–224.

62. Tio RA, Tkebuchava T, Scheuermann TH, et al. Intramyocardial gene therapy with naked DNA encoding vascular endothelial growth factor improves collateral flow to ischemic myocardium. Hum Gen Ther 1999;10:2953–2960.

63. Schwartz ER, Speakman MT, Patterson M, et al. Evaluation of the effects of intramyocardial injection of DNA expressing vascular endothelial growth factor (VEGF) in a myocardial infarction model in the rat—angiogenesis and angioma formation. J Am Coll Cardiol 2000;35:1323–1330.

64. Lee RJ, Springer ML, Blanco-Bose WE, Shaw R, Ursell PC, Blau HM. VEGF gene delivery to myocardium: deleterious effects of unregulated expression. Circulation 2000;102:898–901.

65. Lee M, Rentz J, Bikram M, Han S, Bull DA, Kim SW. Hypoxia-inducible VEGF gene delivery to ischemic myocardium using water-soluble lipopolymer. Gene Ther 2003;10:1535–1542.

66. Wright MJ, Wightman LM, Lilley C, de Alwis M, Hart SL, Miller A, et al. In vivo myocardial gene transfer: optimization, evaluation and direct comparison of gene transfer vectors. Basic Res Cardiol 2001;96(3):227–236.

67. Lee LY, Patel SR, Hackett NR, Mack CA, Polce DR, El-Sawy T, et al. Focal angiogen therapy using intramyoca rdial delivery of an adenovirus vector coding for vascular endothelial growth factor 121. Ann Thorac Surg 2000;69(1):14–24.

68. Mack CA, Patel SR, Schwartz EA, et al. Biological bypass with the use of adenovirus-mediated gene transfer of the complementary deoxyribonucleic acid for vascular endothelial growth factor 121 improves myocardial perfusion and function in the ischemic porcine heart. J Cardiovasc Surg 1998;115:168–177.

69. Safi J, DiPaula AF, Riccioni T, et al. Adenovirus-mediated acidic fibroblast growth factor gene transfer induces angiogenesis in the nonischemic rabbit heart. Microvasc Res 1999;58:238–249.

70. Svensson EC, Marshall DJ, Woodard K, Lin H, Jiang F, Chu L, et al. Efficient and stable transduction of cardiomyocytes after intramyocardial injection or intracoronary perfusion with recombinant adeno-associated virus vectors. Circulation 1999;99(2):201–205.

71. Horvath KA, Doukas J, Lu CY, Belkind N, Greene R, Pierce GF, et al. Myocardial functional recovery after fibroblast growth factor 2 gene therapy as assessed by echocardiography and magnetic resonance imaging. Ann Thorac Surg 2002;74(2):481–487.

72. Miyagawa S, Sawa Y, Taketani S, Kawaguchi N, Nakamura T, Matsuura N, et al. Myocardial regeneration therapy for heart failure: hepatocyte growth factor enhances the effect of cellular cardiomyoplasty. Circulation 2002;105(21):2556–2561.

73. Aoki M, Morishita R, Taniyame Y, et al. Angiogenesis induced by hepatocyte growth factor in non-infarcted myocardium and infarcted myocardium: up-regulation of essential transcription factor for angiogenesis, etc. Gene Ther 2000;7:417–427.

74. Losordo DW, Vale PR, Symes JF, Dunnington CH, Esakof DD, Maysky M, et al. Gene therapy for myocardial angiogenesis: initial clinical results with direct myocardial injection of phVEGF165 as sole therapy for myocardial ischemia. Circulation 1998;98(25):2800–2804.

75. Symes JF, Losordo JW, Vale PR, et al. Gene therapy with vascular endothelial growth factor for inoperable coronary artery disease. Ann Thorac Surg 1999;68:830–837.

76. Rosengardt TK, Lee LY, Patel SR, Sanborn TA, Parikh M, Bergman W, et al. Angiogenesis gene therapy: Phase I assessment of direct intramyocardial administration of an adenovirus vector expressing VEGF 121 cDNA to individuals with clinically significant severe coronary artery disease. Circulation 1999;100:468–474.

77. Schumacher B, Pecher P, von Specht BU, Stegman T, Induction of neoangiogenesis in ischemic myocardium by human growth factors: first clinical results of a new treatment of coronary heart disease. Circulation 1998;97:645–650.

78. Kornowski R, Fuchs S, Tio FO, Pierre A, Epstein SE, Leon MB. Evaluation of the acute and chronic safety of the Biosense injection catheter system in porcine hearts. Catheter Cardiovasc Interv 1999;48(4):447–455.

79. Kornowski R, Leon MB, Fuchs S, Vodovotz Y, Flynn MA, Gordon DA, et al. Electromagnetic guidance for catheter-based transendocardial injection: a platform for intramyocardial angiogenesis therapy. Results in normal and ischemic porcine models. J Am Coll Cardiol 2000;35(4):1031–1039.

80. Fuchs S, Baffour R, Zhou YF, Shou M, Pierre A, Tio FO, et al. Transendocardial delivery of autologous bone marrow enhances collateral perfusion and regional function in pigs with chronic experimental myocardial ischemia. J Am Coll Cardiol 2001;37(6):1726–1732.

81. Park SW, Gwon HC, Jeong JO, Byun J, Kang HS, You JR, et al. Intracardiac echocardiographic guidance and monitoring during percutaneous endomyocardial gene injection in porcine heart. Hum Gene Ther 2001;12(8):893–903.

82. Chazaud B, Hittinger L, Sonnet C, Champagne S, Le Corvoisier P, Benhaiem-Sigaux N, et al. Endoventricular porcine autologous myoblast transplantation can be successfully achieved with minor mechanical cell damage. Cardiovasc Res 2003;58(2):444–450.

83. Kawamoto A, Tkebuchava T, Yamaguchi J, Nishimura H, et al. Intramyocardial transplantation of autologous endothelial progenitor cells for therapeutic neovascularization of myocardial ischemia. Circulation 2003;107:461–468.

84. Vale PR, Losordo DW, Milliken CE, McDonald MC, et al. Randomized single-blind, placebo-controlled pilot study of catheter-based myocardial gene transfer for therapeutic angiogenesis using left ventricle electromechanical mapping in patients with chronic myocardial ischemia. Circulation 2001;103:2138–2143.

85. Losordo DW, Vale PR, Hendel RC, Milliken CE, Fortuin FD, Cummings N, et al. Phase 1/2 placebo-controlled, double-blind, dose-escalating trial of myocardial vascular endothelial growth factor 2 gene transfer by catheter delivery in patients with chronic myocardial ischemia. Circulation 2002;105(17):2012–2018.

86. Fuchs S, Satler LF, Kornowski R, Okubagzi P, Weisz G, Baffour R, et al. Catheter-based autologous bone marrow myocardial injection in no-option patients with advanced coronary artery disease: a feasibility study. J Am Coll Cardiol 2003;41(10):1721–1724.

87. Perin EC, Dohmann HFR, Bororjevic R, Silva SA, Sousa ALS, et al. Transendocardial, autologous bone marrow cell transplantation for severe, chronic ischemic heart failure. Circulation 2003;107:2294–2302.

88. Naimark WA, Lepore JJ, Klugherz BD, Wang Z, Guy TS, Osman H, et al. Adenovirus-catheter compatibility increases gene expression after delivery to porcine myocardium. Hum Gene Ther 2003;14(2):161–166.

89. Lederman RJ, Guttman MA, Peters DC, Thompson RB, Sorger JM, Dick AJ, et al. Catheter-based endomyocardial injection with real-time magnetic resonance imaging. Circulation 2002;105(11):1282–1284.

90. Hill JM, Dick AJ, Raman VK, et al. Serial cardiac magnetic resonance imaging of injected mesenchymal stem cells. Circulation 2003;108:1009–1014.

91. Rezaee M, Yeung AC, Altman P, Lubbe D, Takeshi S, Schwartz RS, et al. Evaluation of the percutaneous intramyocardial injection for local myocardial treatment. Catheter Cardiovasc Interv 2001;53(2):271–276.

92. Rezaee M, Yeung AC, Altman P, et al. Percutaneous intramyocardial delivery is an efficient modality for local myocardial treatment. J Am Coll Cardiol 2001;37(Suppl 1):1157–1128 (Abstr).

93. Grube E, Gerckens U, Altman PA, Rosenman DC, Rezaee M. The helical infusion catheter: first clinical evaluation for local intramyocardial therapeutics. Am J Cardiol 2002;90(Suppl 6A):120H.

94. St. John ME, Xie J, Heldman AW, et al. Catheter-based percutaneous cellular cardiomyoplasty using allogeneic bone marrow derived mesenchymal stem cells. J Am Coll Cardiol 2003;41(Suppl A):1176 (Abstr).

95. Price ET, Ikeno F, Fenn RC, et al. Percutaneous endocardial versus selective coronary venous cellular delivery: comparisons of transplant efficiency, distribution, and efficacy in reducing infarct size and improving myocardial function. J Am Coll Cardiol 2003;41(Suppl A):1176–174 (Abstr).

96. Ujhelyi MR, Hadsall KZ, Euler DE, Mehra R. Intrapericardial therapeutics: a pharmacodynamic and pharmacokinetic comparison between pericardial and intravenous procainamide delivery. J Cardiovasc Electrophysiol 2002;13(6):605–611.

97. Hou D, Rogers PI, Toleikis PM, Hunter W, March KL. Intrapericardial paclitaxel delivery inhibits neointimal proliferation and promotes arterial enlargement after porcine coronary overstretch. Circulation 2000;102(13):1575–1581.

98. Waxman S, Moreno R, Rowe KA, Verrier RL. Persistent primary coronary dilation induced by transatrial delivery of nitroglycerin into the pericardial space: a novel approach for local cardiac drug delivery. J Am Coll Cardiol 1999;33(7):2073–2077.

99. Baek SH, Hrabie JA, Keefer LK, Hou D, Fineberg N, Rhoades R, et al. Augmentation of intrapericardial nitric oxide level by a prolonged-release nitric oxide donor reduces luminal narrowing after porcine coronary angioplasty. Circulation 2002;105(23):2779–2784.

100. Lopez JJ, Edelman ER, Stamler A, Hibberd MG, Prasad P, Thomas KA, et al. Angiogenic potential of perivascularly delivered aFGF in a porcine model of chronic myocardial ischemia. Am J Physiol 1998;274(3 Pt 2):H930–H936.

101. Harada K, Grossman W, Friedman M, Edelman E, Prasad PV, Keighley CS, Manning WJ, Sellke FW, Simons M. Basic fibroblast growth factor improves function in chronically ischemic porcine hearts. J Clin Invest 1994;94:623–630.

102. Pecher P, Schumacher BA. Angiogenesis in ischemic human myocardium: clinical results after 3 years. Ann Thorac Surg 2000;69:1414–1419.

103. Laham RJ, Sellke FW, Edelman ER, Pearlman JD, Ware JA, Brown DL, et al. Local perivascular delivery of basic fibroblast growth factor in patients undergoing coronary bypass surgery: results of a phase I randomized, double-blind, placebo-controlled trial. Circulation 1999;100(18):1865–1871.

104. Ruel M, Laham RJ, Parker JA, et al. Long-term effects of surgical angiogenic therapy with FGF-2 protein. J Thorac Cardiovasc Surg 2002;124:28–34.

105. Griscelli F, Belli E, Opolon P, Musset K, Connault E, Perricaudet M, et al. Adenovirus-mediated gene transfer to the transplanted piglet heart after intracoronary injection. J Gene Med 2003;5(2):109–119.

106. Laham RJ, Rezaee M, Post M, Xu X, Sellke FW. Intrapericardial administration of basic fibroblast growth factor: myocardial and tissue distribution and comparison with intracoronary and intravenous administration. Catheter Cardiovasc Interv 2003;58(3):375–381.

107. Lopez JJ, Laham RJ, Stamler A, Pearlman JD, Bunting S, Kaplan A, et al. VEGF administration in chronic myocardial ischemia in pigs. Cardiovasc Res 1998;40(2):272–281.

108. Lazarous DF, Shou M, Stiber JA, Hodge E, Thirumurti V, Goncalves L, et al. Adenoviral-mediated gene transfer induces sustained pericardial VEGF expression in dogs: effect on myocardial angiogenesis. Cardiovasc Res 1999;44(2):294–302.

109. Ikeno F, Lyons J, Rezaee M, et al. A novel method for delivering cell therapy to the heart: safety and feasibility of periadventitial delivery via the EndoBionics MicroSyringe infusion catheter. Am J Cardiol 2003; Abstract 222:98L.

110. Battler A, Scheinowitz M, Bor A, Hasdai D, Vered Z, Di Segni E, et al. Intracoronary injection of basic fibroblast growth factor enhances angiogenesis in infarcted swine myocardium. J Am Coll Cardiol 1993;22:2001–2006.

111. Horrigan M, MacIsaac A, Nicolini F, et al. Reduction in myocardial infarct size by basic fibroblast growth factor after temporary coronary occlusion in a canine model. Circulation 1996;94:1927–1933.

112. Rajanayagam S, Shou M, Thirumurti V, et al. Two intracoronary doses of basic fibroblast growth factor enhance collateral blood flow in dogs. J Am Coll Cardiol 1996;27(Suppl A):36A (Abstr).

113. Banai S, Jaklitsch MT, Shou M, Lazarous DF, Scheinowitz M, Biro S, et al. Angiogenic-induced enhancement of collateral blood flow to ischemic myocardium by vascular endothelial growth factor in dogs. Circulation 1994;89(5):2183–2189.

114. Donahue JK, Kikkawa K, Johns DC, Marban E, Lawrence JH. Ultrarapid, highly efficient viral gene transfer to the heart. Proc Natl Acad Sci USA 1997;94(9):4664–4668.

115. Shah AS, White DC, Emani S, Kypson AP, Lilly RE, Wilson K, et al. In vivo ventricular gene delivery of a beta-adrenergic receptor kinase inhibitor to the failing heart reverses cardiac dysfunction. Circulation 2001;103(9):1311–1316.

116. Davidson MJ, Jones JM, Emani SM, Wilson KH, Jaggers J, Koch WJ, et al. Cardiac gene delivery with cardiopulmonary bypass. Circulation 2001;104(2):131–133.

117. Boekstegers P, von Degenfeld G, Giehrl W, Heinrich D, Hullin R, Kupatt C, et al. Myocardial gene transfer by selective pressure-regulated retroinfusion of coronary veins. Gene Ther 2000;7(3):232–240.

118. Giordano FJ, Ping P, McKirnan D, Nozaki S, DeMaria A, Dillman WH, Mathieu-Costello O, Hammond K. Intracoronary gene transfer of fibroblast growth factor-5 increases blood flow and contractile function in an ischemic region of the heart. Nat Med 1996;2:534–539.

119. McKirnan MD, Lai NC, Waldman L, et al. Intracoronary gene transfer of fibroblast growth factor-4 increases regional contractile function and responsiveness to adrenergic stimulation in heart failure. Cardiac Vasc Regen 2000;1:11–21.

120. Emani SM, Shah AS, Bowman MK, Emani S, Wilson K, Glower DD, et al. Catheter-based intracoronary myocardial adenoviral gene delivery: importance of intraluminal seal and infusion flow rate. Mol Ther 2003;8(2):306–313.

121. Logeart D, Hatem SN, Heimburger M, Le Roux A, Michel JB, Mercadier JJ. How to optimize in vivo gene transfer to cardiac myocytes: mechanical or pharmacological procedures? Hum Gene Ther 2001;12(13):1601–1610.

122. Simons M, Annex BH, Laham RJ, Kleiman N, Henry T, Dauerman H, Udelson JE, Gervino EV, Pike M, Whitehouse MJ, Moon T, Chronos NA. Pharmacological treatment of coronary artery disease with recombinant fibroblast growth factor-2: double-blind, randomized, controlled clinical trial. Circulation 2002;105:788–793.

123. Grines CL, Watkins MW, Helmer G, Penny W, et al. Angiogenic gene therapy (AGENT) trial in patients with stable angina pectoris. Circulation 2002;105:1291–1297.

124. Hendel RC, Henry TD, Rocha-Singh K, Isner JM, Kereiakas DJ, Giordano FJ, Simons M, Bonow RO. Effect of intracoronary recombinant human vascular endothelial growth factor on myocardial perfusion: evidence for dose-dependent effect. Circulation 2000;101:118–121.

125. Hedman M, Hartikainen J, Syvanne M, et al. Safety and feasibility of catheter-based local intracoronary vascular endothelial growth factor gene transfer in the prevention of postangioplasty and in-stent restenosis and in the treatment of chronic

myocardial ischemia: phase II results of the Kuopio Angiogenesis Trial (KAT). Circulation 2003;107:2677–2683.

126. Wang JS, Shum-Tim D, Chedrawy E, Chiu RC. The coronary delivery of marrow stromal cells for myocardial regeneration: pathophysiological and therapeutic implications. J Thorac Cardiovasc Surg 2001;122(4):699–705.

127. Suzuki K, Murtuza B, Suzuki N, Smolenski RT, Yacoub MH. Intracoronary infusion of skeletal myoblasts improves cardiac function in doxorubicin-induced heart failure. Circulation 2001;104(12 Suppl 1):I213–I217.

128. Strauer BE, Brehm M, Teus T, Kostering M, Hernandez A, Sorg RV, Kogler G, Wernet P. Repair of infarcted myocardium by autologous intracoronary mononuclear bone marrow cell transplantation in humans. Circulation 2002;106:1913–1918.

129. Assmus B, Schachinger V, Teupe C, Britten M, et al. Transplantation of progenitor cells and regeneration enhancement in acute myocardial infarction (TOPCARE-AMI). Circulation 2002;106:3009–3017.

130. Pratt FH. The nutrition of the heart through the vessels of Thebesius and the coronary veins. Am J Physiol 1898;1:86–103.

131. Meerbaum S. Coronary venous retroperfusion delivery of treatment to ischemic myocardium. Herz 1986;11(1):41–54.

132. Mohl W. The momentum of coronary sinus interventions clinically. Circulation 1988;77(1):6–12.

133. Ruengsakulrach P, Buxton BF. Anatomic and hemodynamic considerations influencing the efficiency of retrograde cardioplegia. Ann Thorac Surg 2001;71(4):1389–1395.

134. Mohl W. The relevance of coronary sinus interventions in cardiac surgery. Thorac Cardiovasc Surg 1991;39(5):245–250.

135. Mohl W. Retrograde cardioplegia via the coronary sinus. Ann Chir Gynaecol 1987;76(1):61–67.

136. Gabriele OF. Pacing via coronary sinus. N Engl J Med 1969;280(4):219.

137. Hunt D, Sloman G. Long-term electrode catheter pacing from coronary sinus. BMJ 1968;4(629):495–496.

138. Gerber TC, Kantor B, Keelan PC, Hayes DL, et al. The coronary venous system: an alternative portal to the myocardium for diagnostic and therapeutic procedures in invasive cardiology. Curr Interv Cardiol Rep 2000;2:27–37.

139. Sayad DE, Sawer A, Curkovic V, Gallardo I, Barold SS. Simple access to the coronary venous system for left ventricular pacing. Pacing Clin Electrophysiol 2003;26:1856–1858.

140. Walker S, Levy TM, Coats AJ, Peters NS, Paul VE. Bi-ventricular pacing in congestive cardiac failure: current experience and future directions. Eur Heart J 2000;21:884–889.

141. Karagueuzian HS, Ohta M, Drury JK, Fishbein MC, Meerbaum S, Corday E, et al. Coronary venous retroinfusion of procainamide: a new approach for the management of spontaneous and inducible sustained ventricular tachycardia during myocardial infarction. J Am Coll Cardiol 1986;7(3):551–563.

142. Uriuda Y, Wang QD, Li XS, et al. Coronary venous drug infusion in the ischaemic-reperfused isolated rat heart. Cardiovasc Res 1996;31(1):82–92.

143. Tadokoro H, Miyazaki A, Satomura K, et al. Infarct size reduction with coronary venous retroinfusion of diltiazem in the acute occlusion/reperfusion porcine heart model. J Cardiovasc Pharmacol 1996;28(1):134–141.

144. Hatori N, Miyazaki A, Tadokoro H, et al. Beneficial effects of coronary venous retroinfusion of superoxide dismutase and catalase on reperfusion arrhyth-

mias, myocardial function, and infarct size in dogs. J Cardiovasc Pharmacol 1989;14(3):396–404.

145. Haga Y, Uriuda Y, Bjorkman JA, Hatori N, et al. Ischemic and nonischemic tissue concentrations of felodipine after coronary venous retroinfusion during myocardial ischemia and reperfusion: an experimental study in pigs. J Cardiovasc Pharmacol 1994;24:298–302.

146. Hatori N, Tadokoro H, Satomura K, Miyazaki A, Fishbein MC, et al. Beneficial effects of coronary venous retroinfusion but not left atrial administration of superoxide dismutase on myocardial necrosis in pigs. Eur Heart J 1991;12:442–450.

147. Pakalska E, Kolff WJ. Anatomical basis for retrograde coronary vein perfusion. Venous anatomy and veno-venous anastomoses in the hearts of humans and some animals. Minn Med 1989;63(11):795–801.

148. Chen SG, Chang BL, Meerbaum S, et al. The pattern of delivery and distribution of coronary venous retroinfusate in canine hearts. Proc Chin Acad Med Sci Peking Union Med Coll 1989;4(1):19–25.

149. Hochberg MS, Austen WG. Selective retrograde coronary venous perfusion. Ann Thorac Surg 1980;29(6):578–578.

150. Punzengruber C, Maurer G, Chang BL, Ong K, Meerbaum S, Corday E. Factors affecting penetration of retrograde coronary venous injections into normal and ischemic canine myocardium: assessment by contrast echocardiography and digital angiography. Basic Res Cardiol 1990;85(1):21–32.

151. Oh BH, Volpini M, Kambayashi M, et al. Myocardial function and transmural blood flow during coronary venous retroperfusion in pigs. Circulation 1992;86(4): 1265–1279.

152. Herity NA, Lo ST, Oei F, Lee DP, Ward MR, Filardo SD, et al. Selective regional myocardial infiltration by the percutaneous coronary venous route: a novel technique for local drug delivery. Catheter Cardiovasc Interv 2000;51(3):358–363.

153. Vicario J, Piva J, Pierini A, Ortega HH, Canal A, Gerardo L, et al. Transcoronary sinus delivery of autologous bone marrow and angiogenesis in pig models with myocardial injury. Cardiovasc Radiat Med 2002;3:91–94.

154. Rezaee M, Herity N, Lo S, et al. Therapeutic angiogenesis by selective delivery of basic FGF in the anterior interventricular vein. J Am Coll Cardiol 2001;37(2):47A (Abstr).

155. Hou D, Maclaughlin F, Thiesse M, Panchal VR, Bekkers BC, Wilson EA, et al. Widespread regional myocardial transfection by plasmid encoding Del-1 following retrograde coronary venous delivery. Catheter Cardiovasc Interv 2003;58(2): 207–211.

156. Farcot JC, Barry M, Bourdarias JP, et al. New catheter-pump system for diastolic synchronized coronary sinus retroperfusion. Med Prog Technol 1980;8(1):29–37.

157. Chang BL, Drury JK, Meerbaum S, et al. Enhanced myocardial washout and retrograde blood delivery with synchronized retroperfusion during acute myocardial ischemia. J Am Coll Cardiol 1987;9(5):1091–1098.

158. Villanueva FS, Spotnitz WD, Glasheen WP, et al. New insights into the physiology of retrograde cardioplegia delivery. Am J Physiol 1995;268(4 Pt 2):H1555–H166.

159. Boekstegers P, Diebold J, Weiss C. Selective ECG synchronized suction and retroinfusion of coronary veins; first results of studies in acute myocardial ischemia in dogs. Cardiovasc Res 1990;24:456–464.

160. Boekstegers P, Giehrl W, von Degenfeld G, Steinbeck G. Selective suction and pressure-regulated retroinfusion: an effective and safe approach to retrograde protection against myocardial ischemia in patients undergoing normal and

high risk percutaneous transluminal coronary angioplasty. J Am Coll Cardiol 1998;31(7):1525–1533.

161. Fitzgerald PJ, Hayase M, Yeung AC, et al. New approaches and conduits: in situ venous arterialization and coronary artery bypass. Curr Interv Cardiol Rep 1999;1:127–137.

162. Oesterle SN, Reifart N, Hayase M, et al. Catheter-based coronary bypass: a development update. Catheter Cardioasc Interv 2003;58:212–218.

163. Oesterle SN, Reifart N, Hauptmann E, Hayase M, Yeung AC. Percutaneous in situ coronary venous arterialization: report of the first human catheter-based coronary artery bypass. Circulation 2001;103:2539–2543.

164. Thompson CA, Nasseri BA, Makower J, Houser S, McGarry M, Lamson T, et al. Percutaneous transvenous cellular cardiomyoplasty. A novel nonsurgical approach for myocardial cell transplantation. J Am Coll Cardiol 2003;41(11):1964–1971.

165. Kar S, Nordlander R. Coronary veins: an alternate route to ischemic myocardium. Heart Lung 1992;21(2):148–157.

166. Menasche P, Piwnica A. Cardioplegia by way of the coronary sinus for valvular and coronary surgery. J Am Coll Cardiol 1991;18(2):628–636.

167. Mesisel E, Pfeiffer D, Engelmann L, et al. Investigation of coronary venous anatomy by retrograde venography in patients with malignant ventricular tachycardia. Circulation 2001;104:442–447.

168. Lawrie A, Brisken AF, Francis SE, Cumberland DC, Crossman DC, Newman CM. Microbubble-enhanced ultrasound for vascular gene delivery. Gene Ther 2000;7(23):2023–2027.

169. Shohet RV, Chen S, Zhou YT, Wang Z, Meidell RS, Unger RH, Grayburn PA. Echocardiographic destruction of albumin microbubbles directs gene delivery to the myocardium. Circulation 2000;101:2554–2556.

170. Beeri R, Guerrero JL, Supple G, Sullivan S, Levine RA, Hajjar RJ. New efficient catheter-based system for myocardial gene delivery. Circulation 2002;106(14):1756–1759.

171. Mukherjee D, Wong J, Griffin B, Ellis SG, Porter T, Sen S, et al. Ten-fold augmentation of endothelial uptake of vascular endothelial growth factor with ultrasound after systemic administration. J Am Coll Cardiol 2000;35(6):1678–1686.

172. Bekeredjian R, Chen S, Frenkel PA, Grayburn PA, Shohet RV. Ultrasound-targeted microbubble destruction can repeatedly direct highly specific plasmid expression in the heart. Circulation 2003;108:1022–1026.

173. Fuchs S, Baffour R, Shou M, Stabile E, Singh S, Schwartz B, et al. Could plasmid-mediated gene transfer into the myocardium be augmented by left ventricular guided laser myocardial injury? Catheter Cardiovasc Interv 2001;54(4):533–538.

174. Bao J, Naimark W, Palasis M, Laham R, Simons M, Post MJ. Intramyocardial delivery of FGF2 in combination with radio frequency transmyocardial revascularization. Catheter Cardiovasc Interv 2001;53(3):429–434.

175. Yamamoto N, Kohmoto T, Roethy W, et al. Histological evidence that basic fibroblast growth factor enhances the angiogenic effects of transmyocardial laser revascularization. Basic Res Cardiol 2000;95:55–63.

176. Sayeed-Shah U, Mann MJ, Martin J, et al. Complete reversal of ischemic wall motion abnormalities by combined use of gene therapy with transmyocardial laser revascularization. J Thorac Cardiovasc Surg 1998;116:763–769.

177. Rezaee M, Mead H, Wohlgemuth J, Quertermous T, Rosenman D, Altman P. Enhanced local uptake of genetic material through intramyocardial electroporation with helix infusion electrode. Mol Ther 2001;13:774 (Abstr).

178. Nugent HM, Edelman ER. Tissue engineering therapy for cardiovascular disease. Circ Res 2003;92(10):1068–1078.
179. Lu Y, Shansky J, DelTatto M, Ferland P, Wang X, Vandenburgh H. Recombinant vascular endothelial growth factor secreted from tissue engineered bioartificial muscles promotes localized angiogenesis. Circulation 2001;104:594–599.
180. Kellar R, Landeen LK, Shepherd BR, Naughton GK, Ratcliffe A, Williams SK. Scaffold-based three-dimensional human fibroblast culture provides a structural matrix that supports angiogenesis in infarcted heart tissue. Circulation 2001;104:2063–2068.
181. Shintani S, Murohara T, Ikeda H, Ueno T, et al. Mobilization of endothelial progenitor cells in patients with acute myocardial infarction. Circulation 2001;103:2776–2779.
182. Seiler C, Pohl T, Wustmann K, Hutter D, Nicolet PA, Windecker S, Eberli FR, Meier B. Promotion of collateral growth by granulocyte-macrophage colony-stimulating factor in patients with coronary artery disease: a randomized double-blind, placebo-controlled study. Circulation 2001;104:2012–2017.
183. Gill M, Dia S, Hattori K, et al. Vascular trauma induces rapid but transient mobilization of VEGFR2+AC133+ endothelial precursor cells. Circ Res 2001;88:167–174.
184. Asahara T, Takahashi T, Masuda H, et al. VEGF contributes to postnatal neovascularization by mobilizing bone marrow-derived endothelial progenitor cells. EMBO J 1999;18:3964–3972.
185. Vasa M, Fichtscherer S, Adler K, Aicher A, Martin H, Zeiher AM, Dimmeler S. Increase in circulating endothelial progenitor cells by statin therapy in patients with stable coronary artery disease. Circulation 2001;103:2885–2890.

6

Imaging Angiogenesis
A Guide for Clinical Management and Therapeutic Trials

Justin D. Pearlman, MD, ME, PhD

INTRODUCTION

Rapid advancements in molecular biology have expanded the candidate treatments aiming to modify blood supply without surgery. Laser treatments *(1)*, growth factors, and gene therapies have been touted as capable of improving blood supply sufficient to resolve symptoms and/or reduce the risks of damage. Pro-angiogenic growth factors that induce the growth and development of blood vessels may prove useful in (1) protecting myocardium from cell death, (2) protecting extremities from ischemic ulcers and other damage leading to limb loss, (3) providing relief from ischemic symptoms, and/or (4) improving functional capacity. Antiangiogenic agents may prove valuable in slowing or stopping cancers.

From: *Contemporary Cardiology: Angiogenesis and Direct Myocardial Revasularization*
Edited by: R. J. Laham and D. S. Baim © Humana Press Inc., Totowa, NJ

Unbridled enthusiasm has yielded to the recognition that these biological systems are complex and require very detailed evaluations. Treatment effects can be masked by endogenous inhibitors, by endothelial dysfunction (2), or by various other causes of impaired tissue function such as fibrosis. These complexities can be unraveled by detailed monitoring of multiple relevant parameters of tissue status (3–5). Relevant factors include microvascular development, microvessel maturity, blood delivery, tissue oxygenation, metabolic functions, tissue elasticity, strain development, and systolic and diastolic function.

A therapeutic trial of vessel inhibition around cancer cells (6–10) should consider detrimental effects on the heart and limbs of patients with ischemia. Conversely, trials of angiogenic stimulation should scrutinize for possible effects on cancer development. These concerns support attempts to achieve localized activation of therapy.

Trials that focus only on major endpoints such as heart attack or limb loss or death have limited value because they require very large, costly studies that could be very misleading in the end. Lack of perceived benefit in such trials could relate to complex determinants of outcome, inadequate frequency of treatment, ineffective route of delivery, mitigating sequelae during treatment, changes in progression of underlying disease, or other factors that might have been manageable if recognized. Techniques that identify only late endpoints are confounded by numerous interim changes, which limit their power to discern therapeutic effects. It is vital to understand in detail all the effects of treatment in these complex patients.

The principal alternative to large and long trials with hard endpoints such as death, heart attack, or limb loss is the use of surrogate endpoints. Surrogate endpoints can be equally misleading if they are insensitive to the immediate effects of treatment. It is important to include outcome measures that can identify proximate effects and clarify mechanism of action in clinical trials on complex patients and quantify these effects with high sensitivity and specificity.

Studies of angiogenesis proceed at many levels, including cell cultures (11–13), genetic knockout mice (14–17), many different animal models (18,19). and studies on patients with peripheral ischemia (claudication), cardiac ischemia not resolved by current clinical therapies, other tissue ischemia, or cancer. Technologies include immunohistochemistry (20), electron microscopy (21), optical imaging (22) with fluorescence (23,24), ultrasound (25), laser Doppler (26,27), radionuclide imaging (28), including positron emission tomography (PET) (29,30), x-ray angiography (31), computed tomography (CT) (32,33), and magnetic resonance imaging (MRI) (34–38). These different models afford different opportunities to observe the impact of interventions. For patient studies, the ability to track and quantify changes in microcirculation and vessel development proved challenging but solvable.

The key challenge is the identification of microscopic changes in large targets that may lie deep within tissues. An early accurate definition of the impact of therapy is essential to avoid the mistake of abandoning a therapy that could be very valuable. For example, a therapy that might provide sufficient vascular development to prevent a heart attack, with or without a shift in ischemia threshold, might be deemed a failure if the measure of success rests on elimination of inducible ischemia.

The main candidate techniques for clinical trials when the target may lie deep within the subject are radionuclide imaging (single photon emission computed tomography [SPECT] and PET), CT, and MRI. Radionuclide imaging has primarily focused on blood delivery and recognizing induced ischemia. However, symptom-limited stress studies may show a similar defect extent despite potentially important benefits of treatment, because the subject continues stress until ischemia is produced. Improved exercise tolerance is very difficult to detect owing to training effects, patient bias, high variability in stress tolerance, and other factors. Therefore, it is important to measure vascular effects more directly. PET can measure flow reserve *(30)* but is not widely available. Both MRI and CT can measure blood delivery and the status of vascular development and are increasingly available. Initial experience demonstrates that MRI offers useful diagnostic and therapeutic guidance not available by other techniques *(34–38)*. MRI clarifies the mechanism as well as impact of therapy. Furthermore, it is cost-effective when used efficiently, because its high sensitivity to treatment effects enables smaller trials. Recent advances in molecular and cellular imaging further encourage use of MRI and PET *(4,29)*.

When used effectively, new imaging capabilities can document the status of collateral circulation, tissue jeopardy, neovascular development, tissue viability, and functional impairment, as well as response to stress. New imaging techniques can clarify mechanisms of effect and quantify the impact of therapy. Tailoring the imaging method to different effects of interest can elucidate the relationships between neovascular development, local blood delivery, rest ischemia, inducible ischemia, cell death, local function, arteriogenesis, global function, and clinical outcomes. These relationships are complex and nonlinear *(39)*.

One might argue that only a treatment that produces clear changes in the late sequelae, such as resolution of inducible ischemia, are important. The fallacy of that argument is best illustrated by a counterexample. A treatment that stimulates angiogenesis in the heart may protect the patient from infarction and death and may improve the quality of life, but it may not improve the appearance of stress-induced radionuclide perfusion defects. Treatment may stimulate the development of new vessels, which can play a very important role at rest and normal activity levels, but these immature microvessels may fail to adjust dynamically to maximal stress the same as an entirely normal blood supply. If stress-induced defect size is taken as the primary point of a trial, a potentially life-protecting medical treatment might be discarded.

In therapeutic trials, a technique that may be considered costly and not widely available becomes very cost-effective and highly desirable if it provides early detection with high sensitivity, specificity, and predictive accuracy. The alternative requires much larger trials that greatly limit the ability to explore potentially important variations in treatment approach. The ability to discern differences between placebo and various treatment regimens early after treatment saves money and avoids risk by obtaining useful information quickly from fewer patients. Patient selection criteria and control selection can be more stringent, and various avenues of treatment may be examined in greater depth.

IN VITRO BENCH METHODS

Cell cultures demonstrate organization under the influence of angiogenic factors. Serial microscopic images show progressive organization of cells into vascular elements. Such images can be acquired digitally at regular time intervals by a camera attachment to the microscope. Alternatively, photographs may be obtained optically and subsequently scanned digitally for analysis by software. The goal is to convert the visual record of vascular development to a quantitative measure.

Figure 1 shows micrographs demonstrating the progressive organization of cells into vascular elements. Analysis of such images converts the visual impression of vascular development to a score. The analysis applies methods of morphometrics. First, the image is filtered and mapped to a binary representation (black-and-white image) of borders and spaces. Morphological operations (operations called open and close) fortify the borders to reduce noise and partial volume (faint edge) effects. After completion of the preprocessing, software automatically counts the number of simple closed regions and measures the area and circumference of each. For example, area and perimeter can be combined to a shape index (SI) (40) using the formula $SI = P^2/4\pi A$. For a circle, $P = 2\pi r$, so the SI is 1. With progressive deviations from circular, the SI increases. Examination of micrographs of matured angiogenesis demonstrates the appropriate bounds on A and SI. The number N of regions within those

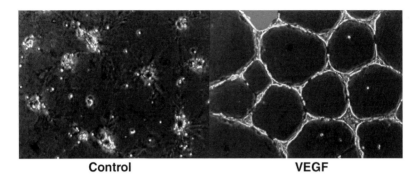

Control   **VEGF**

Fig. 1. Micrographs demonstrating progressive organization of cells into vascular elements. Analysis of such images converts the visual impression of vascular development to a score. VEGF, vascular endothelial growth factor.

bounds, divided by the mean SI of those regions, provides a numerical score that represents a useful measure of vascular development.

A circle can be defined as a closed loop in a plane with the smallest perimeter for the enclosed area. In three dimensions, the corresponding condition produces a sphere. Experimentally, this is demonstrated by releasing a drop of liquid under weightless conditions. The surface tension imposes minimization of surface area for the given volume, and the droplet takes the shape of a sphere. Progressive deviations from circular shape increase the SI.

SI can be applied to hourly images for 24–48 h to establish a curve assessing angiogenic development over time *(41)*. The peak slope, the peak, and the area under the curve are useful indicators of angiogenic response. Area under the curve adds all measurements and is thus noise suppressing. These indices may be used to compare different cell lines for their responsiveness to a fixed angiogenic stimulus and to compare responses of a given cell line to various stimuli to establish and compare dose-response curves. Observation of the changes in these indices in response to alteration of the cell line with inhibitors or knockouts may be used to clarify mechanisms of angiogenic stimulation.

Use of different colored stains provides information about co-localization. For example, superposition of the results from two different stains indicates that macrophages and angiogenic growth factors co-localize, which points to inflammation as an important mediator of angiogenesis. Examination of angiogenesis rates under normal vs ischemic tissues indicates a dramatic increase in ischemic tissue, consistent with the concept that ischemia induces upregulation of the growth factor receptors.

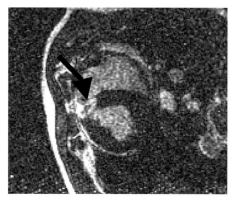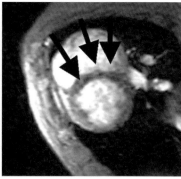

Fig. 2. Cell-labeled ischemic area. (Left) Dark-contrast labeled cells within scar in the anteroseptal wall (arrow). (Right) Single frame from a dynamic image series with additional positive contrast representing tissue perfusion show dark-contrast labeled cells locate throughout ischemic zones (arrows).

CELL TRACKING

Delivery of stem cells to injured tissue has been posited as a possible means to activate lost functionality, with a potential for the undifferentiated cells to assume missing host functions such as contractile muscle and to accelerate formation of vascular elements. To verify delivery of cells and to track their location, cells can be labeled to produce a distinctive signal when the heart is imaged by MRI *(42)*. MRI label options include T1 agents, T2* (susceptibility) agents, and chemical shift agents. T1 agents facilitate change in magnetization and thus increase signal recovery ("positive contrast"). T2* or magnetic susceptibility agents disturb the uniformity of the magnetic field, accelerating signal loss ("negative contrast"). Chemical shift agents change the resonance frequency. Susceptibility agents have been preferred to date because the effect blooms much larger than the target.

Iron-labeled bone marrow and skeletal muscle cells have been injected in the myocardium and successfully imaged with MR after catheter-based delivery *(43–45)* using intracellular magnetic susceptibility, the proportionality between the applied magnetic field strength, and the magnetization established in atoms with an unpaired nucleon. Superparamagnetic iron oxide particles produce a strong augmentation of the local magnetic field. The regional increase in T2 and T2* produces a loss of signal intensity on MR images sensitive to T2* effects.

Figure 2 shows focal hypoenhancement in the heart wall under double contrast imaging (T1 agent in normal tissue, T2* in the labeled cells) demonstrating the location of iron-labeled bone marrow cells in areas of ischemic injury. The use of double agents increased the contrast from $17.58 \pm 8.5\%$ to $27.25 \pm 15.8\%$ ($p < 0.05$) and SNR from $24.87 \pm 9.6\%$ to $35.08 \pm 15.5\%$ ($p < 0.05$).

MOLECULAR IMAGING

As we learn more about signaling pathways and specific regulators and mediators of angiogenesis, the desire to locate and measure specific molecules in the pathway increases. PET, MRI, and optical methods can label a specific molecule to identify its distribution in tissue *(22,46,47)*. Whereas PET studies substitute a positron-emitting isotope for an atom in the target molecule, MRI relies on bulkier attachment of a nanoparticle typically to an antibody fragment or ligand that associates with the target molecule. The techniques can be combined using PET to track agent distribution and MRI to measure effect *(48)*. The size of a molecular tag influences the ability of the agent to enter extravascular tissue, with minimal extravasation occurring at and above 120 kDa *(49)*. In vitro studies demonstrated that cross-linked iron oxide (CLIO), a strong MRI contrast agent, bound to antibody fragments targeted to human E-selectin achieves 100–200 times higher binding to cells stimulated to overexpress E-selectin (human endothelial umbilical vein cells treated with inter-leukin (IL)-1β than control cells *(50)*. In vivo, α(υ)β3-integrin, a biomarker that is highly expressed on activated neovascular endothelial cells and essentially absent on mature quiescent cells, has been tracked in rabbits using paramagnetic nanoparticles to mark the location in MRI and a nonparamagnetic agent to displace the marker *(51)*. Despite their relatively large size, nanoparticles penetrated deep into leaky tumor neovasculature, producing signal changes of 56–126%. Ultrasound contrast agents can also be designed for molecular targets *(52)*. In cancer, molecular markers may vary from case to case, but phage libraries provide a means to screen individual patients for useful markers that can produce a ligand-receptor-based map of the microvasculature *(53)*.

IN VIVO BENCH METHODS

The easiest way to extend bench methods to in vivo studies is to use a gel that can be placed under the abdominal skin of a mouse *(54–56)*. Alternatively, endothelial cells can be grown as a co-culture with fibroblasts *(57)*. Tubular elements form at surfaces and also in three dimensions *(58)*. Such systems are used in knockout mice to clarify the in vivo relevance of angiogenesis regulators such as caveolin-1 *(14)*. Image planes through the structure show circular shapes where the plane intersects a tubule in short axis and elliptical elements where the plane intersects a tubule obliquely. The distribution of shape index values is wider than on a flat dish, but still can monitor vascular development in response to added agents. A chamber can be created for serial optical assessments (59).

Numerous studies that require autopsy for measurement have been performed on small animals to the consternation of animal rights activists. These studies require large numbers in order to generate statistics that overwhelm the variations between individuals. In order to look at different stages of development of angiogenesis by autopsy, cohorts must be treated similarly and sacrificed at different times after intervention. Such methods do not enable tracking the changes in an individual over time. Also, it is very difficult to assess the relationship between demand and response, or even be confident about details of the sequence of events, because of variations between individuals in the severity and timing of injuries and responses.

The ability to follow an individual case over time has tremendous advantages. Each case serves as its own control, dramatically improving the sensitivity of detecting changes over time and in response to treatment. The removal of individual variation as a confounding factor makes the sequence of events and the relationship of response to demand much easier to examine.

In a comparison of cohorts of animals sacrificed under different conditions, the final result is typically a small population difference that attains statistical significance due to very large numbers of sacrificed animals. Such a result leaves us with the question as to whether that small population difference has any biologic significance. An observed population difference may be small on average due to individual variation or very significant for many individuals but with superimposed high variability of disease condition. It could also be a marginal, clinically insignificant but consistent change in each case.

LARGE ANIMAL AND HUMAN ANGIOGENESIS STUDIES

Chronic ischemia is produced by encasing a segment of a proximal coronary artery, e.g., the left circumflex, in ameroid plastic. Tissue reaction and slow progressive swelling of the plastic on absorption of water emulate the slow progression of coronary occlusive disease. Agents known to stimulate neovascular development in the Petri dish may be applied in this model and compared to placebo. Each individual animal is studied in a highly reproducible manner at different stages of treatment, as described below. Microsphere distributions, x-ray angiograms, and histology are also obtained.

Figure 3 shows scout MRI of the heart obtained to determine the precise position and orientation of the heart inside the chest. Successive images are obtained by prescription with respect to the orientation of prior images. The first goal is to establish the orientation of the long axis of the left ventricle, bisecting the base and passing through the apex of the heart.

Figure 4 shows short-axis images perpendicular to the long axis of the left ventricle. These images provide a symmetry that facilitates recognition of abnormalities in wall thickness, motion, and wall thickness change during contraction.

Figure 5 shows a stack of cine images spanning the heart from base to apex. Cine images consist of a series of images of the heart at successive delays into the contraction cycle. Each cine series is obtained in less than 20 s during a breath-hold. We cover the entire heart by obtaining a cine series of 5-cm-thick short-axis sections. The prescription is shifted by 5 mm each time, resulting in a contiguous stack that covers the entire heart without gaps.

Perfusion-Sensitive MRI

Perfusion-sensitive imaging is performed by adjusting imaging parameters so that the heart is dark. Then a series of images are obtained for 40 s following the injection of a contrast agent. As shown in Fig. 5, the arrival of contrast-labeled blood is signaled by a bright signal that arrives first in the right ventricle, then passes through the lungs to fill the left ventricle, then passes to the aorta and coronary arteries to arrive in the myocardium.

Based on either long-axis perfusion-sensitive imaging or prior information, a target level is designated by its fractional distance from base to apex. That target level is studied in particular detail. Perfusion-sensitive short-axis images are obtained specifically at that target short-axis level. At that level and at neighboring levels cine images are obtained that track the out-of-plane motion of the target level resulting from the contraction of the left ventricle. Detailed motion assessment also tracks the twisting motion of the heart from diastole to systole. The tracking is performed both prospectively and retrospectively using the Serial Motion Assessment by Reference Tracking (SMART) technique (60).

Impaired blood arrival to the myocardium is measured by tracking the signal change in every pixel using a space–time map (61). Figure 6 illustrates how the pixels corresponding to the target myocardium are remapped from their annular position around the heart to a vertical stripe so that the views from successive heartbeats may be laid side-by-side to reveal the entire contrast arrival history in a single derived space–time

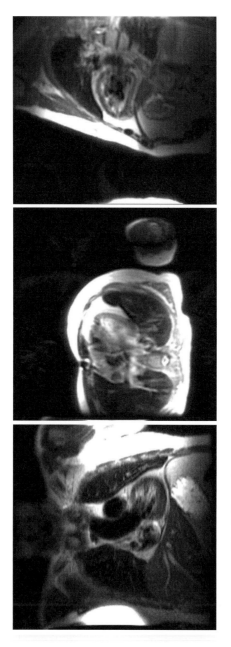

Fig. 3. Scout images show coil placement and cardiac three-dimensional orientation.

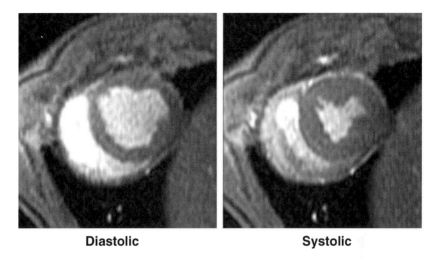

Diastolic   **Systolic**

Fig. 4. A pair of short-axis images perpendicular to the long axis of the left ventricle. These images provide symmetry that facilitates recognition of abnormalities in wall thickness, motion, and wall thickness change between systole and diastole.

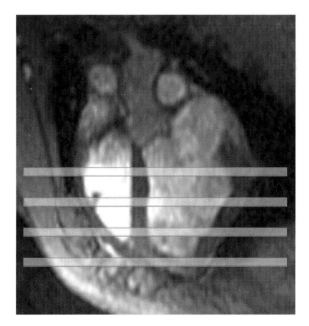

Fig. 5. A stack of images, with each new image perpendicular to the long axis of the heart. A subset is shown for clarity; image typically consists of contiguous slices (no gap) of thickness 3–10 mm as desired. Thinner slices have lower signal:noise ratio.

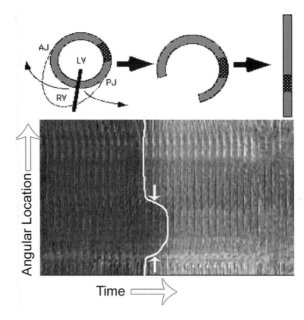

Fig. 6. Space–time map: heart wall is mapped from a closed ring to a vertical bar, with the cut ends corresponding to the posterior third of the interventricular septum and the left edge corresponding to endocardium. The bars are placed one after another corresponding to the time series to display arrival of contrast. Equitime is superimposed. Delayed blood delivery is evident as an indentation to the right, reporting spatial extent (arrows) and also severity by way of the depth of the indentation. Indentation ≥2 bars is abnormal. Inverse delay correlates with flow per gram of tissue. From ref. *61*.

map. The term "space–time map" indicates that the vertical axis of the map reports angular position around the heart and the immediate horizontal position reports position from endocardial layer to epicardial layer (space localization information), whereas the large scale of the horizontal axis represents time (successive heartbeats).

Figure 7 shows examples of space–time maps and the corresponding image frame that best exhibits the pathology. Our software automatically links the two so that placement of the mouse cursor on any point in the space-time map automatically displays the corresponding image frame and location within the myocardium.

Analysis of 30 different methods for analyzing blood arrival to the myocardium revealed the method of greatest accuracy in terms of receiver operator characteristics. The complement of specificity vs sensitivity was plotted for each of the 30 measurement methods. The largest area under the curve corresponds to best performance in terms of best specificity vs sensitivity independent of diagnostic threshold *(62–64)*.

Table 1 summarizes the different methods for assessing blood arrival to tissue. The measurements are based on either the time-intensity relation for pixels in impaired vs normal supply zones or derived time-concentration curves that take into account MRI relaxivity and hematocrit *(65)*. One category of measurements is purely descriptive, focusing, for example, on the upslope or time to peak. Another category of measurements is based on mathematical modeling of contrast arrival based on dye dilution principles of convolution *(66–68)*. A third category is based on a more comprehensive model of blood arrival based on differential equations reflecting multiple pathways, multiple compartments, conservation of mass, and stable exchange rates between compartments *(69,70)*. A major problem with modeling is reliance on simplifying assumptions such as stable exchange rates, assumed details of the pathway distributions, and difficulties accounting for change in hematocrit in the microcirculation. Another problem is noise and error propagation. After substantial experience assessing multicenter preclinical and clinical trials of therapeutic angiogenesis, we devised a new parameter for blood arrival called "Equitime." It combines the strengths of different measurements while minimizing the impact of error and noise propagation.

Figure 8 illustrates the Equitime measurement. Basically, the time-intensity of arrival to the left ventricle provides calibration by specifying the amount of contrast agent available for delivery. Equitime then computes how long it takes for the reference amount to accumulate in the target tissue. For noise suppression, the reference is computed as the integral of signal intensity as it rises from 10 to 90% (from t_1 to t_3 for LV) of baseline to peak. The integral of contrast arrival in the tissue (t_2 to t_4) reduces noise by the effect of ensemble averaging. It combines the effects of slow arrival (low slope), low peak, delayed peak, and other features that distinguish impaired blood delivery from normal.

Receiver operating characteristic (ROC) analysis shows that Equitime proved superior to all other measures for overall detection of impaired blood delivery with respect to the pooled truth from consensus interpretation of microspheres, histology, and angiographic data. A similar analysis comparing different methods in clinical studies with inducible radionuclide defects as standard likewise showed Equitime to be superior to other methods. It offers >95% sensitivity and specificity. In fact, Equitime delay proved equally sensitive as nuclear imaging is identifying impaired blood arrival at rest under stress conditions.

By analogy, consider whether there are enough lunchroom stations to feed the entire staff in 1 h. One could poll the staff to see who went hungry on a calm day. One could also poll the staff on a hectic stressful day when the demand for quick access to lunch is markedly accentuated.

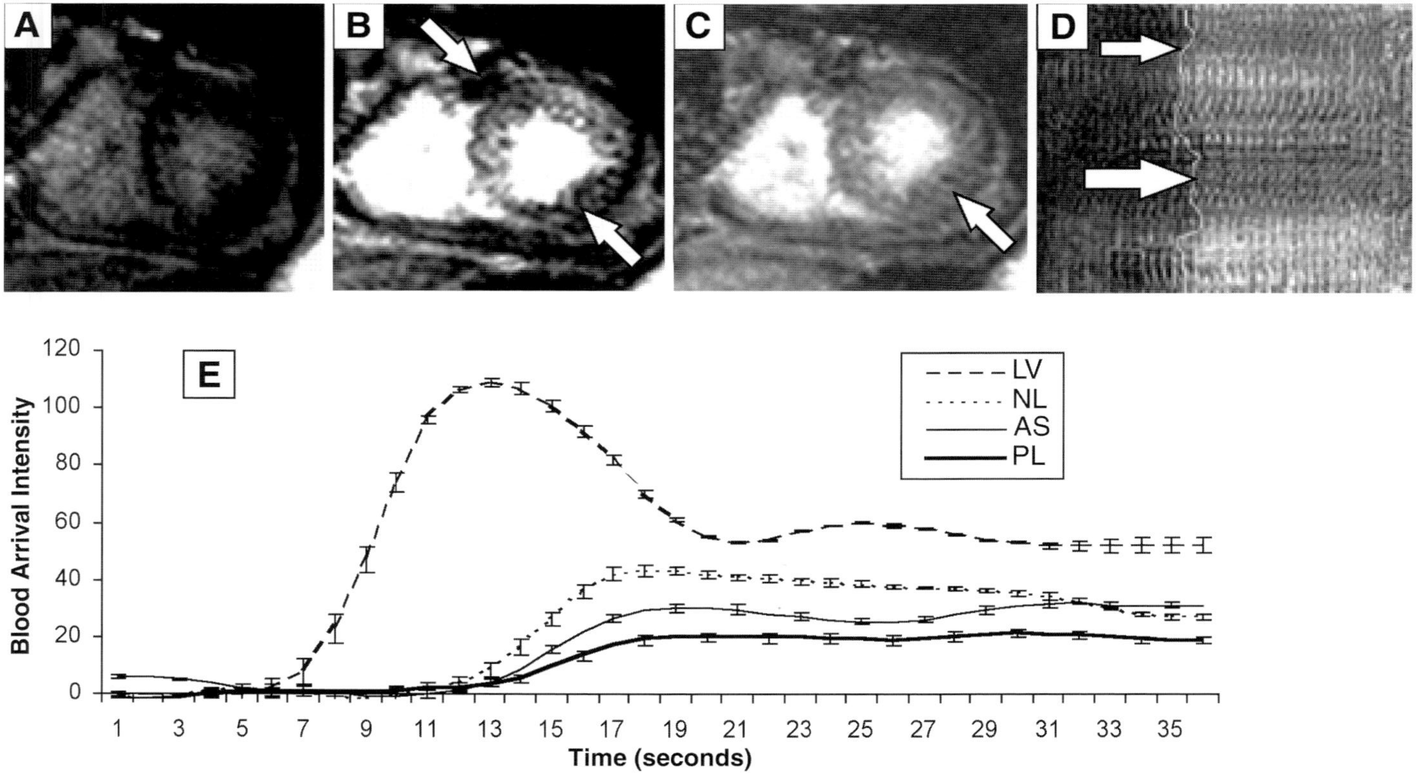
A
B
C
D
E
120
100
80
60
40
20
0
Blood Arrival Intensity
LV
NL
AS
PL
1
3
5
7
9
11
13
15
17
19
21
23
25
27
29
31
33
35
Time (seconds)

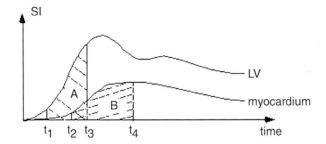

Fig. 8. Equal-time measure of perfusion: area A represents the bolus of contrast agent in the left ventricle (LV). Area B represents equal area of contrast accumulation in a region of myocardium. The time interval t_2-t_4 reports how long it takes to accumulate the designated amount of available bolus of contrast in the region of interest of the myocardium. This measure is noise-reducing, fully automated, and highly sensitive and specific to impaired blood delivery.

Those two polls are comparable to rest and stress nuclear imaging. Are there any areas routinely underfed under calm conditions? Are there any areas of stress-inducible underfeeding? Underfeeding corresponds to ischemia.

Alternatively, one could measure how long it takes to get through the lines in the lunchroom. Prolonged service time identifies a problem even before actual hunger. Foci of delays can identify a problem at rest even if everyone gets fed. Where there are long delays at rest, one can expect inducible problems of feeding at peak demand.

Analogously, delayed Equitime greater than 1 s identifies impaired blood delivery. Impaired delivery present under resting conditions may still suffice to feed the myocardium, albeit just barely, so it does not signify ischemia, just impaired blood arrival. We therefore hypothesized

Fig. 7. *(Opposite page)* Space–time map example: magnetic resonance imaging is performed in a manner that makes the heart wall very dark in the absence of contrast agent arrival (**A**). As the contrast agent arrives, normal zones enhance (**B**), followed by enhancement also of impaired zones (**C**). From the complete time series of images (not shown), the space time map is produced (**D**), in this case demonstrating that the patient has two loci of delayed blood-delivery (arrows, **D**). Pointing to them with a mouse automatically displays the corresponding image frame (**B**) exhibiting lack of contrast in the affected zones when normal zones have accumulated contrast already. Pointing further to the right in D brings up a frame in which contrast agent has had further time to accumulate (**C**). Typically, blood eventually fills in the viable zones, but in this case, there is a persisting deficit in the posterolateral wall indicating a more profound blood-delivery problem in the posterolateral zone.

that regions of impaired blood arrival correspond to regions of inducible ischemia. That hypothesis was tested by comparing impaired blood arrival MRI space–time maps to rest and stress nuclear perfusion study results in a double-blind prospective trial.

Figure 9 shows the results of delayed blood arrival vs rest/stress radionuclide imaging. The rest distribution was assessed by thallium-201. The stress distribution was determined by Tc99m-sestamibi. The myocardium was divided into eight zones starting at the anterior junction of the right and left ventricles. MRI data were evaluated blinded to nuclear data, and vice versa. Deficit of blood distribution was scored 0–3 (0 indicates no reduction, 1 mild, 2 moderate, and 3 severe) by experienced observers blinded to the MRI data and also by automated analysis software.

The results show that impaired blood arrival by Equitime MRI at rest corresponds to zones of inducible ischemia that require stress for detection by radionuclide imaging (Fig. 10). Furthermore, the extent of delay correlates with the severity of defect by stress imaging. Detection of these zones at rest is safer than forcing stress ischemia on patients and is also likely to prove more reproducible. The phrase "zones of impaired blood delivery" should be used, rather than "ischemic zones," to accurately reflect the method. We have determined that a delay of greater than two or more cardiac cycles corresponds to inducible abnormalities.

Technically there are two basic approaches to perfusion-sensitive MRI. The fundamental goal is to establish a distinction between signal intensity at baseline vs when contrast-labeled blood arrives to the target tissue. That is accomplished by adjusting the imaging conditions so that the myocardium is dark and becomes bright when contrast-labeled blood arrives in the tissue. The reverse is also possible—starting bright and aiming for darkening—but there are technical disadvantages. One method of setting the baseline myocardium dark is to use saturation to remove longitudinal magnetization from the tissue just prior to imaging. An alternative is to invert magnetization and then acquire the imaging signal just as the magnetization flips from negative towards positive ("zero-crossing"). These two methods are called saturation recovery and inversion recovery, respectively.

Saturation recovery is easier to perform than inversion recovery. It can be set up as "one size fits all" without specific adjustment for the individual study. It is relatively easy to set up a multislice saturation recovery, so that a plurality of cross sections of the heart may be imaged concurrently during a single bolus transit of injected contrast agent.

Inversion recovery is more complicated. The strength and duration of the preparation pulse must be adjusted to the T1 relaxation of the myocardium and the partial saturation affects that depend on heart rate and

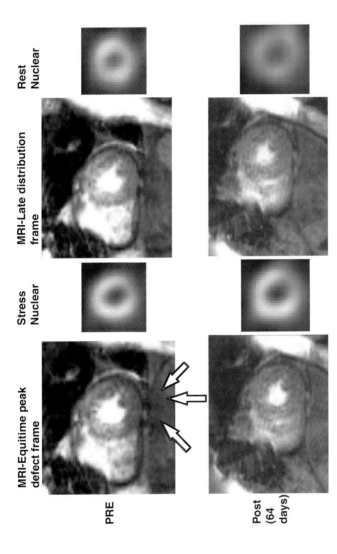

Fig. 9. Comparison of magnetic resonance imaging (MRI) Equitime to stress/rest single photon emission computed tomography (SPECT) imaging before and after angiogenesis therapy. (Top) MRI shows a large posterolateral defect (arrows) that fills in subsequently. Stress SPECT shows inducible ischemia in the same zone that fills at rest. (Bottom) Two months after angiogenic therapy, MRI shows substantial improvement in blood delivery, but stress SPECT still shows inducible ischemia in the posterolateral wall. Quantitation and even recognition of improvement is very difficult with SPECT because the patient felt much better and exercised much more vigorously on the second visit. MRI is not subject to volitional and placebo effects because the Equitime deficit is measured at rest on both visits. MRI Equitime identifies the defects that show up as stress-inducible ischemia by SPECT, but without requiring the exercise demand and its confounding impact on assessment of improvement.

159

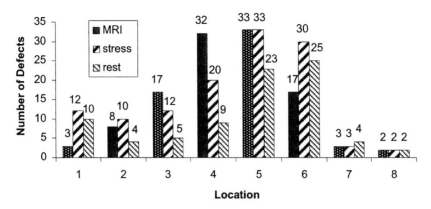

Fig. 10. Comparison of Equitime magnetic resonance imaging (MRI) and stress/rest single photon emission computed tomography (SPECT). Defects from Equitime MRI at rest correspond to stress SPECT defects; MRI detects defects at rest that are not evident by rest SPECT. MRI has the advantage that the rest condition is more reproducible, and thus much more sensitive to improvements following angiogenic therapy. In the membranous septum area (6), automated SPECT analysis appears to overestimate defects.

details of the pulse sequence. However, inversion recovery offers better contrast. Direct comparison in clinical application from our experience shows that inversion recovery offers a mean contrast of 35%, whereas saturation recovery offers 25%, a difference of practical importance.

Angiogenesis-Sensitive MRI

In the course of performing blood arrival imaging in a porcine model of chronic ischemia for an angiogenesis trial, we encountered the "case of the missing heart." MRI showed chest wall, but the chest cavity and upper abdomen were blacked out. Investigation revealed that the animal had swallowed a magnetic beebee, a small sphere that emanated magnetic fields erasing signals from the abdomen and chest. On removal of the beebee, the heart returned. We reasoned that if a small beebee could have such a powerful effect at a distance, perhaps that effect could be scaled down to provide a marker for microvascular development.

We devised a phantom representing microvessels in a tissue background and designed a pulse sequence that maximized the dark flare due to magnetic susceptibility disturbances of contrast agent arrival analogous to the effect of the magnetic beebee destroying signal coherence from the entire heart (Fig. 11). On arrival of a clinically approved MRI contrast agent, gadolinium DPTA, to the microtubules, susceptibility imaging produced a signal void visible by T2*-sensitive MRI. We then

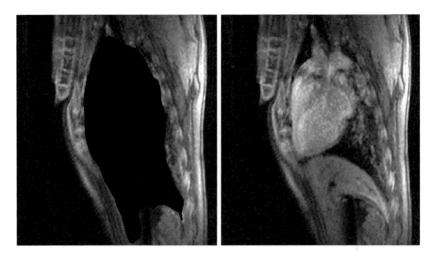

Fig. 11. Magnetic resonance imaging of the chest failed to show the heart in a live pig that had swallowed a small magnetic beebee. Magnetic field disturbance from the 2-mm metal sphere erased signals from the chest. This strong effect at a distance from a small source proved useful in the development of angiogenesis imaging and cell tracking.

applied similar technique to study animals using echo-planar for pure T2* sensitivity. The results were mixed: as constrast agent arrived in a zone of neovascular development, there was a distinctive dark flare that demarcated the extent of neovascular development, as desired. However, when the contrast agent filled the left ventricle, there was a much wider flare that erased the signals from the entire heart (Fig. 12). Only after washout from the left ventricle was the neovascular zone measurable. This partial success meant that early stages of neovascular development could be detected and measured, but if blood delivery improved the arrival time would occur during the blackout of the heart and thus be undetectable. We then invented a novel form of MRI, a T2*/T1 spatial frequency hybrid that applies different contrast mechanisms at different spatial frequencies. We reasoned that the left ventricle constitutes a large fraction of the field of view and therefore affects low spatial frequencies (multiply the image by a slow-changing sine wave to describe the signal distribution), whereas microvascular dark flare is confined to the wall of the heart, requiring a high spatial frequency (multiply the signal pattern by a fast changing sine wave to fit the pattern of bright-dark signal changes). Therefore, a spatial frequency hybrid could minimize the effect of left ventricular filling and amplify the effect of contrast arrival to neovascular development zones. This invention worked and was

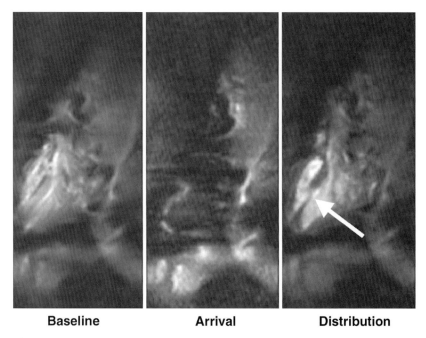

Baseline   **Arrival**   **Distribution**

Fig. 12. Echo-planar magnetic resonance imaging (MRI) eliminates T1-sensitivity. When contrast agent fills the heart, T2* effect (magnetic susceptibility) reduces signal from the region, blotting out the adjacent heart wall. During distribution it may still identify abnormal zones (arrow), but a crucial time period was blanked out that could mask early disease. (Echo-planar MR images [925/28] matrix of 128*128, triggering delay of 0 second, flip angle of 900.)

awarded a US patent as well as National Institutes of Health (NIH) grant support. This new MRI method was validated by microsphere methods and histology. To improve comparative resolution, we came up with another invention, elastic match imaging, which provides a means for submillimeter definition of collateral-dependent myocardium as an independent measure of neovascular development.

Elastic match imaging compares two volumes to identify what is distinct. Elastic match CT of angiogenesis is analogous to shadow microspheres *(71)*, which identify collateral-dependent myocardium surviving because of angiogenesis. If one volume is obtained on injecting iodinated contrast while the territory beyond an obstruction is pressurized with saline and a second image volume is obtained during injection without the backpressure, the difference identifies the zone of collateral-dependent myocardium *(72)*. Figure 13 shows an example. The results of high-resolution CT and MRI methods agree well (*r* = 0.95) *(73)*.

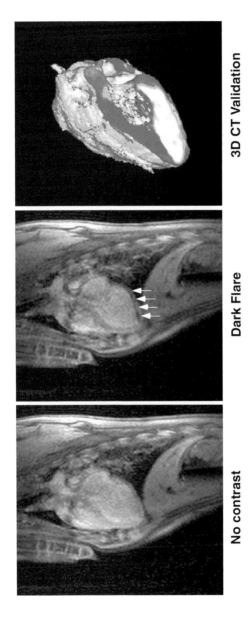

No contrast **Dark Flare** **3D CT Validation**

Fig. 13. Validation of hybrid angiogenesis-sensitive magnetic resonance (AS-MR) with elastic match computed tomography (EM-CT). EM-CT compares distribution of contrast when distal vessel beyond blockage has high backpressure, or not, to eliminate flow through microvessel collaterals and define from the difference the collateral dependent zone(s). AS-MR exhibits angiogenesis zones by a transient dark flare in hybrid T1-T2* imaging. The zones and percent myocardium and histology agree ($r = 0.95$). MR image was obtained by hybrid T2*-T1 imaging with TR/TE 5.6/2.0, flip angle 8-12, slice thickness 5 mm, matrix 256×256. CT was obtained with 180 mA, 120 kV, 1-mm section thickness, matrix of 512×512. From ref. 73.

163

Angiogenesis imaging is crucial to the identification of effective agents, routes of delivery, and regimens to achieve therapeutic angiogenesis as a means of "bypassing bypasses" and providing new vascular supply to jeopardized myocardium. These methods are also relevant to tumor angiogenesis, where they may provide bench-to-bedside transition for therapies aimed at impeding tumor angiogenesis to rob cancers of their blood supply.

Figures 14 and 15 are examples of angiogenesis-sensitive (AS)-MRI. Figure 14 shows AS-MRI before and after laser treatment. Note the punctate zones of dark flare. These findings are consistent with angiogenesis induced by focal inflammatory response to the laser-induced tissue damage. The results are spotty and associated with tissue damage, suggesting that laser revascularization has limited value. Also, the regions of myocardium behind the papillary muscles are not treated. Figure 15 shows AS-MRI before and after treatment with basic fibroblast growth factor (bFGF)-2. Note the dark flare indicating zones of neovascular development in the anteroseptal and posterolateral walls, both of which had exhibited impaired blood delivery prior to treatment. At 1 and 2 mo after treatment, angiogenesis dark flare shows progression inwards from the outer aspects of the ischemic territory, associated with progressive improvement in blood delivery.

Peripheral artery disease can be assessed without contrast agents by observing a series of cross sections under conditions in which stationary tissues deplete longitudinal magnetization ("saturation") while arterial vessels with untapped magnetization produce bright signals (time-of-flight, or TOF, enhancement). This is a form of "arterial spin labeling" (ASL), so named because the signal sources for MRI are known as "spins." Figure 16 shows such images, in which arterial sections appear as bright dots in the short-axis views. Measuring the brightness and size of the vascular elements provides a measure of vascularity that can be followed over time. Such data can be acquired with an electrocardiogram (ECG) EKG trigger so that the inflow is consistent in relation to the pulse, but that slows down the acquisition time. If the data are acquired quickly without pulse synchrony, the images show a series of bright dots aligned with each vessel in the phase-cycle-encoded direction, an effect known as "pulsation artifact." Although pulsation artifact can interfere with visualization and with quantification of vascularity, our lab has shown that the artifact can be converted to useful information that improves the accuracy of assessing vascularity (unpublished data). The data can be decomposed into a sum $Kb + Kv f$, where Kb is the Fourier transform of background tissue, Kv is the Fourier transform of the arterial vessel sections, and f is a filter representing the pulsation enhance-

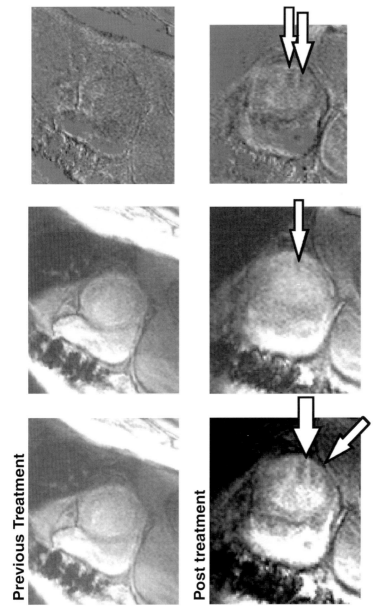

Previous Treatment

Post treatment

Fig. 14. Laser Treatment-collateral extension: (top) previous treatment; (bottom) posttreatment.

165

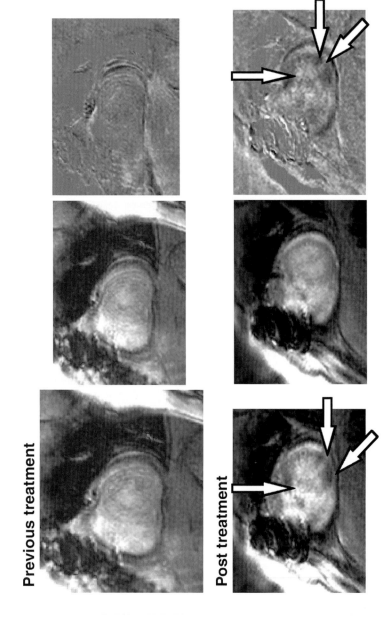

Previous treatment

Post treatment

Fig. 15. Intracoronary fibroblast growth factor (FGF)—Collat Extent: (top) previous treatment; (bottom) posttreatment.

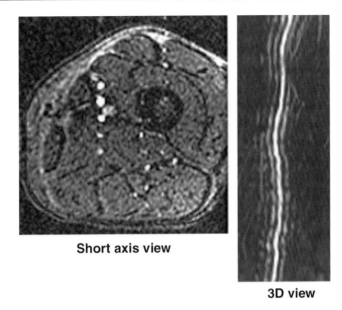

Short axis view

3D view

Fig. 16. Pulsation artifact in time-of-flight magnetic resonace angiography (MRA) of peripheral vasculature. Short-axis imaging (left) shows that a pulsatile vessel appears replicated in the phase-encoded direction (arrow). This produces ghosts in the three-dimesional (3D) view (right). The 3D view is a projection from a series of contiguous short-axis slices.

ment, analogous to a comb filter. Inverting *f* eliminates the artifact and remaps the displaced signal to the arterial segments. Figure 17 shows TOF-MRI short-axis views without ghost artifact from a mouse, assessing vascular development over time after femoral artery occlusion followed by angiogenic stimulation. The left femoral supply disappears postocclusion but is replaced in time by smaller vessels. The right side was not occluded.

Functional Consequences

The consequences of improved blood supply are improved function of the tissue supplied under stress or rest conditions. Regional cardiac function is typically measured as radial wall motion and wall thickening. There are two basic approaches. The fixed approach chooses an image plane of interest. The heart may be imaged in a long-axis view (the long axis of the left ventricle bisects the mitral valve hinge points and passes through the apex). Short-axis views are perpendicular to the long axis and show a cross section of the left ventricle typically as a bagel or doughnut shape, with the right ventricle wrapped around that as a cres-

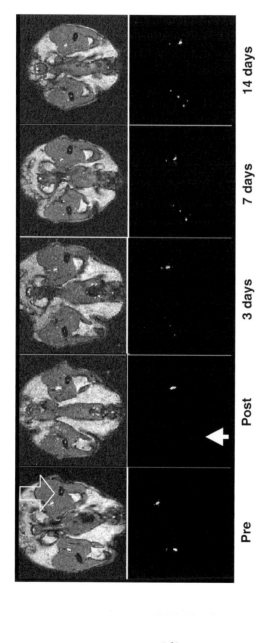

Pre   **Post**   **3 days**   **7 days**   **14 days**

Fig. 17. Time-of-flight magnetic resonance imaging (TOF-MRI) in mouse. MRI is performed such that blood inflow produces a bright signal that can be identified and isolated to produce the lower image series. The preocclusion image shows a left and right femoral artery. The postocclusion image shows occlusion of the left femoral (above the white arrow). Within 2 wk after angiogenic therapy, the left develops new smaller vessels. The dark zone with central fat signal is the femur (hollow arrow). Data from ref. 81.

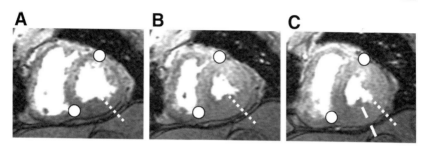

Fig. 18. Short axis images for Serial Motion Assessment by Reference Tracking (SMART) tracking: (**A**) end-diastole; (**B**) same level at peak systole; (**C**) tracked level at peak systole. The white dots mark the junctions of right and left ventricles. The dotted lines mark the position of the radial through the center of the maximum perfusion deficit in diastole. The dashed line in **C** shows where the corresponding radial moved during systole, based on SMART tracking. These images are from the same case as shown in Figs. 3 and 4. Technique: TR/TE = 10.7/6.2 ms, matrix = 256 × 256, FOV = 360 × 360 mm. Data from ref. *60.*

cent. Fixed-plane function is typically assessed by choosing a particular clock face position in a short-axis view to compare radial distance from the center to inner wall (radial length), and from the inner to outer wall (wall thickness) at end-diastole (maximal dilation) and peak systole (maximal contraction). Both radial motion and wall thickening are expressed as the change from diastole to systole divided by the diastolic dimension. Alternatively, wall thickness change can be reported as thickness release—the change from diastole to systole divided by the systolic dimension. Wall thickness release represents the metabolically active component of the cycle (ATP is consumed to enable relaxation), and the values are less subject to noise because the denominator is larger.

Figure 18 illustrates the primary problem with fixed measurements. As the heart contracts, the base approaches the apex, the axis tilts, and the heart rotates. Fixed measurements fail to take those movements into account and end up comparing different regions at systole vs diastole. Tracking the motion (SMART measurement) *(60)* takes these motions into account when calculating radial motion and wall thickness release. We have found that SMART measurement is twice as sensitive to impairments of motion and thickness release, and its greater sensitivity and specificity doubles the power to discern treatment effect resulting from angiogenesis (Fig. 19).

Nuclear Imaging

Nuclear imaging injects a radioactive isotope and then identifies its distribution in tissue, e.g., in heart muscle. Areas that are ischemic and

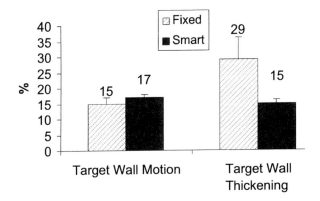

Fig. 19. Wall motion and thickening for fixed vs Serial Motion Assessment by Reference Tracking (SMART) measurements. The bar graph shows motion (left pair) and thickening (right pair) from SMART measurements of ischemic myocardium (right bar of each pair) vs fixed-plane, fixed-radial measurements (left bar of each pair). SMART reports significantly lower values, providing a greater distinction from normal myocardium.

have impaired blood delivery are identified by relative reduction in the uptake of tracer by heart muscle. The earliest clinical methods established thallium-201 scintigraphy as a means of identifying inducible ischemia and infarction. One of the key limitations remains its poor spatial resolution (~10 mm). The limit of resolution approximates the thickness of a normal heart, which is larger than the expected changes from angiogenesis. As a result, significant but smaller changes in perfusion may well be missed. In 121 patients examined by thallium and x-ray angiography, Freedman et al. found that thallium scans had poor predictive value regarding the presence or absence of angiographically demonstrable collaterals *(74)*.

By rotating a collimated array of detectors and applying computer reconstructions analogous to those used by CT, SPECT imaging enables resolution of the isotope distribution to select planes and three-dimensional (3D) summaries, rather than just a volume projection. Also, the use of technetium-99m (Tc-99m) sestamibi instead of thallium-201 allows higher dosage and thus better image quality.

Thallium-201 (Tl-201), a group IIIa transitional metal, is handled by cells similar to potassium. Half of Tl-201 uptake is blocked by Na/K ATPase inhibitors such as digoxin. An additional 15% is blocked by Na/K/Cl co-transport inhibitors. The remaining 35% of uptake does not depend on active transport. Tl-201 uptake is roughly proportional to flow, but it underestimates the extremes. Typically, 2% of the thallium dose accumulates in the heart 10 min after an intravenous bolus. Normal myocytes extract 90% of the available Tl-201 on the first pass, whereas ischemic cells under the same conditions of flow extract less (75%). Thus, uptake can be reduced by a stenosis to a greater extent than predicted by flow alone. Subsequently, thallium washes out fastest where flow is highest, independent of ischemia, plus there is continued uptake from recirculating thallium, resulting in equalization of counts in viable myocardium. That process is called redistribution. Uptake is typically equal in all viable myocardium at 4 h (early redistribution), but viable tissue with obstructed blood supply can require 24 h to achieve equal counts (late redistribution). Alternatively, late redistribution can be accelerated by a second injection of thallium to boost the blood levels. Persisting defects indicate scar (infarction). Partial thickness hyperemia overlaying ischemic subendocardium can mask an ischemic zone at peak stress and reveal it later due to fast washout from the hyperemic region, a situation called reverse redistribution. Reverse redistribution can be seen in an acute subendocardial infarction after thrombolysis. Reverse redistribution also occurs in multivessel disease when enhanced washout in zones of mixed scar and viable tissue are compared to zones that are ischemic. It can also occur by excess background subtraction or by changes in extracardiac attenuation (liver dome, breast).

Thus, thallium scans are interpreted by looking for regions of relatively low uptake, called defects. If defects occur at stress and not at rest, they signify induced ischemia or extracardiac attenuation ("breast artifact" or "liver dome/diaphragm attenuation"). If defects occur both at stress and rest, scar is implicated, but this should be confirmed by examining again after reinjection or at 24 h. If defects occur only at rest, they likely represent extracardiac attenuation or a processing artifact, but that could also represent partial thickness ischemia and hyperemia or multivessel balanced disease (reverse redistribution).

Tl-201 decays by electron capture, when an orbital electron combines with a proton in the nucleus to form a neutron, releasing characteristic x-rays and an Auger electron. The half-life of thallium-201 is 73 h. Thallium has characteristic photopeaks at 135 and 167 keV and emits mercury x-rays from 69 to 83 keV during imaging. The image resolution is 1 cm, the thickness of a normal heart, so thallium imaging is not able to discern the partial-thickness improvements that occur with angiogenesis. Thallium is difficult to quantify. Its primary value is an all-or-none determination as to whether maximally tolerated stress has induced ischemia in a large region of the heart and whether early and/or late redistribution images demonstrate viability in a large region of concern. The viability assessment is imperfect, as even severely injured cells exhibit uptake due to the nonspecific, energy-independent binding. Thus, it is no surprise that thallium imaging was unable to identify collateral development *(74)*.

Tc-99m sestamibi is a lipophilic isonitrile complex that carries a +1 charge. Tc-99m is meta-stable, decaying to Tc-99 by emission of 140-keV γ-rays with a half-life of 6 h. Both the short half-life and the absence of Auger electron emission reduce the biohazard such that much higher dosages of Tc-99m sestamibi than thallium-201 can be given (30 vs 4 mCi), resulting in better image quality. However, there are important biological differences. With Tl-201, uptake is roughly proportional to flow and redistribution indicates viability. Tc-99m uptake is limited by an earlier plateau at 2 mg/mL/min (dilated coronary arteries normally exceed 4 mg/mL/min). Also, redistribution is negligible, and so Tc-99m fails to report viability if the delivery is impaired. Uptake of Tc-99m sestamibi requires a negative potential at the cell membrane (*Em*) and across the inner mitochondrial membrane ($\Delta P\Psi = -150$ to -200 mV). The mitochondria concentrate the sestamibi relative to cytosol, and that which stays in the cytosol is effectively irreversibly bound to cytosolic proteins. It follows, therefore, that cells with high negative *Em* and $\Delta\Psi$; e.g., heart, liver, and certain tumors, accumulate more sestamibi. Sestamibi uptake has the advantage of no nonspecific component as seen with Tl-201. High uptake is not proportional to flow or to accumulated delivery. Ischemic cells depolarize (lose transmembrane potential), as do the mitochondria within ischemic cells, and recovery of transmembrane potential is slow. Thus, after a region undergoes an ischemic insult, it exhibits reduced sestamibi uptake.

Approximately 2.8% of a dose injected at rest and 3.2% of a dose injected during peak stress concentrates in the myocardium, whereas 90% of the injected dose clears from the body in 5 min. Liver uptake is considerable, but that substantively clears within 1 h of injection. Myocardial uptake half-time is 9.5 min. The sestamibi retained by the myocardium clears in approx 25 h, which is slower than its radioactive half-life (~6 h). Thus, imaging may take place anytime between 40 min after injection and approx 12 h later. Typically rest imaging is performed first at one-quarter dose, or one may use a 2-d protocol full dose each, or one may combine sestamibi for stress and thallium for rest and redistribution.

Like thallium, sestamibi imaging is interpreted by looking for large regions of relatively low uptake within the heart muscle (excluding the membranous septum). A defect at stress only generally indicates that ischemia was induced. A matched defect at stress and rest suggests scar or extracardiac attenuation. Unlike thallium, a rest defect suggests artifact only because of the negligible redistribution of sestamibi. Even though the signal is stronger because sestamibi is more efficient and uses a higher dosage of tracer, it is still difficult to quantify, and it is insensitive to gradations of improvement that one expects with ongoing angiogenesis. The primary use is to determine if maximally tolerated physical or pharmaceutical stress can induce ischemia in a quadrant of the heart. Also, because of the negligible redistribution, sestamibi may be injected during a bout of severe chest pain, e.g., in the emergency room or in prison, followed by imaging up to 12 h later to determine if there was regional impaired uptake of the tracer.

In summary, nuclear imaging by thallium or sestamibi identifies regions of relatively low uptake representing induced ischemia, infarction, or artifact. Image resolution is poor, and results are not sensitive to partial thickness progressive changes, but rather focus on all-or-none determination of inducible ischemia at maximally tolerated stress. Although maximal stress defect definition is very useful clinically, it is not ideal for angiogenesis studies, because successful angiogenesis can produce neovascular elements that protect tissue and even improve exercise tolerance, without necessarily abolishing inducible ischemia. Instead of always testing for maximal stress, one might aim for a fixed stress level, for example, matching baseline exercise peak. That, however, is impractical, because stress is not accurately reproducible as a result of conditioning, medications, hormonal effects, fluid loading, and other variables. The data establishing the diagnostic value of thallium and sestamibi are based on maximal stress. Also, radionuclide methods have intrinsically low resolution; angiogenesis occurs on a scale two orders of magnitude smaller than the resolution of these methods. Experience with SPECT imaging in clinical trials of therapeutic angiogenesis and laser revascu- larization have cast doubt on the ability of nuclear imaging to quantify the progressive changes due to therapeutic angiogenesis.

PET uses a distinct form of radioactive decay to map out the location of tracers. Positron emitters release a particle that collides with an electron within a millimeter or so of the source. The collision results in the emission of a pair of γ-rays nearly 180° apart. Detection of paired γ emissions, each at 511 keV, identifies a line from the collision, and relative times of detection can indicate where along the line the collision occurred. The collision loci are mapped to produce a low-resolution image indicating the approximate location of the positron emissions. The paired emissions improve specificity over SPECT and obviate filtering of backscatter, which greatly improves sensitivity. PET studies have proven very useful in mapping specific molecule distributions. For example, distribution of oxygen-15 provides information about perfusion, fractional volume of distribution of water, and blood volume (75).

Fluorodeoxyglucose (FDG) is commonly used in PET studies to trace glucose metabolism and has been applied to demonstrate correspondence between angiogenesis-induced increases in microvasculature and glucose utilization *(76,77)*. The great sensitivity of PET is useful for mapping the tissue distribution of angiogenic agents *(29)*. PET can be applied to clarify ligand-receptor interactions, including receptors essential to angiogenesis *(78)*. Unfortunately, PET has limitations in assessing response to therapy over time *(46)*. Positron-emitting isotopes are produced in a cyclotron, an expensive instrument that accelerates particles close to the speed of light. The short half-life of most positron emitters requires that they be produced near the scanner. This factor makes PET costly and limits its availability.

In practice, three agents are used at sites that cannot afford to maintain their own cyclotron: germanium-68, fluorine-18, and rubidium-82. Germanium-68 is a long-lived PET calibration source (270.8 d). It lasts too long to be used in vivo (too much exposure), but it can be used for transmission imaging to compute attenuation corrections. Fluorodeoxyglucose utilizes fluorine-18, which has a physical half-life of 1.83 h, so it can be shipped from a production site at an increased dose a few hours away from the scanner and used in vivo. Fluorine is relatively easy to use as a marker on specific molecules of interest to angiogenesis *(79)*. Rubidium-82, a potassium analog, has a half-life of 1.273 min, too short to be shipped from another site, but it does not require a local cyclotron because it can be produced fresh from a relatively inexpensive strontium-82 generator, which has a half-life of 25.5 d. Rubidium-82, like thallium and Tc-99m sestamibi, exhibits high uptake in normal myocardium.

SMALL ANIMAL ANGIOGENESIS STUDIES

Radiology has promoted the development of many useful imaging techniques. Although these have been developed primarily for application to humans, most can be scaled down and applied to mice as well, including x-ray, radionuclide imaging, MRI, and CT. To the extent that all aspects may be scaled down together, the resultant capabilities are quite comparable in small animal applications as in imaging patients. In the case of MRI applied to mice, for example, the field of view is on the order of 300 cm for patients and 3 cm for mice. Thus, image resolution ranges from 1 to 10 mm for human patients and 10 to 100 μm for mice (Fig. 20).

The principal difficulty in imaging mice is heart rate. Whereas patients have a heart rate of 50–100 beats per minute (bpm), the mouse rate is 250–650 bpm, and young mice have heart rates that exceed 600 bpm.

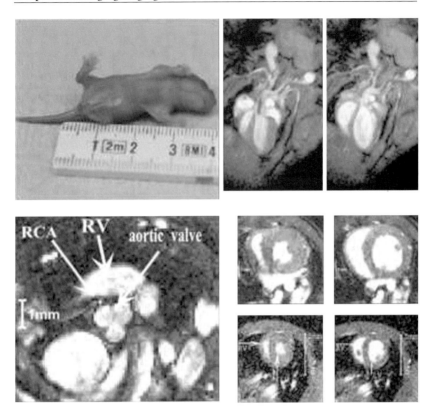

Fig. 20. Mouse magnetic resonance imaging (MRI). Images of live mice (upper left) with weights ranging from 2 to 20 g were obtained on a 7 T Bruker MRI micro-imaging scanner using gradients capable of 870 mT/m with 280 μS rise time. The MRI used a FLASH imaging sequence with flow compensation, TR/TE 4/1.6 mS, field of view 3 cm, acquisition time 100 s *(43)*. (Upper right) long-axis images of the heart with blood supply white and heart wall and other tissues gray. (Lower left) short-axis view through the aortic root showing the three leaflets of the aortic valve and the right coronary artery (RCA). (Lower right) short-axis images of two levels: systole on the left and diastole on the right. Data from ref. *80*.

The corresponding cycle length (time interval from beat to beat) is computed by 600/HR, where HR is the heart rate in bpm. The short cycle length for mice requires adaptations to the imaging methods.

The primary imaging methods of interest in the evaluation of angiogenesis are those that identify impaired blood delivery, the status of neovascular development, and its consequences. These methods are, respectively, perfusion-sensitive imaging, collateral-sensitive imaging, and functional imaging.

Functional imaging of the heart requires comparison of peak systole to end-diastole. Imaging of patients typically applies 50 ms per data collection, making it easy to collect 12 frames, and as many as 60, per cardiac cycle. The result is a sequence of 12–60 image frames played repeatedly as a loop to portray the contraction cycle. Systole is taken as the smallest volume and end-diastole as the largest. Functional imaging of mice requires a different approach. Fewer data are acquired for each image, and typically only one or two phases in the cardiac cycle are acquired at field strengths of 4–9 T. With imaging of just one phase of the cardiac cycle, the trigger-delay, or time after the R-wave of the ECG for initiation of imaging in each cycle, must be adjusted to correspond to peak systole and again to correspond to end-diastole. Unlike imaging in patients, where a delay of zero practically guarantees a good end-diastolic image frame, diastolic imaging in mice should apply a delay past the T-wave of the ECG because there is not enough time immediately after the R-wave to complete diastolic data collection by the usual methods. Recent advances in magnet technology allow imaging at 14 T and higher, which provides much more signal per unit time of acquisition. Combining that with recent advances in fast imaging may enable imaging thin short-axis sections of the mouse heart every heartbeat, a major advantage for perfusion-sensitive and AS-MRI in mice.

The usual methods for perfusion-sensitive imaging of the heart acquire diastolic images repeatedly over time as a bolus of contrast agent arrives at the myocardium or other tissue of interest. Impaired blood supply can result in a lower rate of rise in signal intensity, a lower peak, and a delayed peak. Using Equitime, the time it takes to accumulate the integrated contrast rise observed in the left ventricle on the first pass proved to be the most sensitive and specific of 30 different measures. That method can be applied to mice, but one must either reduce resolution to enable completing an image with adequate sensitivity to contrast arrival every heartbeat or invoke cross-RR (skip one or more cycles for each cycle imaged) to provide the time needed for image resolution and/or for adequate sensitivity to contrast arrival. (Imaging rapidly shifts the T1 sensitivity of the images, which can reduce sensitivity to contrast agent arrival.) While skipping one cycle for each cycle imaged (RR × 2) is tolerable even when imaging patients, as one extends the time between images to increase resolution and/or contrast, the ability to discern differences in the timing of blood arrival between normal and impaired zones is reduced.

Angiogenesis-sensitive imaging uses a hybrid of T1 and T2* with the demarcation of neovascular development occurring as a dark flare by T2* contrast at the time of contrast agent arrival at the zone of neovascular

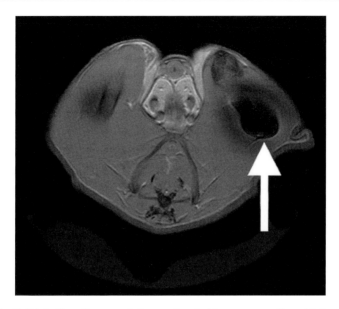

Fig. 21. Cell labeling. Iron particles are loaded into stem cells, which are then injected into the animal with targeting to specific disease. Focal blackout blooms much larger than cell size. The size of the blooming can be adjusted down as desired by T1-T2* hybrid imaging. Bovine smooth muscle cells were expanded in culture and labeled with iron oxide nanoparticles (ferumoxides solution). Transfection agent poly-L-lysine facilitated the uptake of iron oxide at 5.5 µg/ mL of media. The imaging parameters were: TR/TE = 800/40 ms; NEX = 1; slice thickness 3 mm; flip angle = 90; matrix 512×512.

development *(73)*. Reduced recovery time between cycles is less of a problem for AS-MRI because short recovery primarily affects T1 sensitivity. T2*-T1 hybrid imaging can also be used in cell tracking (Fig. 21) to adjust the size of dark flare for conspicuity of labeled cells at the desired scale.

Our laboratory also uses projection x-ray angiography (XRA) to document changes in microvessel development. The projection images are analyzed for vascular fraction, fractal dimension, and mean vessel diameter serially over time with angiogenic treatment or control. Figure 22 shows an example of mouse XRA, exhibiting small vessel recruitment/ redevelopment a week after unilateral femoral artery occlusion (arrow).

CONCLUSIONS

Imaging strategies for therapeutic angiogenesis are now available to measure angiogenic responses over time, including molecular markers,

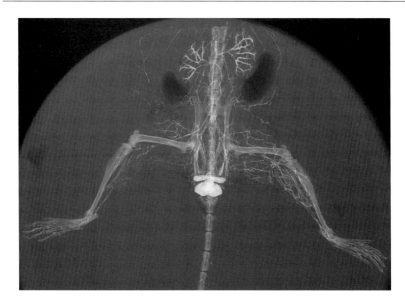

Fig. 22. Mouse angiogram. Serial imaging after femoral artery occlusion shows small collaterals that develop in conjunction with ischemia-induced angiogenesis. Resolution: 1.3 μm; magnification: ×0.167; matrix = 2652 × 3160; field of view = 93 × 109 mm.

vessel leakiness, microvessel volume, and metabolic and functional correlates. In vitro techniques offer microscopic views that assess vascular element formation in response to different agents and different doses. The techniques extend to in vivo models, especially useful in conjunction with genetic knockouts. Large animal and patient studies of angiogenesis have been examined most effectively by MRI and PET using methods such as angiogenesis-sensitive MRI (a T2*-T1 spatial frequency hybrid), blood arrival imaging (during first pass of an injected contrast agent), SMART assessment to track wall motion and wall thickening, cell tracking, and use of molecular tracers. MRI perfusion-sensitive imaging is best accomplished by inversion-recovery and limited to three injections within one session. Equitime reports how long it takes for specified zones to accumulate the contrast agent available on the first pass with high sensitivity and specificity. There are numerous other methods, but they performed less well by ROC analyses. Stress studies before and after angiogenic treatments evaluate inducible ischemic wall motion and wall thickness release abnormalities and/or changes in blood distribution ("flow reserve") to document the consequences of changes in microvascular blood supply. Vasodilator studies identify flow reserve but can underestimate angiogenesis because new microvessels do not exhibit a mature vasodilator response. AS-MRI and Equitime are performed at rest, which improves the ability to detect changes over time. These techniques are more accurate in measuring serial changes following therapeutic angiogenesis than prior alternatives such as sestamibi imaging and XRA.

SUMMARY

When blood supply is impaired and cannot be repaired, angiogenesis, or new vessel development, can offer a vital alternative to severe ischemia and tissue death. Clinically, we infer the presence of angiogenesis when we observe that tissue is alive and functional distal to an occluded artery, because collateral blood supply is not seen without angiogenesis. The basic goal of therapeutic angiogenesis is to make this occurrence more common and more effective. Recognition of angiogenesis and tissue viability are important guides to intervention, and also can help identify medications and activities that help or hurt the cause.

Advances in imaging technologies offer many ways to evaluate microvascular development anywhere in the body. New evolving capabilities include neovascular-sensitive MRI, which identifies the tissue zones supplied by neovascular elements, focal high-resolution vascular imaging, optical systems, molecular imaging to identify the locations of proteins selectively expressed in new vessels and the location and prevalence of receptors that activate angiogenesis, and methods that identify microvascular density and numerous parameters of vascular structure and blood delivery. In addition there have been significant improvements in methods to assess tissue viability and improved methods to quantify blood delivery, assess inducible ischemia, and evaluate tissue function.

If prevention of heart attacks or resolution of inducible ischemia were the only measures of success, tissue protection and improved exercise tolerance might be overlooked because of residual inducible ischemia. Studies designed to look at late consequences are confounded by the interim progression of other diseases. Use of exercise tolerance and symptom history as surrogate endpoints for treatment benefit are unreliable because of subjectivity, bias toward success, and high variability. However, new advanced imaging methods provide means to identify early changes that occur within tissue owing to angiogenesis. These methods report the status of neovascular microcirculatory development more directly than previously possible. Techniques initially considered cost prohibitive have turned out to have a cost advantage because they markedly reduce the number of studies needed to identify treatment effects. In addition to methods that can identify neovascular development in the heart and other tissues, there are now also methods to identify the prevalence and location of the growth factor receptors and other surface proteins that play key roles in angiogenesis.

REFERENCES

1. Bortone AS, D'Agostino D, Schena S, et al. Inflammatory response and angiogenesis after percutaneous transmyocardial laser revascularization. Ann Thorac Surg 2000;70(3):1134–1138.
2. Ruel M, Sellke FW. Angiogenic protein therapy. Semin Thorac Cardiovasc Surg 2003;15(3):222–235.
3. Pearlman JD, Laham RJ, Post M, et al. Medical imaging techniques in the evaluation of strategies for therapeutic angiogenesis. Curr Pharm Des 2002;8(16):1467–1496.
4. Neeman M. Functional and molecular MR imaging of angiogenesis: seeing the target, seeing it work. J Cell Biochem Suppl 2002;39:11–17.
5. McDonald DM, Choyke PL. Imaging of angiogenesis: from microscope to clinic. Nat Med 2003;9(6):713–725.
6. Scappaticci FA. Mechanisms and future directions for angiogenesis-based cancer therapies. J Clin Oncol 2002;20(18):3906–3927.
7. Christofferson R, Claesson-Welsh L, Muhr C. [Anti-angiogenic drugs probable complement in cancer therapy]. Lakartidningen 2002;99(42):4138–4139,4142–4148.
8. Cristofanilli M, Charnsangavej C, Hortobagyi GN. Angiogenesis modulation in cancer research: novel clinical approaches. Nat Rev Drug Discov 2002;1(6):415–426.
9. Weber WA, Haubner R, Vabuliene E, et al. Tumor angiogenesis targeting using imaging agents. Q J Nucl Med 2001;45(2):179–182.
10. Anderson H, Price P, Blomley M, et al. Measuring changes in human tumour vasculature in response to therapy using functional imaging techniques. Br J Cancer 2001;85(8):1085–1093.
11. Nagatoro T, Fujita K, Murata E, Akita M. Angiogenesis and fibroblast growth factors (FGFs) in a three-dimensional collagen gel culture. Okajimas Folia Anat Jpn 2003;80(1):7–14.
12. Montanez E, Cassaroli-Marano RP, Vilaro S, Pagan R. Comparative study of tube assembly in three-dimensional collagen matrix and on Matrigel coats. Angiogenesis 2002;5(3):167–172.
13. Go RS. Ritman EL, Owen WG. Angiogenesis in rat aortic rings stimulated by very low concentrations of serum and plasma. Angiogenesis 2003;6(1):25–29.
14. Woodman SE, Ashton AW, Schubert W, et al. Caveolin-1 knockout mice show an impaired angiogenic response to exogenous stimuli. Am J Pathol 2003;162(6):2059–2068.
15. Duff SE, Garland JM, Kumar S. CD105 is important for angiogenesis: evidence and potential applications. FASEB J 2003;17(9):984–992.
16. Berglin L, Sarman S, van der Ploeg I, et al. Reduced choroidal neovascular membrane formation in matrix metalloproteinase-2-deficient mice. Invest Ophthalmol Vis Sci 2003;44(1):403–408.
17. Cattelino A, Liebner S, Gallini R, et al. The conditional inactivation of the beta-catenin gene in endothelial cells causes a defective vascular pattern and increased vascular fragility. J Cell Biol 2003;162(6):1111–1122.
18. Kusters B, de Waal RM, Wesseling P, et al. Differential effects of vascular endothelial growth factor A isoforms in a mouse brain metastasis model of human melanoma. Cancer Res 2003;63(17):5408–5413.
19. Winter PM, Morawski Am, Caruthers SD, et al. Molecular imaging of angiogenesis in early-stage atherosclerosis with alpha(v)beta3-integrin-targeted nanoparticles. Circulation 2003;108(18):2270–2274.

20. Fanelli M, Locopo N, Gattuso D, Gasparini G. Assessment of tumor vascularization: immunohistochemical and non-invasive methods. Int J Biol Markers 1999;14(4):218–231.
21. Chang CS, Su CY, Lin TC. Scanning electron microscopy observation of vascularization around hydroxyapatite using vascular corrosion casts. J Biomed Mater Res 1999;48(4):411–416.
22. Lin, P.C. Optical imaging and tumor angiogenesis. J Cell Biochem 2003;90(3): 484–491.
23. Stanton AW, Drysdale SB, Patel R, et al. Expansion of microvascular bed and increased solute flux in human basal cell carcinoma in vivo, measured by fluorescein video angiography. Cancer Res 2003;63(14):3969–3979.
24. Yang M, Jiang P, Moossa AR, Penman S, Hoffman RM. Dual-color fluorescence imaging distinguishes tumor cells from induced host angiogenic vessels and stromal cells. Proc Natl Acad Sci USA 2003;100:14,259–14,262.
25. Krix M, et al. Comparison of intermittent-bolus contrast imaging with conventional power Doppler sonography: quantification of tumour perfusion in small animals. Ultrasound Med Biol 2003;29(8):1093–103.
26. Shoji T, Yonemitsu Y, Komori K, et al. Intramuscular gene transfer of FGF-2 attenuates endothelial dysfunction and inhibits intimal hyperplasia of vein grafts in poor-runoff limbs of rabbit. Am J Physiol Heart Circ Physiol 2003;285(1):H173–H182.
27. Newton DJ, Khan F, Belch JJ, Mitchell MR, Leese GP. Blood flow changes in diabetic foot ulcers treated with dermal replacement therapy. J Foot Ankle Surg 2002;41(4):233–237.
28. Blankenberg FG, Eckelman WC, Strauss HW, et al. Role of radionuclide imaging in trials of antiangiogenic therapy. Acad Radiol 2000;7(10):851–867.
29. Gupta N, Price PM, Aboagye EO. PET for in vivo pharmacokinetic and pharmacodynamic measurements. Eur J Cancer 2002;38(16):2094–2107.
30. Schmidt MA, Chakrabarti A, Shamim-Uzzaman Q, Kaciroti N, Koeppe RA, Rajagopalan S. Calf flow reserve with H(2)(15)O PET as a quantifiable index of lower extremity flow. J Nucl Med 2003;44(6):915–919.
31. Gibson CM, Ryan K, Sparano A, et al. Angiographic methods to assess human coronary angiogenesis. Am Heart J 1999;137(1):169–179.
32. Wang ZQ, Li JS, Lu GM, Zhang XH, Chen ZK, Meng K. Correlation of CT enhancement, tumor angiogenesis and pathologic grading of pancreatic carcinoma. World J Gastroenterol 2003;9(9):2100–2104.
33. Maehara N. Experimental microcomputed tomography study of the 3D microangioarchitecture of tumors. Eur Radiol 2003;13(7):1559–1565.
34. Pearlman JD, Laham RJ, Simons M. Coronary angiogenesis: detection in vivo with MR imaging sensitive to collateral neocirculation—preliminary study in pigs. Radiology 2000;214(3):801–807.
35. Bremer C, Mustafa M, Bagdanov A Jr, Ntziachristos V, Petrovsky A, Weissleder R. Steady-state blood volume measurements in experimental tumors with different angiogenic burdens a study in mice. Radiology 2003;226(1):214–220.
36. Muhling O, Jerosch-Herold M, Nabauer M, Wilke N. Assessment of ischemic heart disease using magnetic resonance first-pass perfusion imaging. Herz 2003;28(2):82–89.
37. Turetschek K, Praeda A, Flyod E, et al. MRI monitoring of tumor response following angiogenesis inhibition in an experimental human breast cancer model. Eur J Nucl Med Mol Imaging 2003;30(3):448–455.
38. Bhujwalla ZM, Artemov D, Natarajan K, Solaiyappan M, Kollars P, Kristjansen PE. Reduction of vascular and permeable regions in solid tumors detected by macromolecular contrast magnetic resonance imaging after treatment with antiangiogenic agent TNP-470. Clin Cancer Res 2003;9(1):355–362.

39. Herbst RS, Mullani NA, Davis DW, et al. Development of biologic markers of response and assessment of antiangiogenic activity in a clinical trial of human recombinant endostatin. J Clin Oncol 2002;20(18):3804–3814.

40. Pearlman JD, Southern JF, Ackerman JL. Nuclear magnetic resonance microscopy of atheroma in human coronary arteries. Angiology 1991;42(9):726–733.

41. Ashton AW, Yokota R, John G, et al. Inhibition of endothelial cell migration, intercellular communication, and vascular tube formation by thromboxane A(2). J Biol Chem 1999;274(50):35562–35570.

42. Hawrylak N, Ghosh P, Broadus J, Schlueter C, Greenough WT, Lauterbur PC. Nuclear magnetic resonance (NMR) imaging of iron oxide-labeled neural transplants. Exp Neurol 1993;121(2):181–192.

43. Garot J, Unterseeh T, Teigher E, et al. Magnetic resonance imaging of targeted catheter-based implantation of myogenic precursor cells into infarcted left ventricular myocardium. J Am Coll Cardiol 2003;41(10):1841–1816.

44. Kraitchman DL, Heldman AW, Atalar E, et al. In vivo magnetic resonance imaging of mesenchymal stem cells in myocardial infarction. Circulation 2003;107(18):2290–2293.

45. Hill JM, Dick AJ, Raman VK, et al. Serial cardiac magnetic resonance imaging of injected mesenchymal stem cells. Circulation 2003;108(8):1009–1014.

46. Spence AM, Muzi M, Krohn KA. Molecular imaging of regional brain tumor biology. J Cell Biochem Suppl 2002;39:25–35.

47. Neeman M, Dafni H. Structural, functional, and molecular MR imaging of the microvasculature. Annu Rev Biomed Eng 2003;5:29–56.

48. Jayson GC, Zweit J, Jackson A, et al. Molecular imaging and biological evaluation of HuMV833 anti-VEGF antibody: implications for trial design of antiangiogenic antibodies. J Natl Cancer Inst 2002;94(19):1484–1493.

49. Weissleder R, Bogdanov A, Jr, Tung CH, Weinmann HJ. Size optimization of synthetic graft copolymers for in vivo angiogenesis imaging. Bioconjug Chem 2001;12(2):213–219.

50. Kang HW, Weissleder R, Bogdanov A, Jr. Magnetic resonance imaging of inducible E-selectin expression in human endothelial cell culture. Bioconjug Chem 2002;13(1):122–127.

51. Winter PM, Caruthers SD, Kassner A, et al. Molecular imaging of angiogenesis in nascent Vx-2 rabbit tumors using a novel alpha(nu)beta3-targeted nanoparticle and 1.5 tesla magnetic resonance imaging. Cancer Res 2003;63(18):5838–5843.

52. Hall CS, Marsh JN, Scott MJ, Gaffney PJ, Wickline SA, Lanza GM. Time evolution of enhanced ultrasonic reflection using a fibrin-targeted nanoparticulate contrast agent. J Acoust Soc Am 2000;108(6):3049–3057.

53. Zurita AJ, Arap W, Pasqualini R. Mapping tumor vascular diversity by screening phage display libraries. J Control Release. 2003;91(1–2):183–186.

54. Ito Y, Twamoto Y, Tanaka K, Okuyama K, Sugioka Y. A quantitative assay using basement membrane extracts to study tumor angiogenesis in vivo. Int J Cancer 1996;67(1):148–152.

55. Colorado PC, Torre A, Kamphaus G, et al. Anti-angiogenic cues from vascular basement membrane collagen. Cancer Res 2000;60(9):2520–2526.

56. Akhtar N, Dickerson EB, Auerbach R. The sponge/Matrigel angiogenesis assay. Angiogenesis 2002;5(1–2):75–80.

57. Donovan D, Brown NJ, Bishop ET, Lewis CE. Comparison of three in vitro human 'angiogenesis' assays with capillaries formed in vivo. Angiogenesis 2001;4(2):113–121.

58. Maniotis AJ, Folberg R, Hess A, et al. Vascular channel formation by human melanoma cells in vivo and in vitro: vasculogenic mimicry. Am J Pathol 1999;155(3):739–752.

59. Kragh M, Hjarnaa PJ, Bramm E, Kristjansen PE, Rygaard J, Binderup L. In vivo chamber angiogenesis assay: an optimized Matrigel plug assay for fast assessment of anti-angiogenic activity. Int J Oncol 2003;22(2):305–311.

60. Pearlman JD, Gertz ZM, Wu Y, Simons M, Post MJ. Serial motion assessment by reference tracking (SMART): application to detection of local functional impact of chronic myocardial ischemia. J Comput Assist Tomogr 2001;25(4):558–562.

61. Pearlman JD, Hibberd MG, Chuang ML, et al. Magnetic resonance mapping demonstrates benefits of VEGF-induced myocardial angiogenesis. Nat Med 1995;1(10): 1085–1089.

62. Hanley JA, McNeil BJ. The meaning and use of the area under a receiver operating characteristic (ROC) curve. Radiology 1982;143(1):29–36.

63. McNeil BJ, Hanley JA. Statistical approaches to the analysis of receiver operating characteristic (ROC) curves. Med Decis Making 1984;4(2):137–150.

64. Ackerman DL, Greenland S, Bystritsky A. Use of receiver-operator characteristic (ROC) curve analysis to evaluate predictors of response to clomipramine therapy. Psychopharmacol Bull 1996;32(1):157–165.

65. Vallee JP, Lazeynas F, Kasuboski L, et al. Quantification of myocardial perfusion with FAST sequence and Gd bolus in patients with normal cardiac function. J Magn Reson Imaging 1999;9(2):197–203.

66. Bassingthwaighte JB, Ackerman FH. Mathematical linearity of circulatory transport. J Appl Physiol 1967;22(5):879–888.

67. Bassingthwaighte JB. Physiology and theory of tracer washout techniques for the estimation of myocardial blood flow: flow estimation from tracer washout. Prog Cardiovasc Dis 1977;20(3):165–189.

68. Bassingthwaighte JB, Sparks HV. Indicator dilution estimation of capillary endothelial transport. Annu Rev Physiol 1986;48:321–334.

69. Beard DA, Bassingthwaighte JB. The fractal nature of myocardial blood flow emerges from a whole-organ model of arterial network. J Vasc Res 2000;37(4):282–296.

70. Beard DA, Bassingthwaighte JB. Advection and diffusion of substances in biological tissues with complex vascular networks. Ann Biomed Eng 2000;28(3):253–268.

71. Pearlman JD, Laham RJ, Simons M, Gladstone S, Raptopoulos V. Extent of myocardial collateralization: determination with three-dimensional elastic-subtraction spiral CT. Acad Radiol 1997;4(10):680–686.

73. Pearlman JD, Gao L, Simons M. Magnetic resonance imaging of angiogenesis. In (Fuster V, Chronos N, eds.) Cardiovascular Magnetic Resonance, Established and Emerging Applications. Martin Dunitz Ltd., Taylor and Francis Group PLC, New York: 2003.

74. Freedman SB, Dunn RF, Bernstein L, et al. Influence of coronary collateral blood flow on the development of exertional ischemia and Q wave infarction in patients with severe single-vessel disease. Circulation 1985;71(4):681–686.

75. Anderson H, Yapp JT, Wells P, et al. Measurement of renal tumour and normal tissue perfusion using positron emission tomography in a phase II clinical trial of razoxane. Br J Cancer 2003;89(2):262–267.

76. Aronen HJ, Pardo FS, Kennedy DN, et al. High microvascular blood volume is associated with high glucose uptake and tumor angiogenesis in human gliomas. Clin Cancer Res 2000;6(6):2189–2200.

77. Veronesi G, Landoni C, Pelosi G, et al. Fluoro-deoxi-glucose uptake and angiogenesis are independent biological features in lung metastases. Br J Cancer 2002;86(9): 1391–1395.

78. Hutchinson OC, Collingridge DR, Barthel H, Price PM, Aboagye EO. Pharmaco-dynamics of radiolabelled anticancer drugs for positron emission tomography. Curr Pharm Des 2003;9(11):931–944.

79. Haubner R, Wester HJ, Weber WA, et al. Noninvasive imaging of alpha(υ)beta3 integrin expression using 18F-labeled RGD-containing glycopeptide and positron emission tomography. Cancer Res 2001;61(5):1781–1785.

80. Ruff J, Weismann F, Hiller KH, et al. Magnetic resonance microimaging for noninvasive quantification of myocardial function and mass in the mouse. Magn Reson Med 1998;40(1):43–48.

81. Tirziu DC, Chittenden TW, Moodie KL. Adenoviral PR39 gene transfer in normocholesterolemic and hypercholesterolemic mice. American Heart Association, Scientific Sessions 2003, November 9–12, 2003, Orlando, Florida.

7 Myocardial Angiogenesis
Protein Growth Factors

Kwang Soo Cha, MD, Robert S. Schwartz, MD, and Timothy D. Henry, MD

CONTENTS

INTRODUCTION
VASCULAR ENDOTHELIAL GROWTH FACTORS
    AND FIBROBLAST GROWTH FACTORS
PRECLINICAL STUDIES USING GROWTH FACTORS
    FOR MYOCARDIAL ANGIOGENESIS
CLINICAL STUDIES USING GROWTH FACTORS
    FOR MYOCARDIAL ANGIOGENESIS
SELECTED ISSUES
SUMMARY

INTRODUCTION

Improvements in pharmacological therapy and revascularization procedures have greatly increased the life expectancy of patients with coronary artery disease (CAD) in the last few decades. As a result of these improvements in cardiovascular care and the aging of the population, an increasing number of patients have incomplete revascularization or recurrent myocardial ischemia and are suboptimal candidates for surgical (coronary artery bypass grafting [CABG]) or percutaneous (percutaneous coronary intervention [PCI]) revascularization *(1,2)*. In an analysis of 500 consecutive patients at a tertiary referral center, 12% had myocar-

From: *Contemporary Cardiology: Angiogenesis and Direct Myocardial Revasularization*
Edited by: R. J. Laham and D. S. Baim © Humana Press Inc., Totowa, NJ

dial ischemia and were not optimal candidates for CABG or PCI *(3)*. In patients with two- and three-vessel CAD, complete revascularization was successful in only 23% and 9% of cases, respectively *(2)*. In fact, up to 20–37% of patients with CAD are either poor candidates for CABG or PCI or receive incomplete revascularization with current revascularization strategies *(4–6)*. As a result, many of these patients have residual symptoms and limited quality of life despite maximal medical therapy (frequently described as "refractory angina pectoris") *(7,8)*. Therefore, an alternative revascularization strategy is required and has stimulated intense interest in and excitement about novel approaches to myocardial revascularization.

Angiogenesis, the sprouting of new vessels from pre-existing blood vessels *(9)*, is essential for the proper development of the vascular system not only in physiological situations, including wound healing and ovulation, but also in pathological conditions such as retinopathies, vascular disease, and tumor growth *(9–12)*. Angiogenesis is a natural biological response of a tissue to hypoxia or ischemia and is modulated by the release of endogenous growth factors *(13,14)*. Frequently this compensatory response to the hypoxic stimulus is insufficient in magnitude to return perfusion levels to normal *(15)*. Furthermore, chronic hypoxia results in a reduction in the ability of cells to produce growth factors in response to further episodes of hypoxia and may, in part, be responsible for inadequate compensatory angiogenesis *(16)*. Supplementing a deficient endogenous growth factor response with angiogenic proteins or genes encoding these growth factors may induce neovascularization adequate to reconstitute the ischemic tissue to its state of normal perfusion, a concept known as therapeutic angiogenesis.

Angiogenesis is a complex process that begins with the stimulation of endothelial cell proliferation and migration, followed by the breakdown of the matrix of vessel structures and the formation of new vascular structures. Stimulation of smooth muscle cell proliferation and migration surrounding the new vascular structure enables the formation of mature vessels *(9,17–20)*. A number of growth molecules are involved in this process, which is modulated by the balance between proangiogenic molecules and inhibitors of angiogenesis *(20,21)*. The goal in therapeutic angiogenesis is to increase proangiogenic signals in order to alter the balance to favor new blood vessel growth and vascular remodeling. The ideal agent for therapeutic angiogenesis would be safe, effective, easy to administer, and cost-effective (Table 1). It would stimulate angiogenesis in the targeted ischemic tissue without systemic effects and provide adequate exposure and retention time to maximize angiogenesis to have a sustained clinical benefit.

Table 1
Characteristics of an Ideal Therapeutic Angiogenic Agent

Potent angiogenesis
Sustained clinical benefit
Specific to targeted ischemic tissue
No acute side effects
Absence of unwanted angiogenesis
High local concentration and retention
Adequate exposure time
Non- or less invasive method of delivery (oral or intravenous)
Readministration feasible
Inexpensive (cost-effective)

Adapted from ref. *33*.

Many angiogenic growth factors have been identified. Among these, the vascular endothelial growth factor (VEGF) and fibroblast growth factor (FGF) families are the most widely studied, have induced successful angiogenesis in a number of animal models *(17,19,22)*, and have been utilized in the majority of clinical trials *(23–27)*. In this chapter we review the results of preclinical studies and clinical trials using VEGF and FGF proteins and address the significant challenges ahead in an attempt to provide an alternative method of myocardial revascularization.

VASCULAR ENDOTHELIAL GROWTH FACTORS AND FIBROBLAST GROWTH FACTORS

VEGFs are a family of glycoproteins, of which VEGF-1 (also known as VEGF-A) has been studied most extensively in preclinical and clinical trials of therapeutic angiogenesis. The other VEGFs, which share structural homology with VEGF-1, include VEGF-2 (VEGF-C), VEGF-3 (VEGF-B), VEGF-D, VEGF-E, and placental growth factor *(28–31)*. Seven isoforms of VEGF-1, each the result of alternative splicing, have been identified, having 121, 145, 148, 165, 183, 189, and 206 amino acids per isoform. $VEGF_{165}$ is the predominant isoform, but $VEGF_{121}$ and $VEGF_{189}$ are also usually detected in tissues expressing the VEGF gene. $VEGF_{121}$, $VEGF_{165}$, and $VEGF_{189}$ had similar angiogenic potency in a rabbit model of hindlimb ischemia *(32)*. The isoforms vary in permeability and heparin-binding properties *(29–31)*. Of note, all VEGF-1 isoforms and other VEGF family members contain a secretory signal sequence that permits their active secretion from intact cells transfected by the VEGF gene.

A key distinguishing feature of VEGF is that its mitogenic activity is essentially restricted to cells of the endothelial lineage *(31)*. Besides proliferation, endothelial responses to VEGF include migration, tube formation, and the production of proteases such as plasminogen activator and interstitial collagenase, all of which represent steps critical to capillary sprout formation. VEGF can also affect monocytes, triggering migration and the production of tissue factor. Recently, smooth muscle cells have been shown to be an additional target cell type for VEGF action, including cell migration and the production of matrix metalloproteinases. The physiological effect of VEGF includes enhanced vascular permeability and vasodilation induced by nitric oxide. Expression of both the growth factor and its receptors is upregulated by hypoxia and ischemia, allowing a targeted therapeutic response and also limiting the potential for pathological angiogenesis. The major advantage of VEGF seems to be its specificity for endothelial cells, but this may also be a disadvantage if it stimulates the growth of only small, nonmuscular arteries *(33)*. At this time there are clinical experiences with $VEGF_{165}$ and $VEGF_{121}$ as well as VEGF-2.

FGF is a family of polypeptides that are potent stimulants of angiogenesis *(19,34)*. Acidic FGF (FGF-1) and basic FGF (FGF-2) are potent endothelial cell mitogens. FGF is not specific to endothelial cells and binds with receptors on fibroblasts, neuronal cells, and vascular smooth muscle cells. Like VEGF, FGFs also stimulate endothelial cell synthesis of proteases, including plasminogen activator and metalloproteinase, that can digest extracellular matrix *(19,20)*. Like VEGF, FGF produces nitric oxide-mediated vasodilation, but FGF is not associated with vascular permeability. FGF has a role in wound healing, is cardioprotective in acute myocardial infarction, and may have cytoprotective qualities elsewhere (e.g., in the central nervous system). FGF may stimulate the growth of larger, muscularized arteries with increased perfusion capacity, but its lack of specificity may lead to more systemic side effects. There is evidence that FGF and VEGF act synergistically in animal models *(35)*. Unlike VEGF, the common forms of FGF (FGF-1 and FGF-2) lack a secretory signal sequence; clinical trials of FGF gene transfer have therefore required modification of the FGF gene *(36)* or use of another member of the FGF gene family (FGF-4, FGF-5) with a signal sequence *(37,38)*. FGF-1, FGF-2, and FGF-4 have been used in clinical trials.

PRECLINICAL STUDIES USING GROWTH FACTORS FOR MYOCARDIAL ANGIOGENESIS

Most studies of therapeutic angiogenesis in animal models have utilized the canine or swine ameroid constrictor model, which leads to gradual occlusion of the vessel over 2 or 3 wk. In these models, angiogenic proteins have been delivered by various routes (i.e., periadventitial, intracoronary [ic], intravenous [iv], intrapericardial [ip], and intramyocardial [im]), and their effectiveness has been documented by histological assessment of the number and size of capillaries or vessels, quantitation of endothelial cell markers, measurement of resting or vasodilated coronary blood flow, angiography, and measurement of left ventricular function at rest or during stress. Most studies have demonstrated evidence of enhanced angiogenesis (Tables 2 and 3).

Fibroblast Growth Factors

Early studies using a native form of FGF-1 protein delivered by different modalities reported no angiogenic effect, perhaps a result of the very short half-life *(39,40)*. Sustained release periadventitial administration of the S117 mutant of FGF-1 resulted in marked prolongation of the protein half-life *(41)* and led to improved regional flow and function in a porcine chronic ischemia model *(42,43)*. FGF-1, like FGF-2, provides protection against ischemia-reperfusion injury, an effect likely due to the vasodilatory effects of FGF-1 since a nonmitogenic FGF-1 mutant provided similar protection *(44)*.

The ability of FGF-2 to induce significant angiogenesis in mature tissues was suggested by studies in both canine and porcine infarction models. Intracoronary injections of 10 µg FGF-2 in the setting of acute coronary thrombosis in dogs and ic injections of 0.12 µg/kg FGF-2 containing Affigel beads in pigs led to significantly higher vessel count compared with controls *(45,46)*.

Studies of the therapeutic efficacy of FGF-2 in chronic myocardial ischemia have utilized a variety of routes of administration in both canine and porcine models. In a canine model, 18 daily injections of 110 µg of FGF-2 directly into the left circumflex artery distal to an ameroid occluder increased transmural collateral flow and density of distribution vessels within the collateral zone *(47)*. In the same model, daily left atrial injections of 1.74 mg of FGF-2 for 4 wk resulted in marked acceleration of collateral development. However, collateral flow in control dogs improved toward the end of the study, approaching that of treated dogs at the 38-d endpoint. The improvement of collateral flow occurred primarily between the d 7 and 14 of therapy, and the collateral development did not regress after withdrawal of treatment *(48)*. FGF-2 treatment did not induce more collateralization in dogs with mature collateral vessels, underscoring the role of ischemia for FGF-2-induced collateral development *(49)*.

Local perivascular delivery of sustained heparin-alginate FGF-2 was evaluated in a porcine model of chronic ischemia. This form of delivery

Table 2
Preclinical Studies of FGF Proteins for Myocardial Angiogenesis

Authors (ref.)	Animal model	Administration route, dose	Results
FGF-1			
Banai et al., 1991 (39)	Canine ameroid LAD	Periadventitial FGF-1 800 µg	No visible collaterals; smooth muscle cell hyperplasia noted in ischemic territory
Unger et al., 1993 (40)	Canine ameroid LCX	ic FGF-1 30 µg/h for 4 wk	No effect on collateral blood flow
Sellke et al., 1996 (42)	Porcine ameroid LCX	Periadventitial FGF-1 10 µg	Normalized vasomotor responses to β-adrenergic and endothelium dependent mechanisms; ↑myocardial-perfusion to the collateral-dependent myocardium
Lopez et al., 1998 (43)	Porcine ameroid LCX	Periadventitial FGF-1 10 µg	↑ coronary flow, global and regional LV function at rest and with pacing
FGF-2			
Yanagisawa-Miwa et al., 1992 (45)	Canine infarct model	ic FGF-2 10 µg	↑ cardiac systolic function and reduced infarct size; ↑ arterioles and capillaries in infarct zone
Battler et al., 1993 (46)	Porcine infarct model	ic, slow-release by beads FGF-2 0.12 µg/kg	↑ microvessel count in viable and nonviable tissue within infarct area compared with control group; no difference in total regional left ventricular wall motion
Unger et al., 1994 (47)	Canine ameroid LCX	ic FGF-2 110 µg/d for 18 d	↑ collateral flow and increase in density of vessels (>20 µm) in treated group
Lazarous et al., 1995 (48)	Canine ameroid LCX	LA FGF-2 1.74 mg/d for 4 wk and for 9 or 5 wk vs placebo	↑ collateral development in treated group, but collateral flow in control dogs approached treated dogs at 38-d endpoint
Shou et al., 1997 (49)	Canine ameroid LCX	LA FGF-2 1.74 mg/d for 7 d; 2nd course of FGF-2 at 6 mo	No difference in collateral function compared with controls at 6 mo Subsequent course of FGF-2 did not induce further collateralization

Reference	Model	Route/Dose	Results
Harada et al., 1994 (50)	Porcine ameroid LCX	Periadventitial FGF-2 5 μg	↓ infarct size, ↑ coronary perfusion, and ↓ fractional shortening in treated group; with pacing, less rise in LVEDP
Sellke et al., 1994 (51)	Porcine ameroid LCX	Periadventitial FGF-2 5 μg	Normalized vasomotor responses to β-adrenergic and endothelium-dependent mechanisms; ↑ arteriolar density in treated group
Lopez et al., 1997 (52)	Porcine ameroid LCX	Periadventitial FGF-2 10 or 100 μg	↑ angiographic collateral index, TIMI score, and coronary flow; ↑ global and regional function in treated groups; better preservation of regional wall motion in high dose (100 μg)
Laham et al., 1998 (53)	Porcine ameroid LCX	Intrapericardial FGF-2 30 μg or 2 mg	↑ coronary resistance and vasomotor responses to β-adrenergic and endothelium-dependent mechanisms
Laham et al., 2000 (54)	Porcine ameroid LCX	Intrapericardial FGF-2 30 μg, 200 μg, or 2 mg	↑ collaterals and blood flow; ↑ myocardial perfusion and function in ischemic territory; ↑ myocardial vascularity
Sato et al., 2000 (55)	Porcine ameroid LCX	iv, ic FGF-2 2 or 6 μg/kg	↑ collaterals and regional blood flow in higher ic dose; ↑ ejection fraction, regional wall motion, and thickening in higher ic dose; iv and lower ic dose not effective
Rajanayagam et al., 2000 (56)	Canine ameroid LCX	Central venous bolus, iv, pericardial, and ic FGF-2 variable doses	↑ collateral perfusion by ic route; no improvement by central venous, iv, and pericardial injection
Watanabe et al., 1998 (57)	Porcine infarct model	Intramyocardial FGF-2 10 μg	↑ number of arterioles, not capillaries, in normal and infarct border area; potentiated by heparin co-administration
Yamamoto et al., 2000 (58)	Canine ameroid LAD	Transmyocardial channels FGF-2 100 ng/mL per channel	↑ angiogenesis following TMR mainly by increasing the size but not the total number of vessels

(continued)

Table 2 (*Continued*)
Preclinical Studies of FGF Proteins for Myocardial Angiogenesis

Authors (ref.)	Animal model	Administration route, dose	Results
Kawasuji et al., 2000 (59)	Canine infarct model	Intramyocardial FGF-2 100 μg	↑ regional myocardial blood flow; ↓ thinning of infracted region; ↑ ventricular function
Yamamoto et al., 2001 (60)	Canine infarct model	Intramyocardial FGF-2-impregnated microspheres	↑ collateral circulation to the infracted area, but the flow not changed by free-form FGF-2

FGF = fibroblast growth factor; LAD = left anterior descending artery; LIMA = left internal mammary artery; LCX = left circumflex coronary artery; ic = intracoronary; iv = intravenous; LV = left-ventricular; LA = left atrial; LVEDP = left-ventricular end-diastolic pressure; TIMI = thrombolysis in myocardial infarction; TMR; transmyocardial laser revascularization.

Table 3
Preclinical Studies of VEGF Proteins for Myocardial Angiogenesis

Authors (ref.)	Animal model	Administration route, dose	Results
Banai et al., 1994 (62)	Canine ameroid LCX	ic VEGF 45 µg/d for 28 d	↑ development of small coronary arteries; ↑collateral blood flow
Lazarous et al., 1996 (63)	Canine ameroid LCX	LA VEGF 0.72 mg/d for 7 d	No difference in collateral flow vs control; ↑ neointimal thickening after vascular injury
Sellke et al., 1995 (64)	Porcine ameroid LCX	Periadventitial VEGF₁₆₅ 2 µg over 4 wk	50% ↑ in epicardial blood flow at rest; preserved β-adrenergic mediated relaxation of microvessels in the collateral-dependent myocardium
Pearlman et al., 1995 (65)	Porcine ameroid LCX	Perivascular VEGF	↓ in size of collateral-dependent ischemic zone and contrast arrival half-time; ↑ in LVEF and regional wall thickening in collateral-dependent zone
Harada et al., 1996 (66)	Porcine ameroid LCX	Periadventitial VEGF-2 µg for 4 wk by pump	↑ in collateral vessels and improved coronary flow at rest and with pacing; preservation of endothelium-dependent microvessel relaxation and fractional shortening during pacing
Lopez et al., 1998 (67)	Porcine ameroid LCX	ic or periadventitial VEGF 20 µg	↑ in left-to-left collaterals, myocardial blood flow, and coronary vasodilator reserve; ↑ perfusion and regional wall thickening
Hariawala et al., 1996 (69)	Porcine ameroid LCX	ic VEGF 2 mg	↑ coronary flow at 30 d; four of eight pigs died from hypotension during ic VEGF bolus
Sellke et al., 1998 (68)	Porcine ameroid LCX	ic VEGF 20 µg ± transvascular under pressure or perivascular infusion VEGF 20 µg	↑ADP-mediated endothelium-dependent relaxation in vessels with ic not perivascular infusion; normalization of β-adrenergic- and cyclic AMP–mediated relaxation in all VEGF groups

(continued)

Table 3 (*Continued*)
Preclinical Studies of VEGF Proteins for Myocardial Angiogenesis

Authors (ref.)	Animal model	Administration route, dose	Results
Giordano et al., 1998 (*109*)	Porcine ameroid LCX	ic 250 ng/kg/min iv 250 ng/kg/min iv 50 ng/kg/min	↑ wall thickening in LCX region, especially with 250 ng/kg/min dose (ic or iv); no differences in blood flow
Sato et al., 2001 (*72*)	Porcine ameroid LCX	iv (rapid or slow) ic ± L-NAME VEGF$_{165}$ 10 µg/kg	↑ collateral index, myocardial blood flow, and microvascular function in both ic groups, not in iv groups; no improvements in global and regional function in any groups Concomitant administration of L-NAME inhibits VEGF-induced hypotension while preserving VEGF-induced angiogenesis Not effective in augmenting myocardial flow or function by iv infusion
Hughes et al., 2004 (*73*)	Porcine LCX 90% stenosis	iv VEGF$_{165}$ 50 ng/kg/min im VEGF$_{165}$ 15 µg/kg im FGF-2 1.35 µg/kg	↑ myocardial blood flow in im VEGF and im FGF group vs placebo and vehicle at 3 and 6 mo; for iv VEGF only at 6 mo ↑ vascular density at 6 mo for all three groups
Villanueva et al., 2002 (*110*)	Canine ameroid LAD	ic and subcutaneous VEGF$_{121}$ 108 µg and 1 mg	↑ collateral flow and reserve by myocardial contrast echocardiography

VEGF = vascular endothelial growth factor; LAD = left anterior descending artery; LCX = left circumflex coronary artery; ic = intracoronary; iv = intravenous; im = intramyocardial; LVEF = left-ventricular ejection fraction, L-NAME = nitro-L-arginine methyl ester hydrochloride.

is characterized by first-order release kinetics of growth factor from the polymer over a 4- to 5-wk period, ease of implantation, and the absence of any inflammatory reaction associated with polymer placement *(50,52)*. Examination of the effect of progressively larger amounts of FGF-2 (5, 10, and 100 µg) delivered in this manner in a pig model demonstrated improvement in resting coronary flow in FGF-2-treated group compared with controls and an increase in angiographic collaterals *(50,51)*. Analysis of left-ventricular function demonstrated a higher ejection fraction at rest and during pacing in both 10- and 100-µg FGF-2-treated animals compared with controls. Similarly, regional wall motion in the ischemic territory was better preserved at rest in the 10- and 100-µg FGF-2 groups, though during pacing only the 100-µg FGF-2 group maintained normal wall thickening *(52)*.

A single ip bolus delivery of FGF-2 (30 µg or 2 mg) in a porcine model resulted in significant increases in left-to-left collaterals and blood flow, accompanied by improvements in magnetic resonance-measured myocardial perfusion and function in ischemic territory, as well as histological evidence of increased myocardial vascularity *(53,54)*.

In a study of the efficacy of ic and iv infusion of FGF-2 *(55)*, 6 µg/kg ic FGF-2 increased collaterals and regional blood flow and improved cardiac function, but iv FGF-2 and a lower dose (2 µg/kg) of ic FGF-2 were ineffective. Another comparative study of FGF-2 also showed that only ic administration augmented collateral development in dogs, whereas central venous bolus injection, iv infusion, and pericardial injection failed to enhance collateral perfusion *(56)*.

Local im injection of FGF-2 4–5 wk after infarction in pigs resulted in an increase in the number of arterioles but not capillaries compared with control injections. The FGF-2 effect was potentiated by co-administration with heparin *(57)*. In dog models of infarct or chronic ischemia *(58–60)*, FGF-2 increased myocardial blood flow and improved ventricular function. A biodistribution study showed that FGF-2 retention after transendocardial im delivery was significantly higher than previously observed for ic, iv, and ip delivery *(61)*.

Vascular Endothelial Growth Factors

Two early studies with different delivery methods *(62,63)* in a canine ameroid model produced opposite results. Daily ic injections of 45 µg of VEGF over a 28-d period (total dose 900 µg) resulted in faster restoration of collateral zone flow than similar injections of normal saline *(62)*. However, a 7-d course of left atrial infusion of VEGF (0.72 mg/d) failed to increase collateral flow, with potential reasons being VEGF dose, route of administration, and timing and/or duration of treatment *(63)*.

The efficacy of periadventitial delivery of VEGF was tested in a porcine ameroid model *(64,67)*. Treatment with VEGF was associated with better preservation of coronary flow in the ameroid zone during pacing. Magnetic resonance imaging (MRI) demonstrated not only significantly better perfusion of the compromised territory, but also a reduction in size of this territory in VEGF-treated animals *(65)*. The number of collateral vessels were increased nearly fourfold in the VEGF-treated animals *(66)*. Analysis of microvascular function demonstrated significantly better restoration of endothelium-mediated, receptor-dependent relaxation in VEGF-treated animals *(66,68)*.

The feasibility of ic bolus delivery was tested by Hariawala et al. *(69)*, who injected 2 mg of rhVEGF$_{165}$ into the left coronary arteries of eight pigs. Four of the eight animals survived the injection (four died of refractory hypotension); however, 30 d later, the remaining animals demonstrated improved coronary flow compared with the control group. The efficacy of a lower-dose (20 μg) single ic infusion was compared with the same amount of VEGF delivered either perivascularly, ic, or locally using an InfusaSleeve™ catheter in a porcine ameroid model *(67,68)*. Both ic bolus injection and local delivery resulted in significant increase in angiographically visible left-to-left collaterals, and improvement in myocardial blood flow, regional left ventricular function, and microvascular function. No significant hemodynamic compromise was associated with any of these delivery approaches. The hemodynamic effects of VEGF administration are mediated by nitric oxide release and are secondary to microvascular dilation *(70,71)*. Intracoronary VEGF results in a dose-dependent increase in Doppler-measured coronary flow and systemic hypotension, both effects prevented by pretreatment with nitro-L-arginine methyl ester hydrochloride (L-NAME) *(70)*.

An excellent study with 42 pigs using a circumflex ameroid model demonstrated an improvement in myocardial blood flow, microvascular function, and collateral index with ic VEGF but not with iv delivery. There was no impact with regional or global function by MRI, and the hypotensive effects of VEGF were blocked by L-NAME *(72)*.

In another study using the porcine ameroid model, both im FGF-2 and im VEGF$_{165}$ increased myocardial blood flow by positron emission tomography (PET) scan at 3 and 6 mo. Myocardial blood flow was increased at 6 mo, but not 3 mo for iv VEGF$_{165}$. Quantitative vascular density was increased at 6 mo in all three groups over both vehicle and control animals *(73)*. Finally, a small trial using an ameroid porcine model and contrast myocardial echocardiography demonstrated an improvement with collateral flow and collateral flow reserve with a combination of ic and subcutaneous delivery of VEGF$_{121}$ vs placebo 6 wk posttreatment.

In summary, extensive preclinical research in multiple models with both FGF and VEGF protein have demonstrated successful therapeutic angiogenesis. Although there was some variability depending on the method of delivery and dosing schedule, it appears that im and ic delivery are more effective than iv delivery. The only long-term study showed not only sustained improvement at 6 mo, but ongoing improvement from 1 to 6 mo. These trials laid the groundwork for the initial clinical trials.

CLINICAL STUDIES USING GROWTH FACTORS FOR MYOCARDIAL ANGIOGENESIS

Positive preclinical trials led to phase I dose finding trials with FGF-2 and $VEGF_{165}$ as well as two small placebo-controlled trials with FGF-1 and FGF-2 as an adjunct to CABG (Table 4). These trials laid the groundwork for two larger double-blind, placebo-controlled trials of ic FGF-2 (FGF-2 Initiating Revascularization Support Trial, or FIRST) and $VEGF_{165}$ (VEGF in Ischemia for Vascular Angiogenesis, or VIVA) and an ongoing trial using FGF-2 as an adjunct to CABG. These trials have enrolled patients with ongoing myocardial ischemia despite optimal medical management who are suboptimal candidates for PCI or CABG.

Intramyocardial FGF-1

In the first human trial of myocardial angiogenesis *(74,75)*, 40 patients undergoing bypass surgery were injected with FGF-1 (10 µg/kg) vs placebo intramyocardially close to the anastomosis of the internal mammary artery to the left anterior descending artery. The procedure was well tolerated, with no deaths or perioperative myocardial infarctions. Because all patients were bypassed, clinical improvement was not assessed, but follow-up digital subtraction angiography at 12 wk demonstrated the presence of increased capillary filling in patients injected with FGF-1 compared with controls. The 3-yr follow-up on 33 patients demonstrated a consistent increase in vascular density by digital subtraction angiography ($p < 0.005$) *(75)*. There were three deaths (two cerebral ischemia, one unknown) in the FGF-1-treated group and four deaths (one cerebral ischemia, one myocardial infarction, two unknown) in the control group. Patients treated with FGF-1 were more likely to have class I angina (94% vs 75%) and were less likely to require antianginal medications. There was no evidence for uncontrolled or pathological angiogenesis in the FGF-1-treated patients.

Periadventitial FGF-2 With Slow-Release Beads

A similar phase I study enrolled 24 patients undergoing CABG with ungraftable areas of the myocardium using heparin-alginate microcap-

Table 4

Clinical Studies of Recombinant Proteins for Myocardial Angiogenesis

Authors	Protein (ref.)	Administration route	Dose	Treated/ Placebo	Results	Follow-up duration
Schumacher et al., 1998 (111)	FGF-1 + heparin + fibrin glue	Intramyocardial injection during CABG	100 µg/kg	20/20	↑ capillary density vs placebo; ↓ angina and use of antianginal drugs vs placebo	12 wk to 3 yr
Stegmann et al., 2000 (75)					Similar angiographic improvement at 3 yr	
Laham et al., 1999 (76)	FGF-2 + heparin alginate	Periadventitial implantation during CABG	10 or 100 µg total dose of FGF-2 (divided into 10 implants) or placebo	16/8	↑ perfusion on SPECT and exercise capacity	3–32 mo
Ruel et al., 2002 (77)					↓ angina; ↓ defect size by nuclear perfusion and MRI with high dose	
					Maintained improvement long term	
Udelson et al., 2000 (78)	FGF-2	iv (14 patients) or ic (52 patients) injection	Incremental administration to total dose of 0.33–48 µg/kg	66/0	↑ exercise time, quality of life, LV function, nuclear perfusion, and flow on MRI; ↓ angina	1, 2, and 6 mo
Laham et al., 2000 (79)						
Simons et al., 2002 (80) (FIRST study)	FGF-2	ic injection	0.3, 3.0, 30 µg/kg total dose, or placebo	251/86 total	90-d exercise time (65 s vs 45 s with placebo); stress nuclear perfusion results did not differ from placebo group; ↓ angina (p = 0.057); trend toward improved overall result in older and more symptomatic patients	90 d to 6 mo
Hendel et al., 2000 (83)	VEGF₁₆₅	ic injection	5, 17, 50, or 167 ng/kg/min, 10 min each artery	15/0	↓ angina in 13 of 15 patients; ↑ rest nuclear perfusion results with high dose; ↑ col lateral density in 7 of 7	30 and 60 d

Reference	Growth factor	Delivery method	Dose	n	Results	Follow-up
Henry et al., 2001 (84)						
Henry et al., 2000 (31)	VEGF$_{165}$	iv injection	17–100 ng/kg/min over 1–4 h	28/0	Improvement by 2 grades on 40% of rest nuclear perfusion studies and 20% of stress nuclear perfusion studies; 38% increased collaterals	60 d
Henry et al., 2003 (86) (VIVA study)	VEGF$_{165}$	ic injection + iv injection	17 or 50 ng/kg/min ic for 20 min and iv for 4 h on d 3, 6, and 9	115/63	↑ treadmill exercise time, angina class, and quality of life in all three groups at 60 d No difference between group at d 120, loss of benefit in exercise time, angina class, and quality-of-life scores in the placebo group, but significant improvement in angina class and trends in exercise time and angina frequency in the high-dose VEGF group No improvement in nuclear perfusion No difference in clinical event rates across all three groups during 120 d At 1 yr, significant improvement in angina class and decrease events in high-dose VEGF	60 d, 120 d, 1 yr
Henry et al., 2000 (87)						

CABG = coronary artery bypass grafting; FGF-2 = fibroblast growth factor-2; FIRST = FGF-2 Initiating Revascularization Support Trial; LAD = left anterior descending artery; LIMA = left internal mammary artery; LV = left-ventricular; MRI = magnetic resonance imaging; SPECT = single photon emission computed tomography; VEGF = vascular endothelial growth factor; VIVA = VEGF in Ischemia for Vascular Angiogenesis; MI = myocardial infarction; iv = intravenous; ic = intracoronary.

sules, which released FGF-2 protein over 3–4 wk *(76)*. Patients were randomly assigned into one of three groups: 10 µg FGF-2 ($n = 8$), 100 µg FGF-2 ($n = 8$), or placebo ($n = 8$). Mean clinical follow-up was 16 mo with no recurrent angina or repeat revascularization in the 100-µg FGF-2 group compared with three patients with recurrent angina and two repeat revascularization in the control group. Both nuclear perfusion and MRI demonstrated a significant reduction in the size of the target zone in the 100-µg FGF-2 group but not in the 10-µg FGF-2 or control groups. These revascularization effects and clinical benefit were maintained at more than 2 yr *(77)*. This small initial trial demonstrated the safety and feasibility of this method of delivery, and a larger double-blind trial is ongoing.

Intracoronary and Intravenous FGF-2

In an open-label, dose escalation study using recombinant FGF-2 protein *(78,79)*, 52 patients received ic infusions of FGF-2 ranging in dose from 0.33 to 48 µg/kg and 14 patients received iv infusions of 24 and 36 µg/kg FGF-2. FGF-2 infusions were well tolerated with systemic hypotension at 48 µg/kg. By the end of the 6-mo study, the FGF-2–treated patients demonstrated significant improvement in exercise time (633 ± 24 s vs 510 ± 24 s at baseline, $p < 0.001$), as well as significant improvement in quality of life measured by angina frequency on the Seattle Angina Questionnaire (SAQ). MRI perfusion imaging demonstrated a significant reduction in the size of the ischemic territory and improved left ventricular wall thickening in this territory. These results suggested that ic infusions of FGF-2 were safe and may produce clinical improvements in angina and exercise time.

FIRST therefore examined the effectiveness of ic recombinant FGF-2 *(80)*. A total of 337 patients were randomized to 0.3, 3.0, or 30 µg/kg rFGF-2 or placebo by ic administration. The primary endpoint of this study was change in exercise tolerance test time from baseline to 90 d. At 90 d, the improvement in exercise testing with a treadmill (ETT) for FGF did not differ significantly from placebo (65 s vs 45 s; $p = 0.64$) and there was no difference in rest or stress nuclear perfusion. Angina frequency and angina class were improved by rFGF-2 at 90 d ($p = 0.035$, 0.012, respectively), but the difference between the FGF-2–treated and placebo groups was lost at 180 d because of continued improvement in the placebo group.

In *post hoc* analysis, patients with class III or IV angina had a reduction in angina frequency at 90 d after rFGF-2 therapy (overall $p = 0.035$). Patients with a baseline SAQ angina frequency score of ≤40 (high baseline symptom burden) had a significant reduction in angina frequency at 90 d after rFGF-2 therapy (overall $p = 0.02$) that was reduced by 180 d (overall $p = 0.12$). Subgroup analysis suggested that the benefit, defined as improvement in symptoms, exercise time, and reduction in the size of nuclear-imaging determined ischemic zone defect, was most prominent in "sicker" patients as defined by lower baseline exercise capacity, higher baseline symptom frequency, and larger nuclear perfusion defects. There was no excess mortality, sudden death, or malignancy in FGF-2-treated patients, and the overall mortality (2%) was significantly lower than seen in transmyocardial laser revascularization trials *(81,82)*. Overall, the trial demonstrated excellent safety and some evidence of benefit, especially in high-risk patients.

Intracoronary and Intravenous VEGF$_{165}$

Initial clinical VEGF trials were also performed with ic and iv recombinant VEGF$_{165}$ protein *(31,83,84)*. In a phase I dose-escalation trial, 15 patients received two 10-min ic infusions of 5, 17, 50, or 167 ng/kg/min into each of two coronary distributions for a total of 20 min *(84)*. The maximum tolerated dose was identified as 50 ng/kg/min based on a significant decrease of blood pressure with the 167 ng/kg/min dose. On myocardial perfusion imaging, no significant change was seen in the summed stress score at d 60, but there was a significant improvement in the summed rest score in the high-dose VEGF group (14.7 vs 10.7, $p < 0.05$). Five of the six patients receiving the higher doses demonstrated improvement in both stress and resting perfusion in two segments *(83)*. All seven patients with follow-up angiograms had a significant improvement in collateral density score. In addition, 13 of 15 patients had a significant decrease in angina class.

In a second phase I trial, 28 patients received escalating iv doses of VEGF$_{165}$ protein (17–100 ng/kg/min for 1–4 h) *(31)*. Similar to the ic trial, 50 ng/kg/min was identified as the maximally tolerated dose based on the decrease in systolic pressure at 100 ng/kg/min. Myocardial perfusion imaging was improved in at least two segments by two perfusion grades in 54% of patients. As in the ic trial, the improvement was more impressive in resting perfusion (40% of rest defects vs 20% of stress defects improved). An improvement in ejection fraction from 39.8 to 47.8% ($p = 0.09$) was noted at d 60 in the 10 patients who began the study with left-ventricular ejection fraction <50%. A blinded angiographic assessment based on follow-up angiograms at d 60 demonstrated more collateral vessels in 38% of patients *(85)*. In both phase I trials, VEGF$_{165}$ protein was well tolerated with no significant adverse events such as cancer, retinopathy, or angiographic evidence for progression of atherosclerotic disease.

The two phase I trials using VEGF laid the groundwork for the VIVA trial *(86)*. A total of 178 patients were randomized to receive placebo or low-dose (17 ng/kg/min) or high-dose (50 ng/kg/min) $VEGF_{165}$ for 20 min ic, followed by 4-h iv infusions of the same dose on d 3, 6, and 9. The primary study endpoint, change from baseline in ETT time at 60 d, was not different in all three groups. Angina class and quality of life were significantly improved in all three groups at d 60. By d 120, there was a loss of benefit in ETT time, angina class, and quality-of-life scores in the placebo group, whereas the patients receiving high-dose VEGF experienced significant improvement in angina class ($p = 0.05$) and nonsignificant trends in exercise time ($p = 0.15$) and angina frequency ($p = 0.09$) as compared with placebo.

There was no significant improvement in the summed rest or stress scores of nuclear myocardial perfusion at d 60. The drug was well tolerated with no significant adverse effects. In contrast, there were two deaths, three newly diagnosed cancers, and one worsening retinopathy in the placebo group. The results of this trial clearly illustrate the importance of a placebo control in designing subsequent trials in the field of angiogenesis as well as interpreting positive results and potential complications of angiogenic therapy.

In a substudy of the trial, 106 patients remained blinded to treatment assignment for 1 yr to determine the long-term effects of placebo as well as the long-term safety and efficacy of $VEGF_{165}$ protein *(87)*. By one year, angina class in the placebo group was no longer improved from baseline (mean 2.8 ± 0.6 vs 2.4 ± 1.6), whereas the patients treated with high-dose $VEGF_{165}$ protein had persistent improvement from baseline (2.7 ± 0.8 vs 1.9 ± 1.3, $p < 0.001$). Although there was no significant difference in death or myocardial infarction in the three groups, there were fewer overall events in patients treated with $VEGF_{165}$, driven primarily by the need for less subsequent revascularization. Four patients in the placebo group had developed cancer by 1 yr, compared with one patient who received low-dose $VEGF_{165}$ protein.

On the basis of the results of the VIVA trial, it appears that $VEGF_{165}$ protein is safe and well tolerated with no significant adverse effects when followed to 1 yr. Additionally, a significant improvement in angina was demonstrated at both 4 mo and 1 yr, with a trend for improvement in ETT time at 4 mo in the high-dose group.

SELECTED ISSUES

Protein-Based Therapy vs Gene Therapy for Myocardial Angiogenesis

The relative benefits of protein versus gene therapy are outlined in Table 5. The major advantages of protein therapy lie in precise knowledge of delivered dose, a relatively well-understood safety profile, po-

Table 5
Features of Protein and Gene Therapy for Myocardial Angiogenesis

Characteristic	Protein therapy	Gene therapy
Exposure to growth factor	Short-lived, owing to short half-life of protein	Prolonged, owing to sustained protein production
Dose response	Defined	Unpredictable and/or unknown
Dose titration	Titratable dose	Variable gene expression
Serum half-life	Short	Longer
Tissue half-life	Short, subject to engineering	Unpredictable and/or unknown
Slow release	Possible through formulation	Yes
Need for repeated doses	More likely	Less likely
Readministration	Easier; less risk of inflammatory response or immune inactivation	Potential for activation or inflammatory response at readministration for viral vectors
Exposure to foreign genetic material	No	Yes
Inflammatory response	No	Yes with viral vectors
Influence of patient serology	No	Yes with viral vectors
Systemic exposure	Short-term, but higher than gene therapy	Less likely
Targeting	Possible	Possible

tential for readministration, and the potential to combine several proteins into a single therapeutic formulation *(88)*. The major limitation of the protein therapy approach is believed to be the limited tissue half-life of angiogenic proteins. However, a number of approaches are available to extend the tissue half-life. For instance, the serum half-life of FGF-1 in the presence of heparin can be increased from hours to days by a single amino acid mutation *(41)*. Furthermore, extended tissue exposure to the growth factors can be accomplished by a variety of slow-release formulations (e.g., heparin-alginate beads) *(89)*. A single injection of the protein may be limited by the rapid washout of the protein and limited uptake by the ischemic myocardium, although the level of binding to receptor in ischemic myocardium is unknown and potential effects on other mediators of angiogenesis such as endothelial progenitor cells is unknown. Both ic and iv delivery of protein likely result in higher systemic growth factor levels as well.

The use of gene therapy has a number of potential advantages over administration of the recombinant protein. Theoretically, gene therapy allows sustained local production and release of growth factors by the transfected cells *(90,92)*. Although prolonged presence of growth factors may be beneficial, there is no conclusive evidence to support this hypothesis. In fact, prolonged local production of potent growth factors such as VEGF-A and FGF-2 may cause unwanted angiogenesis *(93–95)*. Moreover, the theoretical advantages of gene therapy are dependent on transfectin rates and local gene expression, which are not well characterized in patients and likely produce significant variability in the level and duration of gene expression in different patients *(96,97)*. This is dependent on the vector, the method of delivery, the presence and level of neutralizing antibodies, and the type of tissue transfected (myocardial versus skeletal muscle). For example, a screen of a consecutive series of patients referred for PCI or CABG demonstrated that over 70% of patients possessed neutralizing antibodies to type 5 adenovirus, which in 50% achieved very high titers *(98,99)*. Vectors differ in their efficacy of cell transduction, the type of cells transduced (proliferating vs nonproliferating), and the duration and extent of transgene expression. Plasmid DNA and early generation adenoviral vectors mediate rather short-term (days to weeks) duration expression, while other viral vectors (e.g., retrovirus, lentivirus, adeno-associated virus) can result in a very long (months) duration of expression. Thus, considerable concerns have arisen over inflammatory responses to these vectors, although this remains controversial and inflammatory responses may be more likely in some tissues than in others *(100)*. Limited data are available in humans regarding gene expression.

At this moment, neither has emerged as the superior agent. Both the protein and gene therapy approaches have distinct advantages and disadvantages and have been applied clinically. Although the primary endpoint of exercise time was negative in the two phase II randomized trials, VIVA and FIRST, there was an excellent safety profile and improvement in angina class and quality of life, especially in high-risk subgroups. Therefore, ongoing studies to improve efficacy by altering the dose, method of delivery, or pharmacokinetics are warranted.

Drug Delivery for Protein Growth Factors

The disappointing results of the VIVA and FIRST studies in terms of primary endpoints underscore the concern that the pharmacokinetics of recombinant protein administered into the vascular space may lead to inadequate local delivery and retention of angiogenic growth factor to ischemic myocardium, as suggested by studies using labeled ligand *(101–103)*.

Current techniques under investigation include iv and ic infusions, im injection, local perivascular delivery, ip instillation, and retroinfusion through coronary vein. Both catheter-based approaches (ic infusion and im injection) and surgical procedures (im and local perivascular delivery) are available. The method of delivery must be evaluated in terms of myocardial retention or expression of growth factor as well as systemic exposure. Despite the potent angiogenic effect of the growth factors, an efficient delivery mechanism that could target the protein to the diseased tissue and maintain a local therapeutic concentration for a prolonged period of time may be advantageous.

Although iv and ic deliveries have proven effective in animal models, the effects in humans are unclear. Systemic administration may not provide a therapeutic concentration of the growth factor at the disease site. Furthermore, the growth factor may be rapidly degrading in the circulation (the biological half-life of VEGF is only a few minutes) and may therefore not be available at the target site for long enough to induce and sustain the growth of new collaterals. Intraluminal localized infusion of only simple solutions may not provide therapeutic arterial drug levels for an adequate period of time because of rapid washout (<24 h, with >90% drug leaching out within 30 min) *(104)*. An ic infusion of ^{125}I-FGF-2 resulted in 0.89% cardiac uptake of growth factor at 1 h, which then dropped to 0.05% in 24 h, suggesting an inefficient uptake of protein by the target tissue and a rapid washout effect *(102)*. Repeat or sustained administration may be beneficial as demonstrated in various animal model studies when administered as a continuous iv infusion or given as repeated intramuscular injections over several weeks. An ic administration of VEGF daily for 28 d enhanced collateral function in a canine model of myocardial ischemia. However, reducing the duration of administration to 7 d failed to show any effect, suggesting the importance of the sustained effect of growth factor for therapeutic results. Improvements in blood flow and hemodynamic parameters were achieved with a continuous sustained administration of the growth factor using an Alzet® pump in the ischemic pig myocardium. These studies demonstrate that a sustained presence of a growth factor may be beneficial for a therapeutic angiogenic effect in different animal models. Gene therapy may be superior to protein therapy because the vascular endothelium and/or myocardium can incorporate the gene, allowing sustained production of angiogenic protein.

Local drug delivery may be an important method to ensure high concentration of a protein at the site where angiogenesis is desired. The suboptimal efficacy seen with intravascular delivery of angiogenic proteins may have been because of their short half-life. Direct injection of FGF protein into the myocardium of patients at the time of bypass surgery resulted in angiogenic evidence of enhanced collateral formation, although it was verified by nonrandomized fashion *(74,105)*. Transepicardial or transendocardial injections of ^{125}I-FGF-2 favorably resulted in 25–30% of the injectate being recovered from the myocardium and 5% retained up to 3 d after injection, compared with <0.1% retained in the myocardium 24 h after ic administration *(102)*. Intramyocardial delivery of growth factors may be preferred since it includes the possibility of targeting the desired areas of the heart and has a higher efficiency of delivery and prolonged tissue retention. However, catheter-based transendocardial technique is more invasive and may require specialized NOGA™ Biosense equipment and higher skill level of the operator than needed for ic injection.

Calcium alginate beads were demonstrated to release a growth factor at a constant rate for up to 14 d in vivo, and its mitogenic activity on endothelial cells in culture was found to be three to five times more potent than the same mass of the growth factor added directly to the culture medium *(106)*. Periadventitial (or perivascular) implantation of heparin-alginate pellets containing FGF-2 during bypass surgery may provide a constant concentration of the protein for a prolonged duration enough to improve myocardial perfusion and angina as suggested by initial clinical results *(76,77)*.

Intrapericardial administration showed improved retention of ^{125}I-FGF-2 compared with intravascular techniques, with up to 8% observed at 24 h in the ischemic myocardium *(102)*. However, this technique requires a normal pericardium, so it is limited due to very high (>90%)

frequency of prior bypass surgery in patients enrolling in angiogenesis trials and by technical difficulties required for access of the normal pericardial space. Percutaneous delivery by coronary venous system is under investigation with potential implications for local protein or gene transfer *(107)*.

Because biological instability of protein growth factors in the intravascular system is a major challenge, it is critical to develop an appropriate drug-delivery system, which could provide a therapeutic dose of growth factor in a target tissue for a period of time necessary for therapeutic angiogenic effect. Pharmacokinetic data in patients are limited *(108)*, and unfortunately results in preclinical animal models may not be directly applicable to humans. This represents a major challenge to successful angiogenesis with protein growth factors.

SUMMARY

Therapeutic myocardial angiogenesis has emerged as a potential treatment for patients with severe myocardial ischemia who are suboptimal candidates for standard revascularization techniques. Recent advances in molecular biology have improved our understanding of the complex process of collateral development. Preclinical studies based on these principles using both FGF and VEGF angiogenic proteins demonstrated successful angiogenesis in multiple different animal models using a variety of methods of delivery. These successful preclinical studies led to successful phase I clinical trials with both recombinant FGF-2 and $VEGF_{165}$ protein using an ic delivery method. Encouraging initial results in these phase I trials led to two large phase II randomized trials, FIRST and VIVA. While both trials demonstrated excellent safety and improvement in secondary endpoints of angina class and quality of life, the primary endpoint in both trials, exercise time, was negative, raising questions about the ultimate benefit of recombinant protein therapy for myocardial angiogenesis. Two small placebo-controlled, unblinded trials using im protein as an adjunct to CABG have been positive, and a larger trial is still underway.

There has been considerable discussion of the theoretical advantages versus disadvantages of protein therapy compared to gene therapy or cell therapy for therapeutic myocardial angiogenesis. Unfortunately, there are limited direct data for comparison of the optimal approach. The number of patients with ongoing myocardial ischemia who are not candidates for standard revascularization continues to grow, and our current treatment options remain limited. Therefore, there continues to be intense interest in therapeutic myocardial angiogenesis as a potential treatment for these patients. It is important to realize that therapeutic angiogenesis remains in its infancy with a number of unanswered questions. Well-designed preclinical and clinical trials are needed to build on the excellent safety and promising but modest efficacy to optimize the treatment effect in this challenging group of patients.

REFERENCES

1. Solomon AJ, Gersh BJ. Management of chronic stable angina: medical therapy, percutaneous transluminal coronary angioplasty, and coronary artery bypass graft surgery. Lessons from the randomized trials. Ann Intern Med 1998;128(3):216–223.
2. Bourassa MG, Holubkov R, Yeh W, Detre KM. Strategy of complete revascularization in patients with multivessel coronary artery disease (a report from the 1985–1986 NHLBI PTCA Registry). Am J Cardiol 1992;70(2):174–178.
3. Mukherjee D, Bhatt DL, Roe MT, Patel V, Ellis SG. Direct myocardial revascularization and angiogenesis—how many patients might be eligible? Am J Cardiol 1999;84(5):598–600, A8.
4. Jones EL, Craver JM, Guyton RA, Bone DK, Hatcher CR Jr, Riechwald N. Importance of complete revascularization in performance of the coronary bypass operation. Am J Cardiol 1983;51(1):7–12.
5. Breisblatt WM, Barnes JV, Weiland F, Spaccavento LJ. Incomplete revascularization in multivessel percutaneous transluminal coronary angioplasty: the role for stress thallium-201 imaging. J Am Coll Cardiol 1988;11(6):1183–1190.
6. Glazier JJ, Verwilghen J, Morgan JM, Rickards AF. Outcome following incomplete revascularisation by coronary balloon angioplasty in patients with multivessel coronary artery disease. Ir Med J 1992;85(4):142–144.
7. Mannheimer C, Camici P, Chester MR, et al. The problem of chronic refractory angina; report from the ESC Joint Study Group on the Treatment of Refractory Angina. Eur Heart J 2002;23(5):355–370.
8. Kim MC, Kini A, Sharma SK. Refractory angina pectoris: mechanism and therapeutic options. J Am Coll Cardiol 2002;39(6):923–934.
9. Folkman J. Angiogenesis in cancer, vascular, rheumatoid and other disease. Nat Med 1995;1(1):27–31.
10. Folkman J, Klagsbrun M. Angiogenic factors. Science 1987;235(4787):442–447.
11. Polverini PJ. The pathophysiology of angiogenesis. Crit Rev Oral Biol Med 1995;6(3):230–247.
12. Folkman J, D'Amore PA. Blood vessel formation: what is its molecular basis? Cell 1996;87(7):1153–1155.
13. Kumar S, West D, Shahabuddin S, et al. Angiogenesis factor from human myocardial infarcts. Lancet 1983;2(8346):364–368.
14. McNeil PL, Muthukrishnan L, Warder E, D'Amore PA. Growth factors are released by mechanically wounded endothelial cells. J Cell Biol 1989;109(2):811–822.
15. Baffour R, Berman J, Garb JL, Rhee SW, Kaufman J, Friedmann P. Enhanced angiogenesis and growth of collaterals by in vivo administration of recombinant basic fibroblast growth factor in a rabbit model of acute lower limb ischemia: dose-response effect of basic fibroblast growth factor. J Vasc Surg 1992;16(2):181–191.
16. Levy AP. A cellular paradigm for the failure to increase vascular endothelial growth factor in chronically hypoxic states. Coron Artery Dis 1999;10(6):427–430.
17. Schaper W, Ito WD. Molecular mechanisms of coronary collateral vessel growth. Circ Res 1996;79(5):911–919.

18. Risau W. Mechanisms of angiogenesis. Nature 1997;386(6626):671–674.
19. Ware JA, Simons M. Angiogenesis in ischemic heart disease. Nat Med 1997;3(2):158–164.
20. Carmeliet P. Mechanisms of angiogenesis and arteriogenesis. Nat Med 2000;6(4):389–395.
21. Iruela-Arispe ML, Dvorak HF. Angiogenesis: a dynamic balance of stimulators and inhibitors. Thromb Haemost 1997;78(1):672–677.
22. Folkman J. Angiogenic therapy of the human heart. Circulation 1998;97(7):628–629.
23. Freedman SB, Isner JM. Therapeutic angiogenesis for coronary artery disease. Ann Intern Med 2002;136(1):54–71.
24. Durairaj A, Mehra A, Singh RP, Faxon DP. Therapeutic angiogenesis. Cardiol Rev 2000;8(5):279–287.
25. Harjai KJ, Chowdhury P, Grines CL. Therapeutic angiogenesis: a fantastic new adventure. J Interv Cardiol 2002;15(3):223–229.
26. Laham RJ, Garcia L, Baim DS, Post M, Simons M. Therapeutic angiogenesis using basic fibroblast growth factor and vascular endothelial growth factor using various delivery strategies. Curr Interv Cardiol Rep 1999;1(3):228–233.
27. Post MJ, Laham R, Sellke FW, Simons M. Therapeutic angiogenesis in cardiology using protein formulations. Cardiovasc Res 2001;49(3):522–531.
28. Houck KA, Ferrara N, Winer J, Cachianes G, Li B, Leung DW. The vascular endothelial growth factor family: identification of a fourth molecular species and characterization of alternative splicing of RNA. Mol Endocrinol 1991;5(12):1806–1814.
29. Ferrara N, Davis-Smyth T. The biology of vascular endothelial growth factor. Endocr Rev 1997;18(1):4–25.
30. Ferrara N. Vascular endothelial growth factor: molecular and biological aspects. Curr Top Microbiol Immunol 1999;237:1–30.
31. Henry TD, Abraham JA. Review of preclinical and clinical results with vascular endothelial growth factors for therapeutic angiogenesis. Curr Interv Cardiol Rep 2000;2(3):228–241.
32. Takeshita S, Weir L, Chen D, et al. Therapeutic angiogenesis following arterial gene transfer of vascular endothelial growth factor in a rabbit model of hindlimb ischemia. Biochem Biophys Res Commun 1996;227(2):628–635.
33. Henry TD. Therapeutic angiogenesis. BMJ 1999;318(7197):1536–1539.
34. Coulier F, Pontarotti P, Roubin R, Hartung H, Goldfarb M, Birnbaum D. Of worms and men: an evolutionary perspective on the fibroblast growth factor (FGF) and FGF receptor families. J Mol Evol 1997;44(1):43–56.
35. Asahara T, Bauters C, Zheng LP, et al. Synergistic effect of vascular endothelial growth factor and basic fibroblast growth factor on angiogenesis in vivo. Circulation 1995;92(9 Suppl):II365–II371.
36. Tabata H, Silver M, Isner JM. Arterial gene transfer of acidic fibroblast growth factor for therapeutic angiogenesis in vivo: critical role of secretion signal in use of naked DNA. Cardiovasc Res 1997;35(3):470–479.
37. Giordano FJ, Ping P, McKirnan MD, et al. Intracoronary gene transfer of fibroblast growth factor-5 increases blood flow and contractile function in an ischemic region of the heart. Nat Med 1996;2(5):534–539.
38. McKirnan MD, Guo X, Waldman LK, et al. Intracoronary gene transfer of fibroblast growth factor-4 increases regional contractile function and responsiveness to adrenergic stimulation in heart failure. CVP 2000;1:11–21.
39. Banai S, Jaklitsch MT, Casscells W, et al. Effects of acidic fibroblast growth factor on normal and ischemic myocardium. Circ Res 1991;69(1):76–85.

40. Unger EF, Shou M, Sheffield CD, Hodge E, Jaye M, Epstein SE. Extracardiac to coronary anastomoses support regional left ventricular function in dogs. Am J Physiol 1993;264(5 Pt 2):H1567–H1574.

41. Ortega S, Schaeffer MT, Soderman D, et al. Conversion of cysteine to serine residues alters the activity, stability, and heparin dependence of acidic fibroblast growth factor. J Biol Chem 1991;266(9):5842–5846.

42. Sellke FW, Li J, Stamler A, Lopez JJ, Thomas KA, Simons M. Angiogenesis induced by acidic fibroblast growth factor as an alternative method of revascularization for chronic myocardial ischemia. Surgery 1996;120(2):182–188.

43. Lopez JJ, Edelman ER, Stamler A, et al. Angiogenic potential of perivascularly delivered aFGF in a porcine model of chronic myocardial ischemia. Am J Physiol 1998;274(3 Pt 2):H930–H936.

44. Cuevas P, Carceller F, Lozano RM, Crespo A, Zazo M, Gimenez-Gallego G. Protection of rat myocardium by mitogenic and non-mitogenic fibroblast growth factor during postischemic reperfusion. Growth Factors 1997;15(1):29–40.

45. Yanagisawa-Miwa A, Uchida Y, Nakamura F, et al. Salvage of infarcted myocardium by angiogenic action of basic fibroblast growth factor. Science 1992;257(5075):1401–1403.

46. Battler A, Scheinowitz M, Bor A, et al. Intracoronary injection of basic fibroblast growth factor enhances angiogenesis in infarcted swine myocardium. J Am Coll Cardiol 1993;22(7):2001–2006.

47. Unger EF, Banai S, Shou M, et al. Basic fibroblast growth factor enhances myocardial collateral flow in a canine model. Am J Physiol 1994;266(4 Pt 2):H1588–H1595.

48. Lazarous DF, Scheinowitz M, Shou M, et al. Effects of chronic systemic administration of basic fibroblast growth factor on collateral development in the canine heart. Circulation 1995;91(1):145–153.

49. Shou M, Thirumurti V, Rajanayagam S, et al. Effect of basic fibroblast growth factor on myocardial angiogenesis in dogs with mature collateral vessels. J Am Coll Cardiol 1997;29(5):1102–1106.

50. Harada K, Grossman W, Friedman M, et al. Basic fibroblast growth factor improves myocardial function in chronically ischemic porcine hearts. J Clin Invest 1994;94(2):623–630.

51. Sellke FW, Wang SY, Friedman M, et al. Basic FGF enhances endothelium-dependent relaxation of the collateral-perfused coronary microcirculation. Am J Physiol 1994;267(4 Pt 2):H1303–H1311.

52. Lopez JJ, Edelman ER, Stamler A, et al. Basic fibroblast growth factor in a porcine model of chronic myocardial ischemia: a comparison of angiographic, echocardiographic and coronary flow parameters. J Pharmacol Exp Ther 1997;282(1):385–390.

53. Laham RJ, Simons M, Tofukuji M, Hung D, Sellke FW. Modulation of myocardial perfusion and vascular reactivity by pericardial basic fibroblast growth factor: insight into ischemia-induced reduction in endothelium-dependent vasodilatation. J Thorac Cardiovasc Surg 1998;116(6):1022–1028.

54. Laham RJ, Rezaee M, Post M, et al. Intrapericardial delivery of fibroblast growth factor-2 induces neovascularization in a porcine model of chronic myocardial ischemia. J Pharmacol Exp Ther 2000;292(2):795–802.

55. Sato K, Laham RJ, Pearlman JD, et al. Efficacy of intracoronary versus intravenous FGF-2 in a pig model of chronic myocardial ischemia. Ann Thorac Surg 2000;70(6):2113–2118.

56. Rajanayagam MA, Shou M, Thirumurti V, et al. Intracoronary basic fibroblast growth factor enhances myocardial collateral perfusion in dogs. J Am Coll Cardiol 2000;35(2):519–526.

57. Watanabe E, Smith DM, Sun J, et al. Effect of basic fibroblast growth factor on angiogenesis in the infarcted porcine heart. Basic Res Cardiol 1998;93(1):30–37.
58. Yamamoto N, Kohmoto T, Roethy W, et al. Histologic evidence that basic fibroblast growth factor enhances the angiogenic effects of transmyocardial laser revascularization. Basic Res Cardiol 2000;95(1):55–63.
59. Kawasuji M, Nagamine H, Ikeda M, et al. Therapeutic angiogenesis with intramyocardial administration of basic fibroblast growth factor. Ann Thorac Surg 2000;69(4):1155–1161.
60. Yamamoto T, Suto N, Okubo T, et al. Intramyocardial delivery of basic fibroblast growth factor-impregnated gelatin hydrogel microspheres enhances collateral circulation to infarcted canine myocardium. Jpn Circ J 2001;65(5):439–444.
61. Bao J, Naimark W, Palasis M, Laham R, Simons M, Post MJ. Intramyocardial delivery of FGF2 in combination with radio frequency transmyocardial revascularization. Catheter Cardiovasc Interv 2001;53(3):429–434.
62. Banai S, Jaklitsch MT, Shou M, et al. Angiogenic-induced enhancement of collateral blood flow to ischemic myocardium by vascular endothelial growth factor in dogs. Circulation 1994;89(5):2183–2189.
63. Lazarous DF, Shou M, Scheinowitz M, et al. Comparative effects of basic fibroblast growth factor and vascular endothelial growth factor on coronary collateral development and the arterial response to injury. Circulation 1996;94(5):1074–1082.
64. Sellke FW, Wang SY, Friedman M, et al. Beta-adrenergic modulation of the collateral-dependent coronary microcirculation. J Surg Res 1995;59(1):185–190.
65. Pearlman JD, Hibberd MG, Chuang ML, et al. Magnetic resonance mapping demonstrates benefits of VEGF-induced myocardial angiogenesis. Nat Med 1995;1(10):1085–1089.
66. Harada K, Friedman M, Lopez JJ, et al. Vascular endothelial growth factor administration in chronic myocardial ischemia. Am J Physiol 1996;270(5 Pt 2):H1791–802.
67. Lopez JJ, Laham RJ, Stamler A, et al. VEGF administration in chronic myocardial ischemia in pigs. Cardiovasc Res 1998;40(2):272–281.
68. Sellke FW, Tofukuji M, Laham RJ, et al. Comparison of VEGF delivery techniques on collateral-dependent microvascular reactivity. Microvasc Res 1998;55(2):175–178.
69. Hariawala MD, Horowitz JR, Esakof D, et al. VEGF improves myocardial blood flow but produces EDRF-mediated hypotension in porcine hearts. J Surg Res 1996;63(1):77–82.
70. Lopez JJ, Laham RJ, Carrozza JP, et al. Hemodynamic effects of intracoronary VEGF delivery: evidence of tachyphylaxis and NO dependence of response. Am J Physiol 1997;273(3 Pt 2):H1317–H1323.
71. Yang R, Thomas GR, Bunting S, et al. Effects of vascular endothelial growth factor on hemodynamics and cardiac performance. J Cardiovasc Pharmacol 1996;27(6):838–844.
72. Sato K, Wu T, Laham RJ, et al. Efficacy of intracoronary or intravenous VEGF165 in a pig model of chronic myocardial ischemia. J Am Coll Cardiol 2001;37(2):616–623.
73. Hughes GC, Biswas SS, Yin B, et al. Therapeutic angiogenesis in chronically ischemic porcine myocardium: comparative effects of bFGF and VEGF. Ann Thorac Surg 2004;77(3):812–818.
74. Schumacher B, Pecher P, von Specht BU, Stegmann T. Induction of neoangiogenesis in ischemic myocardium by human growth factors: first clinical results of a new treatment of coronary heart disease. Circulation 1998;97(7):645–650.
75. Stegmann TJ, Hoppert T, Schlurmann W, Gemeinhardt S. First angiogenic treatment of coronary heart disease by FGF-1: long-term results after 3 years. CVR 2000;1:5–10.

76. Laham RJ, Sellke FW, Edelman ER, et al. Local perivascular delivery of basic fibroblast growth factor in patients undergoing coronary bypass surgery: results of a phase I randomized, double-blind, placebo-controlled trial. Circulation 1999;100(18):1865–1871.

77. Ruel M, Laham RJ, Parker JA, et al. Long-term effects of surgical angiogenic therapy with fibroblast growth factor 2 protein. J Thorac Cardiovasc Surg 2002;124(1):28–34.

78. Udelson JE, Dilsizian V, Laham RJ, et al. Therapeutic angiogenesis with recombinant fibroblast growth factor-2 improves stress and rest myocardial perfusion abnormalities in patients with severe symptomatic chronic coronary artery disease. Circulation 2000;102(14):1605–1610.

79. Laham RJ, Chronos NA, Pike M, et al. Intracoronary basic fibroblast growth factor (FGF-2) in patients with severe ischemic heart disease: results of a phase I open-label dose escalation study. J Am Coll Cardiol 2000;36(7):2132–2139.

80. Simons M, Annex BH, Laham RJ, et al. Pharmacological treatment of coronary artery disease with recombinant fibroblast growth factor-2: double-blind, randomized, controlled clinical trial. Circulation 2002;105(7):788–793.

81. Aaberge L, Nordstrand K, Dragsund M, et al. Transmyocardial revascularization with CO2 laser in patients with refractory angina pectoris. Clinical results from the Norwegian randomized trial. J Am Coll Cardiol 2000;35(5):1170–1177.

82. Frazier OH, March RJ, Horvath KA. Transmyocardial revascularization with a carbon dioxide laser in patients with end-stage coronary artery disease. N Engl J Med 1999;341(14):1021–1028.

83. Hendel RC, Henry TD, Rocha-Singh K, et al. Effect of intracoronary recombinant human vascular endothelial growth factor on myocardial perfusion: evidence for a dose-dependent effect. Circulation 2000;101(2):118–121.

84. Henry TD, Rocha-Singh K, Isner JM, et al. Intracoronary administration of recombinant human vascular endothelial growth factor to patients with coronary artery disease. Am Heart J 2001;142(5):872–880.

85. Dauterman KW, Kraimer N, Weisberg S, Pai R, Marble SJ. rh-VEGF administration is associated with a larger improvement in myocardial blush circumference: a VIVA substudy. Circulation 2001;104:II–54.

86. Henry TD, Annex BH, McKendall GR, et al. The VIVA trial: Vascular endothelial growth factor in Ischemia for Vascular Angiogenesis. Circulation 2003;107(10):1359–1365.

87. Henry TD, McKendall GR, Azrin MA, et al. VIVA trial: one year follow up. Circulation 2000;102:II–309.

88. Simons M, Bonow RO, Chronos NA, et al. Clinical trials in coronary angiogenesis: issues, problems, consensus: An expert panel summary. Circulation 2000;102(11):E73–E86.

89. Edelman ER, Mathiowitz E, Langer R, Klagsbrun M. Controlled and modulated release of basic fibroblast growth factor. Biomaterials 1991;12(7):619–626.

90. Melillo G, Scoccianti M, Kovesdi I, Safi J Jr, Riccioni T, Capogrossi MC. Gene therapy for collateral vessel development. Cardiovasc Res 1997;35(3):480–489.

91. Lewis BS, Flugelman MY, Weisz A, Keren-Tal I, Schaper W. Angiogenesis by gene therapy: a new horizon for myocardial revascularization? Cardiovasc Res 1997;35(3):490–497.

92. Tsurumi Y, Takeshita S, Chen D, et al. Direct intramuscular gene transfer of naked DNA encoding vascular endothelial growth factor augments collateral development and tissue perfusion. Circulation 1996;94(12):3281–3290.

93. Schwarz ER, Speakman MT, Patterson M, et al. Evaluation of the effects of intramyocardial injection of DNA expressing vascular endothelial growth factor (VEGF) in a myocardial infarction model in the rat—angiogenesis and angioma formation. J Am Coll Cardiol 2000;35(5):1323–1330.

94. Ribatti D, Gualandris A, Belleri M, et al. Alterations of blood vessel development by endothelial cells overexpressing fibroblast growth factor-2. J Pathol 1999;189(4):590–599.

95. Brown LF, Tognazzi K, Dvorak HF, Harrist TJ. Strong expression of kinase insert domain-containing receptor, a vascular permeability factor/vascular endothelial growth factor receptor in AIDS-associated Kaposi's sarcoma and cutaneous angiosarcoma. Am J Pathol 1996;148(4):1065–1074.

96. Wahlers A, Schwieger M, Li Z, et al. Influence of multiplicity of infection and protein stability on retroviral vector-mediated gene expression in hematopoietic cells. Gene Ther 2001;8(6):477–486.

97. Davis HL, Whalen RG, Demeneix BA. Direct gene transfer into skeletal muscle in vivo: factors affecting efficiency of transfer and stability of expression. Hum Gene Ther 1993;4(2):151–159.

98. Yap J, O'Brien T, Tazelaar HD, McGregor CG. Immunosuppression prolongs adenoviral mediated transgene expression in cardiac allograft transplantation. Cardiovasc Res 1997;35(3):529-535.

99. Gilgenkrantz H, Duboc D, Juillard V, et al. Transient expression of genes transferred in vivo into heart using first-generation adenoviral vectors: role of the immune response. Hum Gene Ther 1995;6(10):1265–1274.

100. Chan SY, Li K, Piccotti JR, et al. Tissue-specific consequences of the antiadenoviral immune response: implications for cardiac transplants. Nat Med 1999;5(10):1143–1149.

101. Lazarous DF, Shou M, Stiber JA, et al. Pharmacodynamics of basic fibroblast growth factor: route of administration determines myocardial and systemic distribution. Cardiovasc Res 1997;36(1):78–85.

102. Laham RJ, Rezaee M, Post M, et al. Intracoronary and intravenous administration of basic fibroblast growth factor: myocardial and tissue distribution. Drug Metab Dispos 1999;27(7):821–826.

103. Stoll HP, Carlson K, Keefer LK, Hrabie JA, March KL. Pharmacokinetics and consistency of pericardial delivery directed to coronary arteries: direct comparison with endoluminal delivery. Clin Cardiol 1999;22(1 Suppl 1):I10–I16.

104. Meyer BJ, Fernandez-Ortiz A, Mailhac A, et al. Local delivery of r-hirudin by a double-balloon perfusion catheter prevents mural thrombosis and minimizes platelet deposition after angioplasty. Circulation 1994;90(5):2474–2480.

105. Stegmann TJ, Hoppert T, Schneider A, et al. [Induction of myocardial neoangiogenesis by human growth factors. A new therapeutic approach in coronary heart disease]. Herz 2000;25(6):589–599.

106. Peters MC, Isenberg BC, Rowley JA, Mooney DJ. Release from alginate enhances the biological activity of vascular endothelial growth factor. J Biomater Sci Polym Ed 1998;9(12):1267–1278.

107. Herity NA, Lo ST, Oei F, et al. Selective regional myocardial infiltration by the percutaneous coronary venous route: a novel technique for local drug delivery. Catheter Cardiovasc Interv 2000;51(3):358–363.

108. Eppler SM, Combs DL, Henry TD, et al. A target-mediated model to describe the pharmacokinetics and hemodynamic effects of recombinant human vascular endothelial growth factor in humans. Clin Pharmacol Ther 2002;72(1):20–32.

109. Giordano FJ, Ross J, Peterson KL, et al. Intravenous or intracoronary VEGF ameliorates chronic myocardial ischemia. Circulation 1998;98:I–455.
110. Villanueva FS, Abraham JA, Schreiner GF, et al. Myocardial contrast echocardiography can be used to assess the microvascular response to vascular endothelial growth factor-121. Circulation 2002;105(6):759–765.
111. Schumacher B, Stegmann T, Pecher P. The stimulation of neoangiogenesis in the ischemic human heart by the growth factor FGF: first clinical results. J Cardiovasc Surg (Torino) 1998;39(6):783–789.

8 Gene Therapy for Angiogenesis in the Treatment of Cardiovascular and Peripheral Arterial Disease

Pinak B. Shah, MD,
Kapildeo Lotun, MD,
and Douglas W. Losordo, MD

INTRODUCTION

Over the last quarter-century, numerous advances have been made in the understanding of the molecular and cellular processes that lead to the development of atherosclerosis. The respective roles of the endothe-

From: *Contemporary Cardiology: Angiogenesis and Direct Myocardial Revasularization*
Edited by: R. J. Laham and D. S. Baim © Humana Press Inc., Totowa, NJ

lium, inflammatory mediators, and thrombosis in the pathogenesis of vascular disease are beginning to be better understood. As more is learned about the initiation of atherosclerotic cardiovascular disease, new targets for systemic therapies are being discovered. Several classes of medications have been shown to be beneficial in preventing adverse cardiovascular events in patients with cardiovascular disease. These medications include platelet inhibitors (aspirin and thienopyridines), angiotensin-converting enzyme inhibitors, and 3-hydroxy-3-methylglutaryl coenzyme A (HMG-CoA) reductase inhibitors ("statins").

In conjunction with the improved understanding of the pathogenesis of vascular disease have occurred improvements in mechanical therapies for vascular disease. Surgical techniques have been perfected so that obstructed arteries can be effectively bypassed (as in coronary artery bypass grafting and lower extremity bypass grafting) or be cleared of obstructive plaque (as in carotid endarterectomy). Revascularization strategies have since moved to less invasive endovascular techniques. Coronary arteries are routinely treated with metallic stents to improve myocardial blood flow and reduce ischemic symptoms. Stents are also routinely placed in iliac arteries for disabling claudication or critical limb ischemia, renal arteries for renovascular hypertension, and, more recently, carotid arteries for the prevention of stroke. Percutaneous therapies are slowly supplanting surgical therapies as the treatment of choice for patients with cardiovascular disease, particularly in those patients with significant comorbidities limiting surgical options.

Ironically, although advancements in therapy have resulted in patients living longer with more severe cardiovascular disease, they have also resulted in a growing population of people who are no longer candidates for conventional therapies for their symptoms. These "no-option" patients live with severe angina, congestive heart failure, or disabling claudication/limb ischemia and are becoming an increasingly larger part of our aging society. The fundamental problem in these patients is a deficiency in the blood supply to the myocardial and lower extremity muscle beds as a result of severe, diffuse, and often totally occlusive vascular disease. The next "holy grail" in cardiovascular medicine is to stimulate the development of new vasculature to ischemic tissue (therapeutic angiogenesis) in order to improve blood flow, improve end-organ function, and relieve symptoms. Gene therapy may prove to be the most effective means of promoting therapeutic angiogenesis. Before a review of gene therapy for cardiovascular disease, a description of vasculogenesis, angiogenesis, and angiogenic growth factors is warranted.

VASCULOGENESIS AND ANGIOGENESIS

In 1971, Folkman and colleagues published their pioneering work on growth factors, suggesting that the establishment and maintenance of a vascular supply is essential for growth of normal as well as neoplastic tissue (1). The establishment of a vascular supply occurs as a result of two main processes: vasculogenesis and angiogenesis. Vasculogenesis is the de novo *in situ* differentiation of endothelial cells (ECs) from mesodermal precursors in the embryo by association of endothelial progenitor cells (EPCs) or angioblasts and their subsequent reorganization into a primary capillary plexus (2). In contrast, angiogenesis is the formation of new blood vessels from pre-existing blood vessels. Angiogenesis is induced by the proliferation and migration of pre-existing, fully differentiated ECs resident within parent vessels in response to stimuli such as hypoxia, ischemia, mechanical stretch, and inflammation (3,4). Angiogenesis can be a normal physiological process (such as wound healing), or a pathological process (such as in neoplasms and proliferative diabetic retinopathy).

Vasculogenesis was previously considered to be restricted to embryonic vascular development, whereas angiogenesis was thought to be responsible for both embryonic vascular development and postnatal neovascularization. Recent evidence, however, suggests that the basis for embryonic as well as therapeutic neovascularization likely encompasses both processes. Circulating CD34 antigen-positive EPCs were recently isolated from adult species and shown to differentiate along an endothelial cell lineage in vitro, thus constituting inferential evidence for the importance of circulating stem cells in angiogenesis (5). In addition, the demonstration that bone marrow-derived EPCs are increased in number in response to tissue ischemia, migrate and incorporate into foci of neovascularization in adult animals, and augment collateral development following ex vivo expansion and transplantation suggests that neovascularization in the adult involves both angiogenesis and vasculogenesis (6–8). Tateishi-Yuyama et al. recently showed the potential of autologous stem cell transplantation to result in angiogenesis in patients with critical limb ischemia (9).

Arteriogenesis has been recognized as a mechanism that probably contributes to collateral vessel formation. A proportion of newly recognized medium-sized arteries may be the result of proliferation of preexisting arteriolar connections into larger collateral vessels by remodeling (10). It is unknown whether such remodeling occurs as a direct result of growth factor modulation or as a flow-mediated maturation of these collateral conduits by a process of "arteriolization" of capillaries.

ANGIOGENIC GROWTH FACTORS

Although many cytokines have angiogenic activity, the best studied in animal models and clinical trials are vascular endothelial growth factor (VEGF) and fibroblast growth factor (FGF).

Vascular Endothelial Growth Factor

The human VEGF proteins that have been identified to date are VEGF-1, VEGF-2 or VEGF-C, VEGF-3 or VEGF-B, VEGF-D, VEGF-E, and placental growth factor (PlGF). All are encoded by different genes and are localized to different chromosomes but share considerable homology. There are four isoforms of VEGF-1 that are the result of alternate splicing and are named according to the number of amino acids: $VEGF_{121}$, $VEGF_{165}$, $VEGF_{189}$, and $VEGF_{206}$. These isoforms of VEGF show similar angiogenic potential in animal models *(11)* but differ in their solubility and heparin-binding capacity accounting for differences in target cell binding. The principal cellular target of VEGF is the EC. There are three known endothelial-specific fms-like tyrosine kinases: VEGFR-1 (Flt-1), VEGFR-2 (Flk-1/KDR), and VEGFR-3. Hypoxia induces the formation of VEGF by the ECs and leads to upregulation of VEGF receptors *(12)*. VEGFR-1 generates signals that organize the assembly of ECs into tubes and functional vessels *(13)*. VEGFR-2 is responsible for EC proliferation and migration *(14,15)*. VEGFR-3 (Flt-4) principally mediates lymphangiogenesis *(16)*.

VEGF possesses several features that facilitate gene transfer. First, VEGF contains a hydrophobic leader sequence, which is a secretory signal sequence that permits the protein to be secreted naturally from intact cells, thus enabling a sequence of additional paracrine effects to be activated *(17)*. Second, its high-affinity binding sites are exclusive to ECs, and, therefore, the mitogenic effects of VEGF are limited to ECs. This is in contrast to acidic and basic FGF, both of which are known to be mitogenic for smooth muscle cells and fibroblasts as well as ECs *(18,19)*. Third, VEGF possesses an autocrine loop that is shared by most angiogenic cytokines and facilitates modulation of EC behavior. When activated under hypoxic conditions, the autocrine loop serves to amplify and thereby protract the response in ECs stimulated by exogenously administered VEGF. Furthermore, factors secreted by hypoxic myocytes upregulate VEGF receptor expression on ECs within the hypoxic milieu. Such localized receptor expressions may explain the finding that angiogenesis does not occur indiscriminately, but relatively limited to sites of tissue ischemia. Recently, an important additional role for VEGF has been described in augmentation of circulating EPC numbers documented in mice and humans following VEGF gene transfer *(20–22)*. These EPCs have been shown to home into areas of myocardial ischemia.

Fibroblast Growth Factor

FGF is a family of nine factors including acidic FGF (FGF-1), basic FGF (bFGF or FGF-2), and FGF 3–9. Acidic FGF and basic FGF are the most extensively characterized members of the FGF family. FGFs are nonsecreted growth factors lacking a signal peptide sequence. The extracellular release of FGF is caused by cell death or damage. It binds to tyrosine kinase receptors via cell-surface heparan sulfate proteoglycans, and as result, FGF is rapidly removed from the circulation and localized to cells and extracellular matrix. Although FGFs are potent EC mitogens, they are not EC specific and also serve as ligands for other cell types, including vascular smooth muscle cells and fibroblasts. At least four high-affinity FGF receptors have been identified, and their cDNAs have been cloned. The FGFs, like VEGF, also stimulate EC synthesis of proteases, including plasminogen activator and metalloproteinases, important for extracellular matrix digestion in the process of angiogenesis *(23)*. Unlike VEGF, however, the common forms of FGF (FGF-1 and -2) lack a secretory signal sequence, and, therefore, clinical trials of FGF gene transfer have required either modification of the FGF gene or use of another of the FGF gene family with a signal sequence *(24–26)*.

THERAPEUTIC ANGIOGENESIS

Angiogenic cytokines may be administered as recombinant protein or as genes encoding for these proteins. Given that both protein and gene-delivery approaches have been relatively well tolerated thus far in clinical trials, ongoing investigations will determine the optimal preparation and delivery strategy for therapeutic neovascularization. Protein therapy remains the more conventional approach, and some investigators have indicated that this strategy is the closest to practical use. Nevertheless, recombinant protein is usually administered systemically, and several issues limit its use. First, high plasma concentrations are required to achieve adequate tissue uptake to translate into a meaningful biological effect. This leads to higher potential for adverse effects. Second, recombinant human protein is difficult to produce and the costs are prohibitive.

Gene transfer allows for high levels of sustained gene expression without provoking adverse host reactions. The efficiency with which the transgene is introduced and expressed into the target cell and the duration of transgene expression determines the success of gene transfer strategies. Transfer vectors facilitate cellular penetration and intracellular trafficking of the transgene, and local delivery systems deliver the vector to the vicinity of the target cells.

There are two major categories of gene transfer systems: viral and nonviral. The most commonly used viral vectors for gene transfer are adenovirus and retrovirus. The nonviral methods for gene transfer include introduction of naked DNA into the target area or the transfer of genetic material via a liposomal vehicle.

Hypoxia stimulates secretion of the angiogenic cytokines and also causes an increased expression of nitric oxide (NO) and VEGF receptors. Thus, ischemic muscle represents a promising target for angiogenic growth factor therapy. Striated and cardiac muscles have been shown to take up and express naked plasmid DNA as well as transgenes incorporated into viral vectors. Moreover, previous studies have shown that the transfection efficiency of intramuscular gene transfer is augmented more than fivefold when the injected muscle is ischemic (27,28). Viral vectors may enhance transfection efficiency and thus yield higher levels of gene expression. In vitro and in vivo models have demonstrated that low-efficiency, but site-specific, transfection (successful transfection in <1% of cells) with a gene (plasmid DNA) encoding for a secreted protein (e.g., VEGF) may overcome the handicap of inefficient transfection (29,30). By secreting adequate protein locally that translates into physiologically meaningful biological effects, therapeutic effects are achieved that are not realized by transfection with genes encoding for proteins that remain intracellular (e.g., bFGF). Furthermore, unlike viral vectors, plasmid DNA does not induce inflammation.

CLINICAL TRIALS OF VEGF PROTEIN AND GENE THERAPY

Peripheral Vascular Disease

The consensus statement of the European Working Group on Critical Limb Ischemia states that no medical treatment has been shown to alter the natural history of critical limb ischemia (31). In a large proportion of patients with critical limb ischemia, the distribution and extent of the arterial occlusive disease makes percutaneous or surgical revascularization impossible. In advanced stages of disease, quality-of-life measures are comparable to those patients with terminal cancer (32). Despite appropriate medical and surgical therapy, the unrelenting course of the disease ultimately leads to amputation. Of patients undergoing one amputation, 10% require a second amputation (33–36).

Despite the associated morbidity and mortality associated with amputation, it is often chosen as first-line therapy. Consequently, the need for alternative treatment strategies in patients with critical limb ischemia is compelling. Significant research has focused on developing angiogenic therapies to provide novel approaches to the treatment of limb ischemia.

Preclinical studies have established proof of principle for the concept that the angiogenic activity of VEGF is sufficiently potent to achieve therapeutic benefit. After intra-arterial administration of recombinant VEGF protein, augmentation of angiographically visible collateral vessels and histologically identifiable capillaries were demonstrated in rabbits with severe, unilateral hindlimb ischemia *(37)*. Evidence that VEGF stimulates angiogenesis in vivo had been developed in experiments performed on other animal models including rat and rabbit cornea, the chorioallantoic membrane, and the rabbit bone graft model *(18,38)*. Intra-arterial gene transfer of phVEGF$_{165}$ in a human patient subsequently demonstrated angiographic and histological evidence of angiogenesis *(39)*.

Intra-arterial delivery, however, has several inherent limitations that could undermine successful growth factor transfer for critical limb ischemia. In the case of recombinant proteins, large doses of protein are necessary to exert a treatment effect in the face of rapid degradation by circulating proteinases. With naked DNA, i.e., DNA unassociated with viral or other adjunctive vectors, cellular uptake is virtually nil when the transgene is directly injected into the arterial lumen, presumably as a result of prompt degradation by circulating nucleases. In addition, the diffuse distribution of neointimal thickening and/or extensive atherosclerotic disease may limit gene transfer to the smooth muscle cells of the arterial media *(40)*.

Preclinical studies of VEGF gene therapy were therefore designed to establish the feasibility of site-specific intramuscular gene transfer of VEGF in critical limb ischemia to promote therapeutic angiogenesis. Meaningful biological outcomes were observed following VEGF gene transfer of naked DNA by direct injection into skeletal muscle of ischemic rabbit hindlimbs as evidenced by increased hindlimb blood pressure ratio, increased Doppler-derived iliac flow, enhanced neovascularity by angiography, and increased capillary density at necropsy *(28,41)*.

Intramuscular gene transfer of 4000 µg naked plasmid DNA encoding VEGF (phVEGF$_{165}$) was utilized to successfully accomplish therapeutic angiogenesis in patients with critical limb ischemia *(42)*. Gene expression was documented by a transient increase in serum levels of VEGF monitored by enzyme-linked immunosorbent assay (ELISA). Meaningful clinical and physiological benefit was demonstrated by regression of rest pain and/or improved limb integrity, increased pain-free walking time, increased ankle-brachial index, newly visible collateral vessels by digital subtraction angiography, and qualitative evidence of improved distal flow by magnetic resonance imaging (MRI).

In a subsequent clinical trial in 55 patients (ages 24–84 yr, $m = 56.7$ yr) with ischemic rest pain ($n = 14$) or ischemic ulcers ($n = 41$) were treated with intramuscular injections of phVEGF$_{165}$. Evidence of clinical improvement was observed in 13 of 14 (72%) patients with rest pain alone and 26 of 41 (63%) patients with ischemic ulcers over a follow-up period of 4–36 mo. For the total cohort of 55 patients, a favorable clinical outcome was achieved in 65.5%. Multiple logistic regression analysis identified rest pain and age <50 yr as significant, independent predictors of a favorable clinical outcome. Diabetes, smoking, hyperlipidemia, hypertension, and phVEGF$_{165}$ dose were not predictors of clinical outcome (43). Complications in these patients have been limited to lower-extremity edema that develops in approximately one-third of patients (44). Edema was either self-limited or required a brief course of diuretic therapy, and it resolved approx 1–2 mo after gene transfer.

A similar treatment strategy was used in 11 patients with Buerger's disease presenting with critical limb ischemia, 9 of whom were successfully treated with intramuscular phVEGF$_{165}$ (45). These patients had resolution of nocturnal rest pain and healing of foot and/or leg ulcers. The ankle-brachial index (ABI) increased by greater than 0.1, and newly formed collateral vessels were seen on magnetic resonance angiography (MRA) and serial contrast angiography.

Preclinical studies from our laboratory demonstrated that VEGF-2 could promote angiogenesis in a rabbit hindlimb ischemia model and stimulate the release of nitric oxide from ECs (46). Based on these preclinical studies, a randomized, double-blind, placebo-controlled, dose-escalating trial to investigate the therapeutic potential of VEGF-2 gene transfer in patients with critical limb ischemia (CLI) was recently completed. Forty-eight patients were enrolled between 1999 and 2000. These patients had Rutherford category 4/5 limb ischemia and no revascularization options. The dose of gene used ranged between 1.0 and 4.0 mg. Patients received eight calf injections and were followed up weekly for 12 wk and then monthly for 3 mo and at visits at 9 and 12 mo. Data from this study are currently being reviewed, and the results are unavailable.

Recently, Nabel et al. published preliminary results of a phase I trial to evaluate the safety of an adenoviral vector encoding VEGF$_{121}$ in patients with disabling peripheral arterial diseases. Intramuscular injections of the adenoviral vector were performed in skeletal muscle of the lower limbs at sites of desired collateral formation. There was a favorable influence on lower extremity endothelial function and flow reserve in five patients treated (47). However, others have reported negative results with adenovirus-encoded $VEGF_{121}$ for peripheral arterial disease. It is felt that the lack of a heparin-binding domain on the 121 isoform potentially limits the effective local delivery of $VEGF_{121}$ (B. Annex, MD, personal communication).

Prevention of Restenosis After Peripheral Angioplasty

In the adductor canal, the superficial femoral artery (SFA) is prone to stenosis, and this represents one of the most common sites of peripheral arterial obstruction. Several postulates have inadequately explained this phenomenon. Percutaneous transluminal coronary angioplasty (PTCA) has been used widely and successfully to treat atherosclerotic obstructions in the peripheral and coronary circulations. However, high rates of restenosis following angioplasty of the SFA/popliteal artery continues to be a vexing and, consequently, expensive complication of this otherwise efficacious intervention. Although immediate procedural success for percutaneous revascularization of lesions in the SFA using conventional guidewires and standard PTA is well in excess of 90%, published reports have established that restenosis may complicate the clinical course of as many as 60% of patients undergoing PTA for SFA stenosis and/or occlusion. Previous strategies to limit the development of restenosis by nonmechanical means have not proved effective. Treatment strategies aimed at specifically restoring endothelial integrity have not been previously explored for restenosis prevention. Animal studies demonstrated that administration of mitogens, such as VEGF, that promote EC migration and/or proliferation might achieve acceleration of reendothelialization and thereby reduce intimal thickening (48–51).

We therefore designed a phase 1, single-site, dose-escalating open-label, unblinded gene therapy trial to accelerate re-endothelialization at the site of PTCA-induced endothelial disruption as a novel means to inhibit restenosis following PTCA. The primary objective of this study was to document the safety of percutaneous catheter-based delivery of the gene encoding VEGF in patients with claudication resulting from SFA obstruction.

Arterial VEGF gene transfer has thus far been performed in 30 patients— 21 males and 9 females—with a mean age of 68 yr. All patients had two or more cardiovascular risk factors. Gene expression was documented by a rise in plasma levels of VEGF. Peak plasma levels were recorded at a mean of 12 d following gene transfer. Mean claudication time increased from 2 min at baseline to 5 min up to 18 mo post-gene transfer. Prior to gene transfer, all patients were classified as Rutherford class 3. At 12–18 mo following gene transfer, 15 patients were asymptomatic and

8 patients were class 1. After an initial improvement in two Rutherford classes following revascularization, six patients returned to class 3. One patient developed critical limb ischemia and required salvage therapy with intramuscular gene transfer of naked plasmid DNA encoding VEGF.

There was a significant and sustained improvement in ABI post–gene transfer compared to baseline. Prior to gene transfer the mean ABI was 0.70, increased to 0.92 18 mo after gene transfer, and was sustained at 0.91 at 48 mo after gene transfer. SFA stenosis in 24 patients dropped from a mean of 94% at baseline to 30% at an average of 9 mo following gene transfer. These results were supported by intravascular ultrasound (IVUS) findings at the time of follow-up angiography. Six patients had evidence of restenosis at angiography performed 6–12 mo following gene transfer. Target vessel revascularization was required in all six patients. Histology from three of four patients undergoing directional atherectomy at the time of repeat revascularization for restenosis demonstrated active smooth muscle cell proliferation and high levels of proliferating cell nuclear antigen, indicating extensive proliferative activity.

Thus, in the 30 patients treated with arterial VEGF gene transfer for prevention of restenosis, VEGF expression has been documented by ELISA. At 48-mo follow-up, 6 of 30 patients (20%) required target vessel revascularization for angiographic and ultrasound evidence of restenosis. When compared to historical controls at 6 mo, restenosis rate was 20% in the gene transfer group, 29% in patients undergoing brachytherapy, and 55% in patients undergoing percutaneous angioplasty alone *(52)*. This preliminary study suggests that gene therapy designed to accelerate reendothelialization at the site of PTCA-induced endothelial disruption can be safely performed. Importantly, no evidence of accelerated atherosclerosis or increase in the restenosis rate was observed following gene transfer.

Myocardial Ischemia

For patients in whom antianginal medications fail to provide sufficient symptomatic relief, other interventions such as angioplasty or bypass surgery may be required. Although both types of intervention have been shown to be effective for various types of patients, a considerable group of patients may not be candidates for either intervention as a result of to the diffuse nature of their coronary artery disease. Moreover, there are many patients in whom recurrent narrowing and/or occlusion of bypass conduits after initially successful surgery has left the patient again symptomatic with no further option for conventional revascularization.

For the purposes of myocardial angiogenesis, $VEGF_{165}$ recombinant protein has been administered via a wide variety of routes. Phase 1 studies of both intracoronary and intravenous injection of $VEGF_{165}$ recombinant protein in patients with symptomatic, inoperable coronary artery disease revealed encouraging improvements in anginal status as well as both rest and stress nuclear perfusion studies (53–55).

The VEGF in Ischemia for Vascular Angiogenesis (VIVA) study was a phase 2, double-blind, placebo-controlled, multicenter, dose-escalating trial of patients with angina and viable myocardium who were not optimal candidates for percutaneous or surgical revascularization. Patients randomized to the treatment group received intracoronary injections and three intravenous infusion injections of VEGF-1 protein (56–59). The doses used were 17 or 50 µg/kg/min via intracoronary route for 20 min and intravenously for 4 h on d 3, 6, and 9. One hundred and fifteen patients received the recombinant VEGF, and 63 patients received the placebo. Patients were followed up at 60 and 120 d and at 1 yr. At 60 d there was a similar increase in exercise time for both the treatment and the placebo group (approx 45 s). Similarly, there were similar decreases in angina and quality of life and no change in perfusion studies. At 120 d, patients who received the high dose had a decrease in angina grade and a trend to increased exercise time. At 1-yr follow-up there were no statistical differences in the clinical and measured parameters, but there was a trend towards decrease angina class in patients receiving the VEGF-1 recombinant protein. Angiographic and single photon emission computed tomography (SPECT)-sestamibi scan did not show any significant change in any group.

The VIVA trial demonstrated that hypotension was a significant limitation in the dose of recombinant VEGF that could be administered intravasculary. This complication of recombinant VEGF therapy was also seen in animal experiments performed in our laboratory utilizing recombinant human VEGF ($rhVEGF_{165}$). Hypotension after systemic administration of recombinant VEGF is believed to be mediated by VEGF-induced release of NO (60). Similar results were reported from other groups utilizing intracoronary injection in the pig and dog (61,62). Other routes of administration of VEGF (intramyocardial, peri-adventitial, and intravenous) have shown limited efficacy (61,63,64), likely due to an inability to administer a sufficient dose of the protein.

Accordingly, it has been hypothesized that local expression of VEGF for a protracted period of 2–3 wk via gene transfer might circumvent the problem of symptomatic hypotension, yet still achieve a reduction in myocardial ischemia. VEGF gene transfer for myocardial ischemia has been performed in animal models using both adenovirus vectors as well as the administration of naked plasmid DNA. Intramyocardial injection of adenovirus encoding $VEGF_{121}$ via thoracotomy in a pig ameroid model improved collateral perfusion and function *(65,66)*. Intracoronary adenoviral gene delivery produced much lower gene and VEGF levels in the myocardium with poor localization *(66)*. Pericardial delivery of adenovirus encoding $VEGF_{165}$ in a dog model did not increase collateral flow *(67)*.

Our center initiated a phase 1, dose-escalating, open-label clinical study to determine the safety and bioactivity of direct myocardial gene transfer of $phVEGF_{165}$ as sole therapy (i.e., without angioplasty, stenting, or bypass graft surgery) for myocardial ischemia. Patients with stable exertional angina refractory to medical therapy, areas of viable but underperfused myocardium on perfusion scanning, and multivessel occlusive coronary artery disease were selected. Preliminary results of this trial suggested that safe and successful transfection could be achieved by this method with a favorable clinical effect *(68,69)*. Thirty patients with mean age of 63 yr were selected. Twenty-nine of 30 patients had CABG, and all had suffered myocardial ischemia. All received $phVEGF_{165}$ administered by direct myocardial injection in four aliquots of 2.0 mL via a minithoracotomy: total dose 125 µg ($n = 10$), 250 µg ($n = 10$), or 500 µg ($n = 10$). Using a stabilizing device that facilitates vascular anastomosis during beating heart bypass, an immobile field for intramyocardial injection was ensured. Continuous transesophageal echocardiographic monitoring was performed throughout the procedure to monitor development of wall motion abnormalities associated with injections and ensure that plasmid DNA was not injected into the left-ventricular (LV) cavity *(70)*. No peri-operative complications occurred. There was no evidence of myocardial damage by cardiac enzyme analysis, and patients maintained LV function. Gene expression was documented by a transient but significant increase in plasma levels of VEGF monitored by ELISA assay. All patients experienced marked symptomatic improvement and/or objective evidence of improved myocardial perfusion. At 360 d, 15 of 30 patients were free of angina. Specifically, sublingual nitrate use fell from 60 to 3/wk at day 360 accompanied by a significant reduction in episodes of angina from 56 to 4/wk at d 360. Exercise time for the group at 360 d increased by 98 s, and exercise time to angina increased by 2.5 min over baseline. There were two late deaths (4.5 and 28.5 mo), and one patient underwent a cardiac transplant at 13 mo *(69)*. Evidence of reduced ischemia on SPECT-sestamibi myocardial perfusion scanning was documented in 22 of 29 patients, with a significant reduction in both stress and rest mean perfusion/ischemia score at d 60. In addition, 22 of 29 patients (76%) improved by two Canadian Cardiovascular Society (CCS) angina classes at 12 mo, and 20 of 28 patients (71%) improved by 2 or more CCS classes at 2 yr.

It is intriguing to note that not only defects observed in the perfusion scans with pharmacological stress, but also those observed at rest, improved post gene transfer. Sequential SPECT scans recorded before and after gene transfer demonstrated partial or complete resolution of fixed defects in four (33%) and five (43%) patients, respectively, in whom defects were present on the initial rest image. This is consistent with the notion that these pre-existing defects constitute foci of hibernating viable myocardium that have resumed or improved contractile activity as a result of therapeutic neovascularization *(71–73)*. This observation was supported by the findings of electromechanical mapping utilized in the final 13 consecutive patients. Resting perfusion defects on the SPECT images corresponded to areas with ischemic characteristics (reduced wall motion with preserved viability) on the endocardial maps. Foci of ischemia were identified preoperatively in all patients with significant improvement in these endocardial wall motion abnormalities at 60 d post gene transfer *(74)*. This study provides the first evidence for a favorable clinical effect of direct myocardial injection of naked plasmid DNA encoding for VEGF as the sole therapeutic intervention.

A similar favorable experience was seen in an open-label, dose-escalating, multicenter clinical trial of VEGF-2 plasmid DNA in 30 patients with end-stage coronary artery disease and refractory class III or IV angina. Twenty-four male patients and six female patients with a mean age of 61 yr were selected. All had previous CABG, and all had sustained one to two episodes of myocardial ischemia. Their medical regimen included more than two antianginal medications. In all patients, there were no procedural adverse events, although there was one death 20 h after surgery. At 12 mo following gene transfer, the mean number of anginal episodes and nitrate tablets consumed per week decreased significantly. By d 90, 21 of 30 (70%) patients improved by more than two CCS angina classes, with an additional 4 patients (25/29 patients or 86%) with similar improvement at 360 d. The mean duration of exercise also increased by more than 2 min (unpublished data).

The other reported study of direct myocardial VEGF gene transfer was with adenoviral-assisted $VEGF_{121}$ injection to patients undergoing bypass graft surgery ($n = 15$), and as sole therapy via minithoracotomy ($n = 6$). Symptoms and exercise duration improved in both bypass surgery and sole therapy groups, but stress-induced nuclear perfusion images remained unchanged. The data in this study are consistent with the concept that adenovirus VEGF$_{121}$ appears to be well tolerated in patients with advanced coronary disease.

The recently reported REVASC trial is the largest clinical trial in humans to date evaluating the efficacy of adenovirus-mediated VEGF (Ad.VEGF$_{121}$) gene therapy for myocardial ischemia *(75)*. In this phase 2, randomized, multicenter trial, 67 patients were randomized to receive AdVEGF$_{121}$ administered by direct intramyocardial injections via a limited thoracotomy or to continue with optimal medical management. At 26 wk, time to ischemia on treadmill testing was significantly increased in the AdVEGF$_{121}$ versus the medical therapy group ($p = 0.024$). There were significant improvements in anginal status as well as in several domains of the Seattle Angina Questionnaire in the AdVEGF$_{121}$ compared to the medical therapy group. Although these data are encouraging, four patients in the AdVEGF$_{121}$ group suffered cardiac complications as a result of the thoracotomy.

Each of the aforementioned studies has one major limitation: the need for thoracotomy for VEGF gene transfer. Thoracotomy has a small but real complication risk that can lead to substantial morbidity, particularly in patients with significant comorbidities. Furthermore, the strategy of gene therapy alone administered via a minithoracotomy does not permit randomization against placebo (untreated controls) or clinical testing of alternative dosing regimens including multiple treatments.

Recent studies have suggested that a less invasive approach to gene transfer using a catheter-based delivery of naked plasmid VEGF$_{165}$ and VEGF-2 is effective in the pig *(76)*. This less invasive approach to intramyocardial gene transfer has been shown to achieve suitable gene expression *(76–79)*. Catheter-based myocardial gene transfer is performed using a previously described navigation system and catheter mapping technology (NOGA™) integrated with an injection catheter (Biosense-Webster), the distal tip of which incorporates a 27-gage needle to inject plasmid into the myocardium. To determine the safety and feasibility of catheter-based gene transfer, Vale et al. used this system to deliver naked plasmid VEGF to the myocardium of normal and ischemic swine *(77)*. Results with methylene blue suggested safe, reliable, and reproducible targeting of endocardial sites. Injection of a reporter gene (pCMV-nls*LacZ*) demonstrated peak β-galactosidase (β-gal) activity in the target area with low-level to negligible activity seen in areas remote from the injection sites, suggesting relatively localized gene transfer. β-Galactosidase activity was greater in ischemic versus nonischemic myocardium indicating enhanced gene transfer in ischemic myocardium. Similar findings were demonstrated by a study utilizing adenovirally assisted gene transfer of a reporter gene *(80)*. These results established that percutaneous myocardial gene transfer could be successfully achieved in normal and ischemic myocardium in a relatively site-specific fashion without significant morbidity or mortality. The mapping capabilities of the NOGA system utilized in this study were useful for demonstrating that gene expression could be directed to predetermined left ventricle sites. This technique clearly may be advantageous for avoiding gene transfer to sites of myocardial scar as well as relocating the tip of the injection catheter to areas of myocardial ischemia (or hibernating myocardium) where gene transfer will be optimized.

Subsequently, we initiated a pilot study of percutaneous, catheter-based VEGF-2 DNA gene transfer or a sham procedure guided by the NOGA mapping system in six patients with nonrevascularizable symptomatic myocardial perfusion *(81)*. VEGF-2 transfected patients reported significant reduction in weekly anginal episodes and nitrate tablet consumption at 12 mo post gene transfer. In contrast, although blinded patients randomized to the control group reported an initial reduction in these parameters, this changed clinical profile was not sustained past 30 d, suggesting that the continued reduction in angina in the VEGF-2–treated group was not a placebo effect. The symptomatic improvement was again accompanied by objective evidence of improved myocardial perfusion by both SPECT-sestamibi perfusion scanning and electromechanical mapping *(81)*. Although the clinical findings of this pilot trial concerning efficacy are similarly encouraging, the number of patients and the single-blinded design preclude firm conclusions in this regard.

Consequently, a multicenter randomized, double-blind, placebo-controlled trial of catheter-based VEGF-2 gene transfer was initiated, and the results were recently published *(82)*. Nineteen patients with chronic myocardial ischemia not amenable to percutaneous or surgical revascularization were randomized in a double-blind fashion to receive six injections of placebo or phVEGF-2. It was planned that 27 patients were to be randomized to receive gene or placebo in a 2:1 ratio. The study was, however, interrupted by the US Food and Drug Administration (FDA) after 19 patients had been enrolled. Twelve patients received the gene product and seven patients were randomized to placebo. A total of 114 injections were delivered through a steerable deflectable 8-french catheter with a 27-gauge needle guided by LV electromechanical mapping (NOGA) mapping. Perioperatively there were no hemodynamic alterations, sustained arrhythmias, myocardial infarction, or ventricular perforation. There was a significant improvement in the CCS angina class at endpoint analysis at 12 wk. Other endpoint analysis studied, including change in exercise duration, functional improvement in CCS by more than two classes, and Seattle Angina Questionnaire data, showed strong trends favoring the efficacy of phVEGF-2 compared to placebo treatment.

These preliminary experiences suggest that it is feasible to supplement or potentially replace currently employed operative approaches with minimally invasive techniques for applications of cardiovascular gene therapy designed to target myocardial function and perfusion. Such an approach may have at least three advantages compared to an operative approach. First, it potentially allows more selective delivery of the transgene to targeted ischemic zones, including sites less accessible by a minithoracotomy. Second, because it obviates the need for general anesthesia and operative dissection through adhesions resulting from prior surgery, the trans-catheter approach facilitates placebo-controlled, double-blind testing of myocardial gene therapy. Third, the intervention can be performed as an outpatient procedure and repeated if necessary.

Prevention of In-Stent Restenosis

Drug-eluting stents are expected to revolutionize interventional cardiology by reducing the incidence of in-stent restenosis from 30% to nearly 10%. However, the agents that have been studied to date as candidate drug coatings delay endothelial recovery. Prior studies have suggested that acceleration of endothelial cell formation following coronary stenting may attenuate the restenosis process. VEGF is a potent stimulator of endothelial cell recovery, and it has been hypothesized that a coronary stent coated with VEGF may have beneficial effects in the prevention of stent thrombosis and prevention of in-stent restenosis. This hypothesis has been tested in a randomized fashion in the rabbit model of atherosclerosis (83). Fifty-four rabbits were treated with either an uncoated coronary stent or a stent coated with phVEGF-2 plasmid. At 3 mo the rabbits treated with the gene-coated stents had significantly larger lumen cross-sectional areas and significantly less cross-sectional narrowing. In addition, there were increased numbers of EPCs and increased EC recovery (as assessed by NO production) in the rabbits treated with the gene-coated stents.

The phase 2 results of the Kuopio Angiogenesis Trial (KAT) were recently reported (84). In this trial, 103 patients with Canadian Cardiovascular Class II or III angina and 60–99% stenosis in a major epicardial artery were enrolled. These patients were then assigned (in a randomized, double-blind fashion) to undergo arterial gene transfer with $VEGF_{165}$ contained within adenovirus, liposomal $VEGF_{165}$, or placebo. Arterial gene transfer was performed using an infusion-perfusion catheter (Dispatcher Catheter, Boston Scientific). The primary endpoints of the study were minimal lumen diameter and percent diameter stenosis measured by quantitative coronary angiography at 6-mo follow-up. All patients were first treated with balloon angioplasty, followed by gene/ placebo transfer, followed by coronary stenting. The treatment was safe in all groups with few adverse events. There were no significant differences in death, acute coronary syndrome, or the development of carcinoma at follow-up between the three groups. All patients underwent angiography at 6 mo after treatment. In the entire cohort, the overall clinical restenosis rate was quite low at 6%. There were no significant differences between the three groups with respect to follow-up minimum lumen diameter and clinical restenosis rate. Interestingly, there was significant improvement in myocardial perfusion score using SPECT-sestamibi scanning in patients receiving VEGF-Adv ($p < 0.05$).

Currently, a phase 1 trial is being designed for evaluating the safety of phVEGF-2-coated stents in humans. Alternative strategies for preventing restenosis are also being evaluated, including using a specialized infiltration catheter to directly deliver plasmid VEGF into coronary plaque prior to stenting.

CARDIOVASCULAR TRIALS OF FGF PROTEIN AND GENE THERAPY

Peripheral Vascular Disease

Several investigators have shown improvements in muscle perfusion in animal models of hindlimb ischemia using recombinant FGF *(85–87)*. The safety of intra-arterial bFGF administration in patients with intermittent claudication was recently demonstrated *(88)*. In this phase 1, double-blind, placebo-controlled clinical trial there was improvement in calf blood flow by strain gauge plethysmography in bFGF-treated patients at 6 mo compared to controls. To date, the Therapeutic Angiogenesis with Recombinant FGF-2 for Intermittent Claudication (TRAFFIC) study is the only clinical trial testing the efficacy of recombinant FGF in humans with peripheral vascular disease *(89)*. A total of 190 patients with intermittent claudication were randomized to receive placebo, a single dose of FGF-2 (30 µg/kg), or two doses of FGF-2. There was a trend towards patients receiving FGF-2 having increases in peak walking time at 90 d (0.60 min in placebo vs 1.77 min in single-dose FGF-2 vs 1.54 min in double-dose FGF-2, $p = 0.075$). There was no significant difference in adverse events between the three groups. The authors concluded that the increase in walking time in patients receiving FGF provided evidence that that recombinant FGF-2 resulted in angiogenesis.

The first clinical trial in human subjects with peripheral vascular disease using FGF gene therapy was conducted on 51 patients with ischemic rest pain or tissue necrosis *(90)*. This was a phase 1 evaluation of naked plasmid DNA encoding for FGF-1 (NV1FGF) administered via intramuscular injection. These patients were deemed to have severe obstructive lower extremity vascular disease not amenable to mechanical revascularization. Patients received either escalating single dose or escalating double dose NV1FGF. Overall, intramuscular injection of NV1FGF was well tolerated. While there were adverse events, none were felt to be due to NV1FGF. Measurements of serum and plasma FGF-1 were made to assess gene expression. The distribution of plasmid in the plasma was limited, presumably due to destruction by endogenous endonucleases. There was no increase in serum FGF-1 levels. In the first 15 patients with completed 6-mo follow-up, there was a significant reduction in pain and ulcer size as well as an increase in transcutaneous oxygen pressure compared to pretreatment values. There was also a significant increase in the ABI in these patients. This study confirmed the safety of NV1FGF for the treatment of inoperable lower extremity peripheral vascular disease. The encouraging clinical results, however, need to be confirmed in larger, double-blind, placebo-controlled trials.

Presently, phase 1/2 clinical trials are ongoing in Europe to evaluate the safety and potential efficacy of FGF-4 delivered via an adenovirus vector (Ad5-FGF4) do the treatment of peripheral vascular disease. These are double-blind, placebo-controlled trials that will enroll up to 130 patients at 10 sites across Europe.

Myocardial Ischemia

A series of animal experiments has demonstrated that intracoronary and local delivery of FGF improves myocardial perfusion and function and increases collateral flow in myocardial ischemia *(91–94)*. Several phase 1 trials have been performed to evaluate the safety of recombinant FGF-1 and FGF-2 for therapeutic angiogenesis in patients with myocardial ischemia *(95–100)*. Each of these small studies showed reductions in anginal status, need for anti-anginal medications, and improvements in nuclear perfusion scanning. These studies, however, were limited by the fact that these patients were all scheduled for coronary artery bypass graft surgery. Therefore, any potential applicability of these approaches would be limited to patients able to undergo thoracotomy. Intravenous and intracoronary administration of recombinant FGF-2 have also been evaluated in phase 1 studies of patients with symptomatic coronary artery disease with mixed results *(100–103)*. Intravenous injection of recombinant FGF-2 was associated with improvements in anginal status, exercise time, and left ventricular function. However, intracoronary administration resulted in no change in exercise time or time to ischemia.

Several patients experienced persistent hypotension for up to 3 d, conduction system disturbances, thrombocytopenia, and proteinuria.

The FGF-2 Initiating Revascularization Support Trial (FIRST) was a phase 2 trial that randomized 337 patients with inoperable coronary artery disease to receive either placebo or one of three doses of intracoronary recombinant FGF-2 (104). The results of this trial did not show dramatic improvements in objective endpoints in patients receiving intracoronary FGF-2. The 90-d exercise time and stress nuclear perfusion results were not significantly different between FGF-2-treated patients and placebo-treated patients. There was a trend toward improved anginal status in patients receiving intracoronary FGF-2, particularly in older and more symptomatic patients.

Results of these phase 1 and 2 trials again point to the potential shortcomings of recombinant protein therapy for therapeutic angiogenesis. FGF gene therapy in animal models of coronary ischemia has shown promise for therapeutic angiogenesis. In a chronic coronary occlusion animal model, human FGF-5 carried by an adenovirus vector (Ad5-FGF5) administered by intracoronary infusion resulted in sustained production of growth factors at 12 wk, effective development of coronary collaterals, and relief of stress-induced ischemia (25,105).

Thus far, only one clinical trial in humans using FGF gene therapy for myocardial ischemia has been reported. Grines et al. conducted the Angiogenic Gene Therapy (AGENT) trial in which 79 patients with chronic stable angina (Canadian Cardiovascular Class II and III) were randomized to receive placebo or one of five escalating doses of Ad5-FGF4 in a double-blind fashion (106). The Ad5-FGF4 was administered by a single intracoronary injection. Overall, patients receiving Ad5-FGF4 tolerated the infusion well with few immediate adverse events. One patient developed a fever during the first day after virus transfer, and two patients had minor, self-limited elevations of liver enzymes. There were no significant differences in adverse events in patients receiving placebo and Ad5-FGF4 at a mean of 311 d of follow-up. Overall, patients receiving Ad5-FGF4 experienced a trend towards increased exercise times at 4 wk. The trial prespecified a subgroup analysis in the 50 patients with baseline exercise times of less than 10 min. There was a significant improvement in exercise time in this more symptomatic subgroup of patients in those who received Ad5-FGF5 (1.6 vs 0.6 min, $p < 0.01$). These data suggest that the intracoronary infusion of Ad5-FGF4 is safe and may be effective at improving hard clinical endpoints in patients with myocardial ischemia. Interestingly, in this study, patients enrolled were not "no-option" patients. The effects of intracoronary Ad5-FGF5 may be more dramatic in no-option patients. The true clinical value of this approach will be evaluated in future clinical trials designed to assess hard clinical endpoints.

SAFETY CONCERNS REGARDING CARDIOVASCULAR GENE THERAPY

Given that the inhibition of angiogenesis may be of value in the treatment of neoplasms, concern has been raised that the administration of angiogenic growth factors could lead to development of tumors. There are neither in vitro nor in vivo data to suggest that either VEGF or FGF increases the risk of neoplastic growth and/or metastases, although longer-term follow-up will be required to address this issue in clinical trials. In our own experience with 88 subjects who have undergone VEGF gene transfer for critical limb ischemia, the cumulative 7-yr incidence of cancer was limited to two patients with bladder cancer and one with liver and brain metastases from unknown primary (107). It was interesting to note that in the VIVA Trial that there was a greater incidence of tumors in the placebo group compared to the VEGF group. This highlights the fact that the age group receiving such therapy will develop some unrelated tumors. Because of the theoretical risk of neoplastic growth, one must be vigilant about the possibility of cancer in patients treated with these angiogenic growth factors. In addition, concerns regarding the development of angiomata were raised in studies involving mice or rats treated with transduced myoblasts or supraphysiological doses of plasmid DNA respectively. Importantly, no other preclinical or clinical reports, including those using adenoviral vectors, have described this complication (108,109).

It is theoretically possible that VEGF may exacerbate proliferative and/or hemorrhagic retinopathy in patients with diabetes in view of the high VEGF levels demonstrated in the ocular fluid of patients with active proliferative retinopathy leading to loss of vision (110). To date, this adverse effect of therapeutic angiogenesis has not been observed. The local delivery of naked plasmid DNA encoding for VEGF-1 or VEGF-2 to more than 100 patients (one third with diabetes and/or remote retinopathy) treated at our institution with up to 4-yr follow-up did not affect the visual acuity or fundoscopic findings as evidenced by serial funduscopic examinations pre- and post-gene transfer by an independent group of retinal specialists.

Experiments in transgenic mice engineered to overexpress VEGF ± angiopoietin have demonstrated the lethal permeability-enhancing effects of VEGF (111). However, even though VEGF has been reported to cause local edema, which manifests as pedal edema in patients treated with VEGF for critical limb ischemia, it responds well to treatment with diuretics *(44)*. As previously described, hypotension has been observed in therapies with recombinant proteins particularly when used systemically and in higher doses *(112,113)*. This is believed to be a result of the fact that VEGF upregulates NO synthesis. This complication, however, has never been described following gene transfer in either animals or humans *(114,115)*.

Moulton et al. recently observed that when hypercholesterolemic, apolipoprotein E-deficient mouse models were treated with inhibitors of angiogenesis (endostatin or TNP-470), there was significant regression of plaque areas and inhibition of intimal neovascularization *(116)*. This and other studies raised concern regarding the potential for VEGF and other proangiogenic therapies to promote atherosclerosis *(92,117,118)*. However, data available from four separate animal studies and two clinical studies of human subjects fail to support the notion that accelerated atherosclerosis is a likely consequence of administering angiogenic cytokines *(48–51,119,120)*. The outcome is quite the opposite, in that administration of VEGF led to a statistically significant reduction in intimal thickening due to accelerated reendothelialization, thereby refuting the notion that acceleration of atherosclerosis will be a consequence of VEGF-induced stimulation of angiogenesis.

CONCLUSIONS

The preliminary effectiveness of gene therapy for therapeutic angiogenesis in patients with critical limb and chronic myocardial ischemia is both encouraging and promising. The different trials using angiogenic protein and transgenes encoding for VEGF and FGF attest to the safety and effectiveness of these strategies. The current clinical strategies employed for critical limb ischemia and chronic myocardial ischemia constitute an extrapolation from initial applications of gene transfer to animal models with limb ischemia. These results, however, likely have generic implications for strategies of therapeutic neovascularization using alternative candidate genes, vectors, and delivery strategies. Preclinical data supporting the use of other VEGF-1 isoforms *(121)* other VEGF genes *(122)*, and FGF *(25,133)* has been reported and are actively being studied in ongoing clinical trials. Furthermore, the relative merits of gene transfer versus recombinant protein administration remain to be clarified. In addition, the ideal vector for gene transfer has yet to be determined. There continues to be concern about potential carcinogenesis in patients treated with retroviral vectors as seen in a recent trial of gene therapy utilizing a retroviral vector for the treatment of severe combined immunodeficiency syndrome (SCIDS) (FDA communication). A naked DNA vector strategy may have safety advantages in the early stages of cardiovascular gene therapy.

The otherwise negative primary endpoint results of the VIVA and FIRST studies using intracoronary ± intravenous protein administration underscore the concern that the pharmacokinetics of recombinant protein administered into the vascular space may lead to inadequate local delivery of angiogenic growth factor within the ischemic myocardium. Additional investigations comparing doses of recombinant protein and routes of delivery will be required to resolve this issue. Until these studies are complete, the ideal method of achieving therapeutic angiogenesis remains unknown. In addition, results of phase 1 studies, designed by definition to assess safety, must be interpreted with caution. Typically, the number of patients enrolled in such trials is relatively small, and for those lacking a control group a placebo effect cannot be excluded. For studies in which recombinant protein or gene is administered in conjunction with conventional revascularization, it may be difficult to determine the relative contributions of the angiogenic agent versus bypass surgery to the symptomatic response.

It is clear, however, that site-specific VEGF gene *transfer* can be used to achieve physiologically meaningful *therapeutic* modulation of vascular disorders and specifically that intramyocardial injection of naked plasmid DNA achieves constitutive overexpression of VEGF sufficient to induce therapeutic angiogenesis in selected patients with critical limb ischemia. Of note, there was no evidence of immunological toxicity in either our intra-arterial animal studies or our human clinical experience utilizing naked plasmid DNA encoding for VEGF. Furthermore, at this early stage of clinical trials into myocardial gene therapy, it has been shown that direct myocardial gene transfer utilizing different doses of naked plasmid DNA encoding for $VEGF_{165}$ and VEGF-2 as well as intracoronary FGF-5 carried by an adenovirus vector can be performed safely with augmentation of myocardial perfusion. The catheter-based delivery of plasmid DNA is an attractive and safe option. In terms of safety, no operative complications and no aggravated deterioration in eyesight due to diabetic retinopathy *(124)* have been observed in patients treated with $phVEGF_{165}$ gene transfer. With specific regard to mortality, it should be noted that the cumulative mortality for the 85 patients with class 3 or 4 angina undergoing operative or percutaneous naked DNA gene transfer of VEGF-1 or VEGF-2 has been 3 of 85 (3.5%) at up to 33 mo follow-up. This compares favorably with an average 11–13% 1-yr mortality for a similar group of almost 1000 patients receiving laser myocardial revascularization or continued medical therapy in five contemporary controlled studies *(125–129)*. Ongoing clinical studies will determine the potential for neovascularization gene therapy to be performed by nonsurgical, catheter-based delivery, although early results are encouraging from a therapeutic standpoint.

For the most part, clinical studies of therapeutic angiogenesis have been restricted to patients with myocardial or limb ischemia who have no other options. Although this is the group to target in the near future, it is not difficult to foresee a time when a significant populations of patients who undergo bypass surgery but are not optimal candidates for that procedure may be eligible for therapeutic angiogenesis. The latter might be performed at an earlier stage of disease, and the potential for repeat treatment may translate into a greater possibility of a successful outcome.

REFERENCES

1. Folkman J. Tumor angiogenesis: therapeutic implications. N Engl J Med 1971;285:1182–1186.
2. Risau W. Differentiation of endothelium. FASEB J 1995;9:926–933.
3. Folkman J, Shing Y. Angiogenesis. J Biol Chem 1992;267:10931–10934.
4. Risau W. Mechanisms of angiogenesis. Nature 1997;386:671–674.
5. Asahara T, Murohara T, Sullivan A, et al. Isolation of putative progenitor endothelial cells for angiogenesis. Science 1997;275:964–967.
6. Takahashi T, Kalka C, Masuda H, et al. Ischemia- and cytokine-induced mobilization of bone marrow-derived endothelial progenitor cells for neovascularization. Nat Med 1999;5:434–438.
7. Asahara T, Masuda H, Takahashi T, et al. Bone marrow origin of endothelial progenitor cells responsible for postnatal vasculogenesis in physiological and pathological neovascularization. Circ Res 1999;85:221–228.
8. Kalka C, Masuda H, Takahashi T, et al. Transplantation of ex vivo expanded endothelial progenitor cells for therapeutic neovascularization. Proc Natl Acad Sci USA 2000;97:3422–3427.
9. Tateishi-Yuyama E, Matsubara H, Murohara T, et al. Therapeutic angiogenesis for patients with limb ischaemia by autologous transplantation of bone-marrow cells: a pilot study and a randomised controlled trial. Lancet 2002;360:427–435.
10. Arras M, Ito WD, Scholz D, Winkler B, Schaper J, Schaper W. Monocyte activation in angiogenesis and collateral growth in the rabbit hindlimb. J Clin Invest 1998;101:40–50.
11. Takeshita S, Weir L, Chen D, et al. Therapeutic angiogenesis following arterial gene transfer of vascular endothelial growth factor in a rabbit model of hindlimb ischemia. Biochem Biophys Res Commun 1996;227:628–635.
12. Brogi E, Schatteman G, Wu T, et al. Hypoxia-induced paracrine regulation of VEGF receptor expression. J Clin Invest 1996;97:469–476.
13. Fong GH, Rossant J, Gertsenstein M, Breitman ML. Role of flt-1 receptor tyrosine kinase in regulating the assembly of vascular endothelium. Nature 1995;376:66–70.
14. Shalaby F, Rossant J, Yamaguchi TP, et al. Failure of blood-island formation and vasculogenesis in Flk-1 deficient mice. Nature 1995;376:62–66.
15. Carmeliet P, Collen D. Molecular analysis of blood vessel formation and disease. Am J Physiol 1997;273:H2091–H2104.

16. Jeltsch M, Kaipainen A, Joukov V, et al. Hyperplasia of lymphatic vessels in VEGF-C transgenic mice. Science 1997;276:1423–1425.

17. Leung DW, Cachianes G, Kuang WJ, Goeddel DV, Ferrara N. Vascular endothelial growth factor is a secreted angiogenic mitogen. Science 1989;246:1306–1309.

18. Ferrara N, Henzel WJ. Pituitary follicular cells secrete a novel heparin-binding growth factor specific for vascular endothelial cells. Biochem Biophys Res Commun 1989;161:851–855.

19. Conn G, Soderman D, Schaeffer M-T, Wile M, Hatcher VB, Thomas KA. Purification of glycoprotein vascular endothelial cell mitogen from a rat glioma cell line. Proc Natl Acad Sci USA 1990;87:1323–1327.

20. Kalka C, Masuda H, Takahashi T, et al. Vascular endothelial growth factor(165) gene transfer augments circulating endothelial progenitor cells in human subjects. Circ Res 2000;86:1198–1202.

21. Asahara T, Takahashi T, Masuda H, et al. VEGF contributes to postnatal neovascularization by mobilizing bone marrow-derived endothelial progenitor cells. EMBO J 1999;18:3964–3972.

22. Kalka C, Tehrani H, Laudenberg B, et al. Mobilization of endothelial progenitor cells following gene therapy with VEGF165 in patients with inoperable coronary disease. Ann Thorac Surg 2000;70:829–834.

23. Carmeliet P. Mechanisms of angiogenesis and arteriogenesis. Nat Med 2000;6:389–395.

24. Tabata H, Silver M, Isner JM. Arterial gene transfer of acidic fibroblast growth factor for therapeutic angiogenesis in vivo: critical role of secretion signal in use of naked DNA. Cardiovasc Res 1997;35:470–479.

25. Giordano FJ, Ping P, McKirnan MD, et al. Intracoronary gene transfer of fibroblast growth factor-5 increases blood flow and contractile function in an ischemic region of the heart. Nat Med 1996;2:534–539.

26. McKirnan MD, Guo X, Waldman LK, et al. Intracoronary gene transfer of fibroblast growth factor-4 increases regional contractile function and responsiveness to adrenergic stimulation in heart failure. Cardiac Vasc Regen 2000;1:11–21.

27. Takeshita S, Isshiki T, Sato T. Increased expression of direct gene transfer into skeletal muscles observed after acute ischemic injury in rats. Lab Invest 1996;74:1061–1065.

28. Tsurumi Y, Takeshita S, Chen D, et al. Direct intramuscular gene transfer of naked DNA encoding vascular endothelial growth factor augments collateral development and tissue perfusion. Circulation 1996;94:3281–3290.

29. Takeshita S, Losordo DW, Kearney M, Isner JM. Time course of recombinant protein secretion following liposome-mediated gene transfer in a rabbit arterial organ culture model. Lab Invest 1994;71:387–391.

30. Losordo DW, Pickering JG, Takeshita S, et al. Use of the rabbit ear artery to serially assess foreign protein secretion after site specific arterial gene transfer in vivo: Evidence that anatomic identification of successful gene transfer may underestimate the potential magnitude of transgene expression. Circulation 1994;89:785–792.

31. Ischemia EWGoCL. Second European consensus document on chronic critical leg ischemia. Circulation 1991;84:IV-1–IV-26.

32. Treat-Jacobson D, Halverson SL, Ratchford A, Regensteiner JG, Lindquist R, Hirsch AT. A patient-derived perspective of health related quality of life with peripheral arterial disease. J Nurs Scholarship 2002;34:55–60.

33. Eneroth M, Persson BM. Amputation for occlusive arterial disease. A multicenter study of 177 amputees. Int Orthop 1992;16:382–387.

34. Campbell WB, Johnston JA, Kernick VF, Rutter EA. Lower limb amputation: striking the balance. Ann Royal Coll Surg Engl 1994;76:205–209.

35. Dawson I, Keller BP, Brand R, Pesch-Batenburg J, Hajo van Bockel J. Late outcomes of limb loss after failed infrainguinal bypass. J Vasc Surg 1995;21:613–622.

36. Skinner JA, Cohen AT. Amputation for premature peripheral atherosclerosis: do young patients do better? Lancet 1996;348:1396.

37. Takeshita S, Zheng LP, Brogi E, et al. Therapeutic angiogenesis: a single intra-arterial bolus of vascular endothelial growth factor augments revascularization in a rabbit ischemic hindlimb model. J Clin Invest 1994;93:662–670.

38. Connolly DT, Hewelman DM, Nelson R, et al. Tumor vascular permeability factor stimulates endothelial cell growth and angiogenesis. J Clinl Invest 1989;84:1470–1478.

39. Isner JM, Pieczek A, Schainfeld R, et al. Clinical evidence of angiogenesis following arterial gene transfer of phVEGF165. Lancet 1996;348:370–374.

40. Feldman LJ, Steg PG, Zheng LP, et al. Low-efficiency of percutaneous adenovirus-mediated arterial gene transfer in the atherosclerotic rabbit. J Clin Invest 1995;95:2662–2671.

41. Rivard A, Silver M, Chen D, et al. Rescue of diabetes related impairment of angiogenesis by intramuscular gene therapy with adeno-VEGF. Am J Pathol 1999;154:355–364.

42. Baumgartner I, Pieczek A, Manor O, et al. Constitutive expression of phVEGF165 following intramuscular gene transfer promotes collateral vessel development in patients with critical limb ischemia. Circulation 1998;97:1114–1123.

43. Rauh G, Gravereaux EC, Pieczek AM, Radley S, Schainfeld RM, Isner JM. Age <50 years and rest pain predict positive clinical outcome after intramuscular gene transfer of phVEGF165 in patients with critical limb ischemia. Circulation 1999;100:I-319.

44. Baumgartner I, Rauh G, Pieczek A, et al. Lower-extremity edema associated with gene transfer of naked DNA vascular endothelial growth factor. Ann Int Med 2000;132:880–884.

45. Isner JM, Baumgartner I, Rauh G, et al. Treatment of thromboangiitis obliterans (Buerger's disease) by intramuscular gene transfer of vascular endothelial growth factor: preliminary clinical results. J Vasc Surg 1998;28:964–975.

46. Witzenbichler B, Asahara T, Murohara T, et al. Vascular endothelial growth factor-C (VEGF-C/VEGF-2) promotes angiogenesis in the setting of tissue ischemia. Am J Pathol 1998;153:381–394.

47. Rajagopalan S, Shah M, Luciano A, Crystal R, Nabel EG. Adenovirus-mediated gene transfer of VEGF(121) improves lower-extremity endothelial function and flow reserve. Circulation 2001;104:753–755.

48. Asahara T, Bauters C, Pastore CJ, et al. Local delivery of vascular endothelial growth factor accelerates reendothelialization and attenuates intimal hyperplasia in balloon-injured rat carotid artery. Circulation 1995;91:2793–2801.

49. Asahara T, Chen D, Tsurumi Y, et al. Accelerated restitution of endothelial integrity and endothelium-dependent function following phVEGF165 gene transfer. Circulation 1996;94:3291–3302.

50. Van Belle E, Tio FO, Couffinhal T, Maillard L, Passeri J, Isner JM. Stent endothelialization: time course, impact of local catheter delivery, feasibility of recombinant protein administration, and response to cytokine expedition. Circulation 1997;95:438–448.

51. Van Belle E, Tio FO, Chen D, Maillard L, Kearney M, Isner JM. Passivation of metallic stents following arterial gene transfer of phVEGF165 inhibits thrombus formation and intimal thickening. J Am Coll Cardiol 1997;29:1371–1379.

52. Minar E, Pokrajac B, Maca T, et al. Endovascular brachytherapy for prophylaxis of restenosis after femoropopliteal angioplasty: results of a prospective randomized study. Circulation 2000;102:2694–2699.

53. Hendel RC, Henry TD, Rocha-Singh K, et al. Effect of intracoronary recombinant human vascular endothelial growth factor on myocardial perfusion: evidence for a dose-dependent effect. Circulation 2000;101:118–121.

54. Henry TD, Abraham JA. Review of prelcinical and clinical results with vascular endothelial growth factors for therapeutic angiogenesis. Curr Intervent Cardiol Rep 2000;2:228–241.

55. Henry TD, Rocha-Singh K, Isner JM, et al. Intracoronary administration of recombinant human vascular endothelial growth factor to patients with coronary artery disease. Am Heart J 2001;142:872–880.

56. Henry TD, Rocha-Singh K, Isner JM, et al. Results of intracoronary recombinant human vascular endothelial growth factor (rhVEGF) administration trial. J Am Coll Cardiol 1998;31:65A.

57. Henry TD, Annex BH, Azrin MA, et al. Final results of the VIVA trial of rhVEGF for human therapeutic angiogenesis. Circulation 1999;100:I-476.

58. Ferguson JJ. Meeting highlights: highlights of the 48th scientific sessions of the American College of Cardiology. Circulation 1999;100:570–575.

59. Henry TD, McKendall GR, Azrin MA, et al. VIVA trial: one year follow up. Circulation 2000;102:II-309.

60. Hariawala MD, Horowitz JR, Esakof D, et al. VEGF improves myocardial blood flow but produces EDRF-mediated hypotension in porcine hearts. J Surg Res 1996;63:77–82.

61. Lopez JJ, Laham RJ, Stamler A, et al. VEGF administration in chronic myocardial ischemia in pigs. Cardiovasc Res 1998;40:272–281.

62. Banai S, Jaklitsch MT, Shou M, et al. Angiogenic-induced enhancement of collateral blood flow to ischemic myocardium by vascular endothelial growth factor in dogs. Circulation 1994; 89:2183–2189.

63. Hughes CG, Biswas SS, Yin B, et al. Intramyocardial but not intravenous vascular endothelial growth factor improves regional perfusion in hibernating porcine myocardium. Circulation 1999;100:I-476.

64. Harada K, Friedman M, Lopez JJ, et al. Vascular endothelial growth factor in chronic myocardial ischemia. Am J Physiol 1996;270:H1791–H1802.

65. Mack CA, Patel SR, Schwarz EA, et al. Biologic bypass with the use of adenovirus-mediated gene transfer of the conplementary deoxyribonucleic acid for vascular endothelial growth factor 121 improves myocardial perfusion and function in the ischemic porcine heart. J Thorac Cardiovasc Surg 1998;115:168–176.

66. Lee LY, Patel SR, Hackett NR, et al. Focal angiogen therapy using intramyocardial delivery of an adenovirus vector coding for vascular endotehlial growth factor 121. Ann Thorac Surg 2000;69:14–24.

67. Lazarous DF, Shou M, Stiber JA, et al. Adenoviral-mediated gene transfer induces sustained pericardial VEGF expression in dogs: effect on myocardial angiogenesis. Cardiovasc Res 1999;44:294–302.

68. Losordo DW, Vale PR, Symes J, et al. Gene therapy for myocardial angiogenesis: initial clinical results with direct myocardial injection of phVEGF165 as sole therapy for myocardial ischemia. Circulation 1998;98:2800–2804.

69. Symes JF, Losordo DW, Vale PR, et al. Gene therapy with vascular endothelial growth factor for inoperable coronary artery disease: preliminary clinical results. Ann Thorac Surg 1999;68:830–837.

70. Esakof DD, Maysky M, Losordo DW, et al. Intraoperative multiplane transesophageal echocardiograpy for guiding direct myocardial gene transfer of vascular endothelial growth factor in patients with refractory angina pectoris. Human Gene Ther 1999;10:2315–2323.
71. Shen Y-T, Vatner SF. Mechanism of impaired myocardial function during progressive coronary stenosis in conscious pigs: hibernation versus stunning? Circ Res 1995;76:479–488.
72. Wijns W, Vatner SF, Camici PG. Hibernating myocardium. N Engl J Med 1998;3:173–181.
73. Dilsizian V, Bonow RO. Current diagnostic techniques of assessing myocardial viability in patients with hibernating and stunned myocardium. Circulation 1993;87:1–20.
74. Vale PR, Losordo DW, Milliken CE, et al. Left ventricular electromechanical mapping to assess efficacy of phVEGF(165) gene transfer for therapeutic angiogenesis in chronic myocardial ischemia. Circulation 2000;102:965–974.
75. Stewart JD. A phase 2 randomized, multicenter, 26-week study to assess the efficacy and safety of BIOBYPASS (adgfVEGF121.10) delivered through maximally invasive surgery versus maximal medical treatment in patients with severe angina, advanced coronary artery disease and no options for revascularization. Circulation 2002;106:2986-a.
76. Vale PR, Milliken CE, Tkebuchava T, et al. Catheter-based gene transfer of VEGF utilizing electromechanical LV mapping accomplishes therapeutic angiogenesis: pre-clinical studies in swine. Circulation 1999;100:I-512.
77. Vale PR, Losordo DW, Tkebuchava T, Chen D, Milliken CE, Isner JM. Catheter-based myocardial gene transfer utilizing nonfluoroscopic electromechanical left ventricular mapping. J Am Coll Cardiol 1999;34:246–254.
78. Deutsch E, Tarazona N, Sanborn TA, et al. Percutaneous endocardial gene therapy: patterns of in-vivo gene expression related to regional myocardial delivery. J Am Coll Cardiol 2000;35:6A.
79. Kornowski R, Fuchs S, Vodovotz Y, et al. Catheter-based transendocardial injection of adenoviral VEGF121 offers equivalent gene delivery and protein expression compared to a surgical-based transepicardial injection approach. J Am Coll Cardiol 2000;35:73A.
80. Kornowski R, Leon MB, Fuchs S, et al. Electromagnetic guidance for catheter-based transendocardial injection: a platform for intramyocardial angiogenesis therapy. J Am Coll Cardiol 2000;35:1031–1039.
81. Vale PR, Losordo DW, Milliken CE, et al. Randomized, placebo-controlled clinical study of percutaneous catheter-based left ventricular endocardial gene transfer of VEGF-2 for myocardial ischemia. Circulation 2002;102:II-563.
82. Losordo DW, Vale PR, Hendel RC, et al. Phase 1/2 placebo-controlled, double-blind, dose-escalating trial of myocardial vascular endothelial growth factor 2 gene transfer by catheter delivery in patients with chronic myocardial ischemia. Circulation 2002;105:2012–2018.
83. Walter DH, Cejna M, Diaz-Sandoval LJ, et al. Local gene transfer of phVEGF-2 plasmid by gene-eluting stents: an alternative strategy for inhibition of restenosis. Circulation 2002;106:II-125.
84. Hedman M, Hartikainen J, Syvanne M, et al. Safety and feasibility of catheter-based local intracoronary vascular endothelial growth factor gene transfer in the prevention of postangioplasty and in-stent restenosis and in the treatment of chronic myocardial ischemia. Circulation 2003;107:2677–2683.

85. Baffour R, Berman J, Garb JL, Rhee SW, Kaufman J, Friedmann P. Enhanced angiogenesis and growth of collaterals by in vivo administration of recombinant basic fibroblast growth factor in a rabbit model of acute lower limb ischemia: dose-response effect of basic fibroblast growth factor. J Vasc Surg 1992;16:181–191.

86. Yang HT, Deschenes MR, Ogilvie RW, Terjung RL. Basic fibroblast growth factor increases collateral blood flow in rats with femoral arterial ligation. Circ Res 1996;79:62–69.

87. Chlegoun JO, Martins RN, Mitchell CA, Chirila TV. Basic FGF enhances the development of collateral circulation after acute arterial occlusion. Biochem Biophys Res Commun 1992;185:510–516.

88. Lazarous DF, Unger EF, Epstein SE, et al. Basic fibroblast growth factor in patients with intermittent claudication: results of a phase I trial. J Am Coll Cardiol 2000;36:1339–1344.

89. Lederman R. Therapeutic angiogenesis with recombinant fibroblast growth factor-2 for intermittent claudication (TRAFFIC). Presented at Late-Breaking Clinical Trials session of 50th annual American College of Cardiology, Orlando, FL, March 19, 2001.

90. Comerota A, Throm R, Miller K, et al. Naked plasmid DNA encoding fibroblast growth factor type 1 for the treatment of end-stage unreconstructible lower extremity ischemia: preliminary results of a phase I trial. J Vasc Surg 2002;35:930–936.

91. Unger EF, Banai S, Shou M, et al. Basic fibroblast growth factor enhances myocardial collateral flow in a canine model. Am J Physiol 1994;266:H1588–H1595.

92. Lazarous DF, Scheinowtiz M, Shou M, et al. Effects of chronic systemic administration of basic fibroblast growth factor on collateral development in the canine heart. Circulation 1995;91:145–153.

93. Lazarous DF, Shou M, Scheinowitz M, et al. Comparative effects of basic fibroblast growth factor and vascular endothelial growth factor on coronary collateral development and arterial response to injury. Circulation 1996;94:1074–1082.

94. Rajanayagam MA, Shou M, Thirumurti V, et al. Intracoronary basic fibroblast growth factor enhances myocardial collateral perfusion in dogs. J Am Coll Cardiol 2000; 35:519–526.

95. Schumacher B, Pecher P, vonSpecht BU, Stegmann T. Induction of neoangiogenesis in ischemic myocardium by human growth factors: first clinical results of a new treatment of coronary heart disease. Circulation 1998;97:645–650.

96. Schumacher B, Stegmann T, Pecher P. The stimulation of neoangiogenesis in the ischemic human heart by the growth factor FGF: first clinical results. J Cardiovas Surg 1998;39:783–789.

97. Stegmann TJ, Hoppert T, Schlurmann W, Gemeinhardt S. First angiogenic treatment of coronary heart disease by FGF-1: long-term results after 3 years. Cardiac Vasc Regen 2000;1:5–10.

98. Sellke FW, Laham RJ, Edelman ER, Pearlman JD, Simons M. Therapeutic angiogenesis with basic fibroblast growth factor: technique and early results. Ann Thorac Surg 1998;65:1540–1544.

99. Laham RJ, Sellke FW, Edelman ER, et al. Local perivascular delivery of basic fibroblast growth factor in patients undergoing coronary bypass surgery: results of a phase 1 randomized, double-blind, placebo-controlled trial. Circulation 1999;100:1865–1871.

100. Stegmann TJ, Hoppert T, Schneider A, et al. Induction of myocardial neoangiogenesis by human growth factors. A new therapeutic option in coronary heart disease. Herz 2000;25:589–599.

101. Udelson JE, Dilsizian V, Laham RJ, et al. Therapeutic angiogenesis with recombinant fibroblast growth factor-2 improves stress and rest myocardial perfusion abnormalities in patients with severe symptomatic chronic coronary artery disease. Circulation 2000;102:1605–1610.

102. Laham RJ, Chronos NA, Pike M, et al. Intracoronary basic fibroblast growth factor (FGF-2) in patients with severe ischemic heart disease: results of a phase 1 open-label dose escalation study. J Am Coll Cardiol 2000;36:2132–2139.

103. Unger E, Goncalves L, Epstein S, et al. Effects of a single intracoronary injection of basic fibroblast growth factor in stable angina pectoris. Am J Cardiol 2000;85:1414–1419.

104. Kleiman NS, Califf RM. Results from late-breaking clinical trials sessions at ACCIS 2000 and ACC 2000. J Am Coll Cardiol 2000;36:310–311.

105. Harada K, Grossman W, Friedman M, et al. Basic fibroblast growth factor improves myocardial function in chronically ischemic porcine hearts. J Clin Invest 1994;94:623–630.

106. Grines CL, Watkins MW, Helmer G, et al. Angiogenic Gene Therapy (AGENT) trial in patients with stable angina pectoris. Circulation 2002;105:1291–1297.

107. Isner JM, Vale PR, Symes JF, Losordo DW. Assessment of risks associated with cardiovascular gene therapy in human subjects. Circ Res 2001;895(5):389–400.

108. Springer ML, Chen AS, Kraft PE, Bednarski M, Blau HM. VEGF gene delivery to muscle: potential role of vasculogenesis in adults. Mol Cell 1998;2:549–558.

109. Schwartz ER, Speakman MT, Patterson M, et al. Evaluation of the effects of intramyocardial injection of DNA expressing vascular endothelial growth factor (VEGF) in a myocardial infarction model in the ratt—ngiogenesis and angioma formation. J Am Coll Cardiol 2000;35:1323–1330.

110. Aiello LP, Avery RL, Arrigg PG, et al. Vascular endothelial growth factor in ocular fluids of patients with diabetic retinopathy and other retinal disorders. N Engl J Med 1994;331:1480–1487.

111. Thurston G, Suri C, Smith K, et al. Leakage-resistant blood vessels in mice transgenically overexpressing angiopoietin-1. Science 1999;286:2511–2514.

112. Hariawala M, Horowitz JR, Esakof D, et al. VEGF improves myocardial blood flow but produces EDRF-mediated hypotension in porcine hearts. J Surg Res 1996;63:77–82.

113. Horowitz JR, Rivard A, van der Zee R, et al. Vascular endothelial growth factor/vascular permeability factor produces nitric oxide-dependent hypotension. Arterioscler Thromb Vasc Biol 1997;17:2793–2800.

114. van der Zee R, Murohara T, Luo Z, et al. Vascular endothelial growth factor (VEGF)/vascular permeability factor (VPF) augments nitric oxide release from quiescent rabbit and human vascular endothelium. Circulation 1997;95:1030–1037.

115. Murohara T, Asahara T, Silver M, et al. Nitric oxide synthase modulates angiogenesis in response to tissue ischemia. J Clin Invest 1998;101:2567–2578.

116. Moulton KS, Heller E, Konerding MA, Flynn E, Palinski W, Folkman J. Angiogenesis inhibitors endostatin and TNP-470 reduce intimal neovascularization and plaque growth in apolipoprotein E-deficient mice. Circulation 1999;99:1726–1732.

117. Inoue M, Itoh H, Ueda M, et al. Vascular endothelial growth factor (VEGF) expression in human coronary atherosclerotic lesions: possible pathophysiological significance of VEGF in progression of atherosclerosis. Circulation 1998;98:2108–2116.

118. Celletti FL, Waugh JM, Amabile PG, Brendolan A, Hilfiker PR, Dake MD. Vascular endothelial growth factor enhances atherosclerotic plaque progression. Nat Med 2001;7:425–429.

119. Vale PR, Wuensch DI, Rauh GF, Rosenfield K, Schainfeld RM, Isner JM. Arterial gene therapy for inhibiting restenosis in patients with claudication undergoing superficial femoral artery angioplasty. Circulation 1998;98:I-66.

120. Laitinen M, Hartikainen J, Hiltunen MO, et al. Catheter-mediated vascular endothelial growth factor gene transfer to human coronary arteries after angioplasty. Human Gene Ther 2000;11:263–270.

121. Takeshita S, Tsurumi Y, Couffinhal T, et al. Gene transfer of naked DNA encoding for three isoforms of vascular endothelial growth factor stimulates collateral development in vivo. Lab Invest 1996;75:487–502.

122. Witzenbichler B, Asahara T, Murohara T, et al. Vascular endothelial growth factor-C (VEGF-C/VEGF-2) promotes angiogenesis in the setting of tissue ischemia. Am J Pathol 1998;153:381–394.

123. Lopez JJ, Edelman ER, Stamler A, et al. Angiogenic potential of perivascularly delivered aFGF in a porcine model of chronic myocardial ischemia. Am J Physiol 1998;274:H930–H936.

124. Vale PR, Rauh G, Wuensch DI, Pieczek A, Schainfeld RM. Influence of vascular endothelial growth factor on diabetic retinopathy. Circulation 1998;17:I-353.

125. Schofield PM, Sharples LD, Caine N, et al. Transmyocardial laser revascularisation in patients with refractory angina: a randomised controlled trial. Lancet 1999;353:519–524.

126. Burkhoff D, Schmidt S, Schulman SP, et al. Transmyocardial laser revascularisation compared with continued medical therapy for treatment of refractory angina pectoris: a prospective randomised trial. Lancet 1999;354:885–890.

127. Allen KB, Dowling RD, Fudge TL, et al. Comparison of transmyocardial revascularization with medical therapy in patients with refractory angina. N Engl J Med 1999;341:1029–1036.

128. Frazier OH, March RJ, Horvath KA, Group FtTCDLRS. Transmyocardial revascularization with a carbon dioxide laser in patients with end-stage coronary artery disease. N Engl J Med 1999;341:1021–1028.

129. Aaberge L, Nordstrand K, Dragsund M, et al. Transmyocardial revascularization with CO_2 laser in patients with refractory angina pectoris: clinical results from the Norwegian randomized trial. J Am Coll Cardiol 2000;35:1170–1177.

9 Therapeutic Angiogenesis in Peripheral Arterial Disease
Current Approaches and Future Directions

Richard E. Waters, MD
and Brian H. Annex, MD

CONTENTS

INTRODUCTION
SCOPE OF CLINICAL PROBLEM
ANGIOGENESIS VS THERAPEUTIC ANGIOGENESIS
ANGIOGENIC GROWTH FACTORS
ANGIOGENIC GROWTH FACTORS: FORMULATIONS
 AND DELIVERY STRATEGIES
PRECLINICAL MODELS OF THERAPEUTIC ANGIOGENESIS
 IN PERIPHERAL ARTERIAL DISEASE
CLINICAL TRIALS OF THERAPEUTIC ANGIOGENESIS
 IN CRITICAL LIMB ISCHEMIA
CLINICAL TRIALS OF THERAPEUTIC ANGIOGENESIS
 IN INTERMITTENT CLAUDICATION
FUTURE DIRECTIONS

INTRODUCTION

Angiogenesis, the growth and proliferation of blood vessels from existing vascular structures, is a tightly regulated process in adult tissues. Abnormalities in angiogenesis are associated with a number of pathological states. Strategies designed to promote angiogenesis to treat disorders of inadequate tissue perfusion, such as occurs in peripheral

From: *Contemporary Cardiology: Angiogenesis and Direct Myocardial Revasularization*
Edited by: R. J. Laham and D. S. Baim © Humana Press Inc., Totowa, NJ

Table 1
Comparison of the Two Major PAD Syndromes

	Intermittent claudication	*Critical limb ischemia*
Relative frequency	Common	Less common
Defining symptoms	Pain with walking	Rest pain, nonhealing ulcers, gangrene
Comorbid disease	Moderate	High
Blood flow	Moderately impaired	Severely impaired
Effective therapy	Revasc (minority) Exercise Atherosclerosis therapy	Revasc (majority)
Goal of therapy	↑PWT, ↑QOL	Limb salvage

PWT = peak walking time on treadmill exercise protocol; QOL = quality of life as assessed by validated questionnaires.

arterial disease, have led to the area of therapeutic angiogenesis. Angiogenic growth factors of varying types and preparations are being investigated to promote therapeutic angiogenesis and reduce the sequelae of atherosclerotic disease. In addition to promoting blood vessel growth, these angiogenic growth factors have the potential to influence important biological processes such as the response to injury and cell survival. This chapter reviews the use of angiogenic growth factors for therapeutic angiogenesis in peripheral arterial disease.

SCOPE OF CLINICAL PROBLEM

Though once viewed by the cardiology community as a disease with an incidence and prevalence markedly lower than coronary artery disease, peripheral artery disease (PAD) is increasingly being viewed as a common and underrecognized clinical syndrome. An estimated 15% of North American adults over the age of 55 yr have detectable hemodynamic impairments attributed to PAD, and the incidence of PAD is very close to that of coronary artery disease *(1,2)*.

Patients with PAD have symptoms that overwhelmingly afflict the lower extremity. PAD has a disease spectrum that ranges from clinically silent, but hemodynamically significant, reductions in the ankle-brachial index (ABI) of systolic blood pressure to obvious limb-threatening ischemia. The two major types of clinical presentations are intermittent claudication and critical limb ischemia (Table 1). In patients with claudication, arterial occlusive disease results in reduced blood flow manifested during exercise. In patients with critical limb ischemia, blood flow is inadequate to meet the resting demands of the limb.

Intermittent claudication (IC), muscular leg discomfort provoked by exercise and promptly relieved by rest, is the most common manifestation of PAD. Intermittent claudication, however, is not merely a disease that limits walking, as these patients actually have marked reductions in walking speed, exercise tolerance, functional status, as well as significant impairments in many quality-of-life measures *(3)*. Critical limb ischemia (CLI) is a less common but more profound manifestation of PAD. It includes a constellation of syndromes: intermittent or unremitting metatarsalgia even at rest (probably representing ischemic neuritis), lower extremity ulcers that fail to heal, or frank gangrene. Compared with patients with IC, patients with CLI tend to be older and have significantly more co-morbidity (especially diabetes mellitus) and more diffuse and distal obstructive atherosclerosis. Lower extremity blood flow is severely impaired in CLI, and limb loss is common without successful revascularization. The mortality rates in this population can approach 40% by 6 mo *(4)*.

The site of vascular obstruction to the lower extremity in PAD is often divided into inflow vessels (aortic and iliac arteries), conduit vessels (fermoropopliteal arteries), and run-off vessels (tibial and pedal arteries). Many patients have more than one level of vascular obstruction. In general, clinical syndromes do not correlate with the location of the obstruction. Additionally, the extent of atherosclerotic disease also does not correlate directly with symptoms. An enormous variability exists in the severity of clinical symptoms associated with a given lesion, and this variability likely can be attributed to one or more of the following: (1) baseline functional status, (2) skeletal muscle metabolic "economy," (3) adaptive collateral artery formation, and (4) other factors. Furthermore, a large number of patients with hemodynamic abnormalities consistent with PAD (i.e., a low ABI) have "atypical" or no leg discomfort with walking but still have marked functional impairment and poor clinical courses *(5)*.

Although the primary pathophysiology of PAD is impaired perfusion to the lower extremity, all conventional PAD treatments such as antiplatelet therapy, angiotensin-cascade antagonists, HMG-CoA-reductase inhibitors, and smoking cessation target general atherosclerotic risk factor reduction (especially smoking cessation). In selected patients, structured exercise (in IC) and limb hygiene (in CLI) are of benefit. At present, pharmacological therapies used in PAD do not improve perfusion. Pentoxifylline, although widely prescribed in the United States, has little or no clinical benefit *(6)*. Cilostazol, a phosphodiesterase inhibitor, offers some clinical efficacy, but its safety in patients with ventricular dysfunction remains in question, and the US Food and Drug

Administration (FDA) has issued a black box warning for patients with any degree of heart failure *(7,8)*. Mechanical revascularization, either surgically or percutaneously, can be beneficial in patients with focal or "single-segment" atherosclerotic obstruction confined to aorto-iliac or femoropopliteal levels. Unfortunately, obstruction at multiple levels is common, and it is often difficult or impossible to perform complete revascularization. Even if the anatomy is amenable to surgical revascularization, perioperative morbidity and mortality, loss of conduit, and graft attrition often make this approach largely justifiable only in cases of limb-threatening ischemia. Overall, surgical bypass using autologous or prosthetic conduits is generally offered only to patients with CLI or severe IC. Percutaneous treatment is feasible in many patients with PAD; however, intermediate-term (6–12 mo) recurrent obstruction is common, especially in the large proportion of patients with diffuse or distal disease. For these reasons, new treatment options such as therapeutic angiogenesis have emerged, and such approaches designed to improve perfusion to the lower extremity have the potential to dramatically impact clinical care in this disease.

ANGIOGENESIS VS THERAPEUTIC ANGIOGENESIS

Over the past two decades, tremendous advances have occurred in the understanding of the basic mechanisms of blood vessel growth and maturation *(9–11)*. Two distinct forms of blood vessel growth have been described: vasculogenesis and angiogenesis. Vasculogenesis occurs through much of embryonic vascular development where there is differentiation of endothelial cells from pluripotent stem cells. Once endothelial cells have developed, they begin to assemble into a primitive vascular network, called the primary capillary plexus. Vascularization of several organs, including the endocardium of the heart and the dorsal aorta, occurs by vasculogenesis. In contrast, the brain, kidneys, and the developing limbs are vascularized by angiogenesis, which is defined as the sprouting of new blood vessels from a pre-existing vascular network. Angiogenesis is likely the primary mechanism for most new blood vessel growth in the adult, whether it is due to physiological or pathological stimuli *(12)*. Additionally, it appears that the same molecular mechanisms that mediate normal embryonic vascular development also play a role in pathological angiogenesis which has led to the use of extreme caution and careful patient selection in human clinical trials *(13)*.

The cellular and molecular mechanisms involved in angiogenesis are quite complex and to this date remain incompletely understood. Even in its simplest form, angiogenesis requires a carefully orchestrated sequence of events, both temporally and spatially, in order to form new blood vessels *(14)*. Conceptually, endothelial and surrounding cells must undergo a series of characteristic responses to varying stimuli including proliferation, migration, adhesion and cell-to-cell and cell-to-matrix interaction, matrix degredation, and capillary lumen formation. Each of the events must be viewed within the context of the associated disease process (e.g., angiogenesis in the process of wound repair and angiogenesis following episodes of arterial occlusion). Finally, angiogenesis is not a unidirectional process, but involves a balance between stimulators, inhibitors, and modulators. Therapeutic angiogenesis seeks to exploit the phenomenon of angiogenesis in order to treat disorders of inadequate tissue perfusion *(15)*. Growth factors known to play a role in angiogenesis were analyzed initially, and they continue to be used as agents for therapeutic angiogenesis.

ANGIOGENIC GROWTH FACTORS

Over the past two decades a large number of cytokine growth factors that stimulate endothelial cell proliferation in vitro and, either directly or indirectly, induce angiogenesis ex vivo, or modulate angiogenesis in vivo, have been identified. A list of some of these angiogenic factors is included in Table 2. The vascular endothelial growth factor (VEGF) and fibroblast growth factor (FGF) families have been the most frequently studied, and these factors may be the most potent. VEGF itself is not one gene, but consists of a family of five different and distinct genes known as VEGF-A, VEGF-B (or VEGF-3), VEGF-C (or VEGF-2), VEGF-D, and VEGF-E, as well as the closely related placental growth factor (PlGF) *(16)*. Of these, VEGF-A is thought to be the most physiologically relevant. Even within the VEGF-A gene there are four or more isoforms. These isoforms are produced by alternate splicing of the VEGF mRNA and differ in their extracellular matrix-binding properties, with the 121 isoform being the weakest heparin-binding factor and the 206 isoform being the strongest. VEGF-A also exists in vivo as dimers—either homodimers (i.e., 121:121) or heterodimers (i.e., 121:165)—and each of the single isoform polypeptide chains can bind to other VEGF genes. The VEGF ligands bind to one of three known VEGF receptors. The complexity of the VEGF system is minimal when compared to the complexity of the FGF family. The FGF family contains at least 20 members, with the most significant factors being acidic FGF (FGF-1) and basic FGF (FGF-2) *(17)*. Other important angiogenic growth factors include platelet-derived growth factor (PDGF), hepatocyte growth factor (HGF), and the angiopoietins.

Table 2
Angiogenic Factors, Their Receptors, and Unique Properties

Growth factor	Full name	Receptor	Properties	Human clinical trials?
VEGF-A (VEGF, VEGF1)	Vascular endothelial growth factor-A	VEGFR1 (*flt-1*), VEGFR2 (*flk-1, kdr*), VEGFR3	Endothelial cell mitogen; required for angio/vasculogenesis; multiple isoforms	Yes
VEGF-B	Vascular endothelial growth factor-B	VEGFR1 (*flt-1*)	Forms dimers with VEGF-A; preferentially expressed in heart and skeletal muscle	Yes
VEGF-C	Vascular endothelial growth factor-C	VEGFR2 (*flk-1, kdr*), VEGFR3	May play role in lymphangiogenesis; not regulated by hypoxia	Yes
aFGF (FGF-1)	Acidic fibroblast growth factor	FGF receptor	Endothelial cell, fibroblast, smooth muscle cell mitogen; isoelectric point 5.6	Yes
bFGF (FGF-2)	Basic fibroblast growth factor	FGF receptor	Endothelial cell, fibroblast, smooth muscle cell mitogen; isoelectric point 9.6	Yes
HIF1α	Hypoxia inducible factor-1 alpha	Hypoxia response elements upstream from VEGF and other genes	Constitutively expressed; binds VEGF promoter inducing VEGF transcription	Yes
HGF (scatter factor, SF)	Hepatocyte growth factor	*c-met* tyrosine kinase	Strongly extracellular matrix bound	Yes
PDGF	Platelet-derived growth factor	PDGF receptor	Currently in topical form	Yes
PlGF	Placental growth factor	VEGFR1 (*flt-1*) neuropilin	Synergistic with VEGF	No
Ang-1	Angiopoietin-1	Tie-2	Vascular branching morphogenesis; potentiates effect of VEGF	No
Ang-2	Angiopoietin-2	Tie-2	Inhibition of vascular stabilization	No

ANGIOGENIC GROWTH FACTORS: FORMULATIONS AND DELIVERY STRATEGIES

To date, attempts to achieve therapeutic angiogenesis have exclusively involved the exogenous administration of angiogenic growth factors through either direct administration of recombinant proteins or the administration of genes that encode the proteins. Protein administration offers more predictable and controllable delivery than gene therapy, but many of the proteins have very short half-lives *(18,19)*. Despite this, single-dose administration of recombinantly manufactured growth factors have been shown to be effective, and the short half-life can be circumvented with repeat dosing or through pharmacological alterations *(20,21)*. Systemic hypotension has been reported with recombinant protein administration, but this can usually be managed with fluid hydration *(22)*.

Gene therapy includes the use of viral or plasmid DNA, with or without liposomal vectors, to promote transfection efficiency. Persistent gene expression leads to prolonged local exposure of the angiogenic growth factor protein, although the precise timing of this expression in human tissues is unknown. Adenoviral vectors are easily produced, have a reasonable transfection efficiency, and are expressed in nonproliferating cells. The deletion of nonessential components of the adenoviral genome prior to administration leads to less host inflammation, which results in more efficient gene delivery and expression. More recent approaches to further reduce host inflammation have included the development of a fully deleted adenoviral vector that uses a helper virus to provide essential replication and packaging proteins, as well as the development of a recombinant adeno-associated virus (AAV) *(23–25)*. The use of nonviral techniques, including plasmid DNA and liposomal vectors, is also associated with less host inflammation. The ease of production of these nonviral vectors is appealing, but they are generally regarded as less efficient than viral agents *(26,27)*.

Although delivery of angiogenic agents to patients with PAD may be viewed as trivial, alternative administration routes exist. Angiogenic agents have been delivered intra-arterially or intramuscularly in preclinical and clinical trials. Intra-arterial delivery of protein produces more systemic growth factor exposure and, in theory, could produce unwanted toxicities. This has yet to be observed clinically. A major advantage of therapeutic angiogenesis approaches in the periphery vs the myocardium is that direct intramuscular delivery to peripheral skeletal muscle is technically simple, feasible for repeated injection strategies, and can be achieved without systemic exposure. However, it

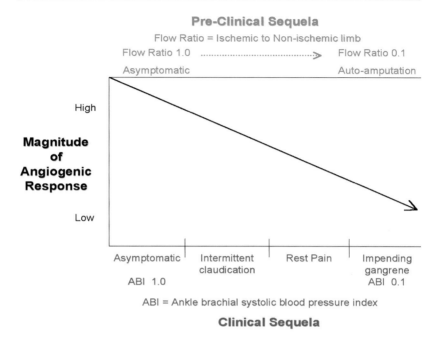

Fig. 1. Angiogenic response to limb ischemia.

remains to be determined whether intramuscular injections will lead to "focal" or "patchy" expression that may limit efficacy.

PRECLINICAL MODELS OF THERAPEUTIC ANGIOGENESIS IN PERIPHERAL ARTERIAL DISEASE

Preclinical models of hindlimb ischemia have been used in an attempt to better understand the angiogenic response in humans with PAD. Before considering the various animal models or approaches, it is critical to recognize that, for the most part, all preclinical ischemia models assess an angiogenic agent's ability to improve upon the extent of endogenous recovery that occurs after arterial ligation. Because of this, the context in which the model is studied is critical (Fig. 1). For example, the endogenous angiogenic response in normal young animals is very robust, and even a complete occlusion (i.e., simple arterial ligation) often results in normal or near-normal limb perfusion in a relatively short period of time. In this setting, the speed and magnitude of the endogenous angiogenic response makes quantitative assessment of potential therapies challenging and may bring their therapeutic/clinical applicability into question. For this reason, preclinical models with a slower and less complete endogenous angiogenic response to ischemia have been developed. Arterial ligation followed by complete excision of the femoral artery produces an ischemic/normal limb flow ratio and a blunted angiogenic response that more closely mimics PAD, and intermittent claudication in particular *(28,29)*. Subsequent administration of angiogenic growth factors or angiogenic gene therapy leads to more rapid and complete recovery, as manifested by enhanced collateral vessel development, increased capillary density, and improved calf blood pressure ratios *(25–27,30–39,51)*. When arterial ligation and excision is applied to animal models with hypercholesterolemia, diabetes or hyperhomocystemia, an even more profound impairment in the endogenous angiogenic response, results, and this scenario is more analogous to critical limb ischemia *(40–44)*. Therapeutic angiogenesis in this setting will seek to prevent limb loss *(40–44)*. All of the angiogenic growth factors that have entered human trials have been successful in some preclinical context (Table 3).

CLINICAL TRIALS OF THERAPEUTIC ANGIOGENESIS IN CRITICAL LIMB ISCHEMIA

The first reports of therapeutic angiogenesis in humans with PAD (CLI) were reported by Isner and colleagues, who described angiographic and histological evidence of angiogenesis after intravascular administration of VEGF plasmid DNA in a single patient with critical limb ischemia *(45)*. This report was followed by a small open-label phase I trial that suggested efficacy following VEGF plasmid DNA administration in nine patients with critical limb ischemia. The authors reported a significant improvement in ABI (0.33 SEM $\pm$ 0.05 to 0.48 SEM $\pm$ 0.03, $p = 0.02$ at 12 wk) as well as new angiographically visible vessels, improved distal flow by magnetic resonance angiography, and enhanced ischemic ulcer healing in the majority of patients *(46)*. Comerota and colleagues published preliminary results of a phase I trial using acidic FGF-1 in patients with critical limb ischemia *(47)*. In this study, 51 patients with unreconstructible peripheral arterial disease and rest pain or tissue necrosis received intramuscular naked plasmid DNA encoding FGF-1 (increasing single and repeated doses). The treatment was well tolerated in all patients. Clinical outcomes in the first 15 patients to complete the 6-mo follow-up study demonstrated a significant reduction in pain ($p < 0.001$) and aggregate ulcer size ($p < 0.01$) that was associated with an increased transcutaneous oxygen pressure ($p < 0.01$) as compared with baseline values. Additionally, a significant increase in ABI ($p < 0.01$) was seen at 8 and 12 wk, but not at 24 wk. Taken together, these

Table 3
Preclinical Studies of Therapeutic Angiogenesis

Factor	Route	Model	Species	Outcome	Ref.
VEGF (protein)	im	LE	Rabbit	↑angio score, ↑flow ratio, ↑CD, ↑BF (microspheres)	30,31
VEGF (protein)	ia	LE	Rabbit	↑angio score, ↑flow ratio, ↑CD	32
VEGF (protein)	iv	LE	Rabbit	↑angio score, ↑flow ratio, ↑CD, ↑max flow reserve	33
VEGF (plasmid)	im	LE	Rabbit	↑BP ratio, ↑flow (microspheres, doppler wire)	26
VEGF (plasmid)	ia	LE	Rabbit	↑angio score, ↑flow ratio, ↑CD	34
VEGF (adenovirus)	im	L[a]	Rat	↑angio score, ↑CD, ↑flow (microspheres)	35
AAV-VEGF (adeno-associated virus)	im	LE	Rat	↑CD, ↑flow (microspheres, infrared thermography)	24,25
VEGF (plasmid-liposome)	im	LE	Rabbit	↑angio score, ↑flow ratio, ↑CD, ↑flow (microspheres)	27
FGF-2 (protein)	im	L	Rabbit	↑CD, ↑recovery TcPO$_2$, ↑muscle viability	36
rFGF-2 (protein)	ia	L	Rat	↑CD, ↑flow (microspheres)	37
HIF-1α/VP16 (hybird gene transfer)	im	LE	Rabbit	↑angio score, ↑flow ratio, ↑CD, ↑flow (microspheres)	51

[a]Ligation in setting of recent ischemia.

im = intramuscular; ia = intra-arterial; iv = intravenous; LE= ligation and excision; L= ligation; CD = capillary density; flow ratio = ratio between ischemic and nonischemic limb.

preliminary trials, although small, provided sufficient evidence for the following studies in intermittent claudication.

CLINICAL TRIALS OF THERAPEUTIC ANGIOGENESIS IN INTERMITTENT CLAUDICATION

The first human studies using basic FGF , or FGF-2, were performed at the National Institutes of Health, where Lazarous and colleagues administered intravascular FGF-2 to 11 patients with claudication and an ABI < 0.8 in a phase I, double-blind, placebo-controlled, dose escalation trial (48). They found FGF-2 to be well tolerated, even at the highest doses, and showed plethysmographic evidence of improved lower extremity blood flow in the treated group.

The Therapeutic Angiogenesis with Recombinant Fibroblast Growth Factor-2 for Intermittent Claudication (TRAFFIC) trial was a phase II, double-blind, placebo-controlled study comparing intra-arterial infusions of recombinant FGF-2 (rFGF-2) with placebo *(49)*. One hundred and ninety patients with moderate-severe intermittent claudication, infra-inguinal obstructive atherosclerosis, and a resting ABI of <0.8 were randomly assigned to receive bilateral infusions of placebo, single-bolus, or double-bolus rFGF-2. All groups demonstrated an increase in the primary endpoint, a change in peak walking time at 90 d, which was significantly greater in the single-bolus group than in the placebo group (1.77 min vs 0.6 min, $p = 0.026$). The addition of a second bolus did not provide additional benefit (1.54 min). The secondary endpoints of quality of life and claudication onset time did not differ significantly between the groups, but there was a trend toward an increase in peak walking time at 180 d and a small but significant increase in ABI among treated patients that was not seen with placebo. TRAFFIC remains the only phase II trial of therapeutic angiogenesis to show benefit in its primary efficacy measure.

The Regional Angiogenesis with Vascular Endothelial Growth Factor in PAD (RAVE) trial was a phase II, double-blind, placebo-controlled trial comparing intramuscular injections of $VEGF_{121}$ adenovirus ($AdVEGF_{121}$) with placebo *(50)*. One hundred and five patients with chronic, stable, predominately unilateral, intermittent claudication, and resting ABI of <0.8 were randomly assigned to receive intramuscular injections of low-dose $AdVEGF_{121}$, high-dose $AdVEGF_{121}$, or placebo. Although all groups demonstrated an increase in the primary endpoint, a change in peak walking time at 12 wk, this change did not differ between the placebo (1.8 ± 3.2 min), low-dose (1.6 ± 1.9 min), and high-dose (1.5 ± 3.1 min) groups. Furthermore, the secondary endpoints of peak walking time at 26 wk, quality-of-life measures, claudication onset time, and ABI also did not differ among the groups.

FUTURE DIRECTIONS

Future approaches to achieve therapeutic angiogenesis in humans can be categorized into four areas: new factors, alternative targets, combinations of factors, and the link to cell therapy. The vast majority of initial human studies have employed single growth factors delivered as a protein or gene product. These cytokine growth factors have generally targeted one receptor or one family of receptors. New targets for therapeutic angiogenesis are emerging, and these include transcription factors that have the potential to modulate a number of downstream gene products; an example of this is hypoxia-inducible factor 1α *(51)*. Angiogenesis is a complex coordinated process that involves multiple growth factors. Asahara and colleagues first demonstrated the synergy between VEGF and basic FGF in models of hindlimb ischemia *(52)*. A recent report by Cao et al. *(53)* demonstrated that PDGF is synergistic with basic FGF, but the synergy did not apply to PDGF and VEGF. Although complexities will exist in translating this into human studies, approaches like this will eventually be employed.

Angiogenic growth factors may also have effects aside from simple proliferation. For example, VEGF is a survival factor for microvascular endothelial cells and can permit the survival of these cells in the face of injury *(54,55)*. A recent study from our group demonstrated that hindlimb ischemia induces apoptosis in peripheral skeletal muscle and angiogenic growth factors may ultimately influence apoptosis and thereby exert beneficial effects in targeted skeletal muscle *(56)*. Finally, the classic study by Asahara and Isner *(57)* demonstrated that circulating cells contribute to the angiogenic response. Currently, it is well established that angiogenic growth factors have some interplay with circulating or bone marrow–derived progenitor cells *(58)*. Initial studies have demonstrated the potential feasibility of cell therapy to mitigate the sequelea of peripheral arterial disease *(59)*, but definitive studies are still pending.

REFERENCES

1. Criqui MH, Fronek A, Barrett-Connor E, et al. The prevalence of peripheral arterial disease in a defined population. Circulation 1985;71:510–515.
2. Hirsch AT, Criqui MH, Treat-Jacobson D, et al. Peripheral arterial disease detection, awareness, and treatment in primary care. JAMA 2001;286:1317–1324.
3. Hiatt WR, Hirsch AT, Regensteiner JG, et al. Clinical trials for claudication. Assessment of exercise performance, functional status, and clinical endpoints. Vascular Clinical Trialist. Circulation 1995;92:614–621.
4. Management of peripheral arterial disease (PAD). TransAtlantic Inter-Society Consensus (TASC). Section D: chronic critical limb ischaemia. Eur J Vasc Endovasc Surg 2000;Suppl A:S144–S243.
5. McDermott MM, Greenland P, Liu K, et al. Leg symptoms in peripheral arterial disease: associated clinical characteristics and functional impairment. JAMA 2001;286:1599–1606.
6. Radack K, Wyderski RJ. Conservative management of intermittent claudication. Ann Intern Med 1990;113:135–146.
7. Money SR, Herd JA, Issacsohn JL, et al. Effect of Cilastazol on walking distances in patients with intermittent claudication caused by peripheral vascular disease. J Vasc Surg 1998;27:267–275.
8. Beebe HG, Dawson DL, Cutler BS, et al. A new pharmacological treatment for intermittent claudication: results of a randomized multicenter trial. Arch Intern Med 1999;159:2041–2050.

9. Carmeliet P, Conway EM. Growing better blood vessels. Nat Biotechnol 2001;19:1019–1020.

10. Conway EM, Collen D, Carmeliet P. Molecular mechanisms of blood vessel growth. Cardiovasc Res 2001;49:507–521.

11. Folkman J. Clinical applications of research on angiogenesis. N Engl J Med 1995;333:1757–1763.

12. Folkman J. Angiogenesis in cancer, vascular, rheumatoid, and other disease. Nat Med 1995;1:27–31.

13. Folkman J. Tumor angiogenesis: therapeutic implications. N Engl J Med 1971;285:1182–1186.

14. Jain RK, Carfmeliet P. Anti- and pro-angiogenesis therapy. Sci Am 2001;285:38–45.

15. Waltenberger J. Modulation of growth factor action: Implications for the treatment of cardiovascular diseases. Circulation 1997;96:4083–4094.

16. Veikkola T, Karkkainen M, Claesson-Welsh L, et al. Regulation of angiogenesis via vascular endothelial growth factor receptors. Cancer Res 2000;60:203–212.

17 Simons M, Annex BH, Laham RJ, et al. Pharmacological treatement of coronary artery disease with recombinant fibroblast growth factor-2: double-blind, randomized, controlled, clinical trial. Circulation 2002;105:788–793.

18. Laham RJ, Rezaee M, Post M, et al. Intracoronary and intravenous administration of basic fibroblast growth factor: myocardial and tissue distribution. Drug Metab Dispos 1999;27:821–826.

19. Eppler SM, Combs DL, Henry TD, et al. A target-mediated model to describe the pharmacokinetics and hemodynamic effects of rhVEGF in humans. Clin Pharmacol Therap 2002;72:20–32.

20. Lopez JJ, Edelman ER, Stamler A, et al. Angiogenic potential of perivasculary delivered aFGF in a porcine model of chronic myocardial ischemia. Am J Physiol 1998;274:H930–H936.

21. East MA, Landis DI, Thompson MA, et al. Effect of single dose of intravenous heparin on plasma levels of angiogenic growth factors. Am J Cardiol 2003;91:1234–1236.

22. Hariawala MD, Horowitz JR, Esakof D, et al. VEGF improves myocardial blood flow but produces EDRF-mediated hypotension in porcine hearts. J Surg Res 1996;63:77–82.

23. Maione D, Della Rocca C, Gianetti P, et al. An improved helper-dependent adenoviral vector allows persistent gene expression after intramuscular delivery and overcomes preexisting immunity to adenovirus. Proc Natl Acad Sci USA 2001;98:5986–5991.

24. Byun J, Heard JM, Huh JE, et al. Efficient expression of the vascular endothelial growth factor gene in vitro and in vivo, using an adeno-associated virus vector. J Mol Cell Cardiol 2001;33:295–305.

25. Shimpo M, Ikeda U, Maeda Y, et al. AAV-mediated VEGF gene transfer into skeletal muscle stimulates angiogenesis and improves blood flow in a rat hindlimb ischemia model. Cardiovasc Res 2002;53:993–1001.

26. Tsurumi Y, Takeshita S, Chen D, et al. Direct intramuscular gene transfer of naked DNA encoding vascular endothelial growth factor augments collateral development and tissue perfusion. Circulation 1996;94:3281–3290.

27. Gowdak LH, Poliakova L, Li Z, et al. Induction of angiogenesis by cationic lipid-mediated VEGF165 gene transfer in the rabbit ischemic hindlimb model. J Vasc Surg 2000;32:342–352.

28. Couffinhal T, Silver M, Zheng LP, et al. Mouse model of angiogenesis. Am J Pathol 1998;152:1667–1679.

29. Hong JH, Bahk YW, Suh JS, et al. An experimental model of ischemia in rabbit hindlimb. J Korean Med Sci 2001;5:630–635.

30. Pu LQ, Sniderman AD, Brassard R, et al. Enhanced revascularization of the ischemic limb by angiogenic therapy. Circulation 1993;88:208–215

31. Takeshita S, Pu LQ, Stein LA, et al. Intramuscular administration of vascular endothelial growth factor induces dose-dependent collateral artery augmentation in a rabbit model of chronic limb ischemia. Circulation 1994;90:II228–II234.

32. Takeshita S, Zheng LP, Brogi E, et al. Therapeutic angiogenesis. A single intrarterial bolus of vascular endothelial growth factor augments revascularization in a rabbit ischemic hind limb model. J Clin Invest 1994;93:662–670.

33. Bauters C, Asahara T, Zheng LP, et al. Site-specific therapeutic angiogenesis after systemic administration of vascular endothelial growth factor. J Vasc Surg 1995;21:314–324.

34. Takeshita S, Weir L, Chen D, et al. Therapeutic angiogenesis following arterial gene transfer of vascular endothelial growth factor in a rabbit model of hindlimb ischemia. Biochem Biophys Res Commun 1996;227:628–635.

35. Mack CA, Magovern CJ, Budenbender KT, et al. Salvage angiogenesis induced by adenovirus-mediated gene transfer of vascular endothelial growth factor protects against ischemic vascular occlusion. J Vasc Surg 1998;27:699–709.

36. Baffour R, Berman J, Garb JL, et al. Enhanced angiogenesis and growth of collaterals by in vivo administration of recombinant basic fibroblast growth factor in a rabbit model of acute lower limb ischemia: dose-response effect of basic fibroblast growth factor. J Vasc Surg 1992;16:181–191.

37. Yang HT, Deschenes MR, Ogilvie RW, et al. Basic fibroblast growth factor increases collateral blood flow in rats with femoral arterial ligation. Circ Res. 1996;79:62–69.

38. Murohara T, Asahara T, Silver M, et al. Nitric oxide synthase modulates angiogenesis in response to tissue ischemia. J Clin Invest 1998;101:2567–2578.

39. Rissanen TT, Markkanene JE, Arve K, et al. Fibroblast growth factor 4 induces vascular permeability, angiogenesis and arteriogenesis in a rabbit hindlimb ischemia model. FASEB J 2003;1:100–102.

40. Rivard A, Silver M, Chen D, et al. Rescue of diabetes-related impairment of angiogenesis by intramuscular gene therapy with adeno-VEGF. Am J Pathol 1999;154:355–363.

41. Van Belle E, Rivard A, Chen D, et al. Hypercholesterolemia attenuates angiogenesis but does not preclude augmentation by angiogenic cytokines. Circulation 1997;96:2667–2674.

42. Duan J, Muohara T, Ikeda H, et al. Hyperhomocysteinemia impairs angiogenesis in response to hindlimb ischemia. Atheriocler Thromb Vasc Biol 200;20:2579–2585.

43. Duan J, Murohara T, Ikeda H, et al. Hypercholesterolemia inhibits angiogenesis in response to hindlimb ischemia; nitric oxide-dependent mechanism. Circulation 2000;102(Suppl III):III370–III376.

44. Couffinhal T, Silver M, Kearney M, et al. Impaired collateral vessel development associated with reduced expression of vascular endothelial growth factor in ApoE-/- mice. Circulation 1999;99:3188–3198.

45. Isner JM, Pieczek A, Schainfeld R, et al. Clinical evidence of angiogenesis following arterial gene transfer of phVEGF165. Lancet 1996;348:370–374.

46. Baumgartner I, Pieczek A, Manor O, et al. Constitutive expression of phVEGF165 after intramuscular gene transfer promotes collateral vessel development in patients with critical limb ischemia. Circulation 1988;97:1114–1123.

47. Comerota AJ, Throm RC, Miller KA, et al. Naked plasmid DNA encoding fibroblast growth factor type I for the treatment of end-stage unreconstructible lower extremity ischemia: preliminary results of a phase I trial. J Vasc Surg 2002;35:930–936.

48. Lazarous DF, Unger EF, Epstein SE, et al. Basic fibroblast growth factor in patients with intermittent claudication: results of a phase I trial. JACC 2000;36:1239–1244.

49. Lederman RG, Mendelsohn FO, Anderson RD, et al. Therapeutic angiogenesis with recombinant fibroblast growth factor-2 for intermittent claudication (the TRAFFIC study): a randomised trial. Lancet 2002;359:2053–2058.

50. Rajagopalan S, Mohler ER, Lederman RJ, et al. A phase II randomized double blind controlled study of adenoviral delivery of VEGF121 in patients with disabling intermittent claudication. Regional angiogenesis with vascular endothelial growth factor (VEGF) in peripheral arterial disease. Circulation 2003 (in press).

51. Vincent KA, Shyu KG, Luo Y, et al. Angiogenesis is induced in a rabbit model of hindlimb ischemia by naked DNA encoding an HIF-1(/VP16 hybrid transcription factor. Circulation 2000;102:2266–2261.

52. Asahara T, Bauters C, Zheng OP, et al. Synergistic effect of vascular endothelial growth factor and basic fibroblast growth factor on angiogenesis in vivo. Circulation 1995;93(9 Suppl):II365–II371.

53. Cao R, Brakenhielm E, Pawliuk R, et al. Angiogenic synergism, vascular stability and improvement of hind-limb ischemia by a combination of PDGF BB and FGF-2. Nat Med 2003;5:604–613.

54. Spyridopolous I, Brogi E, Kearney M, et al. Vascular endothelial growth factor inhibits endothelial cell apoptosis induced by tumor necrosis factor-alpha:balance between growth and death signals. J Mol Cell Cardiol 1997;29:1321–1330.

55. Dimmeler S, Zeiher AM. Endothelial cell apoptosis in angiogenesis and vessel regression. Circ Res 2000;434–439.

56. Dai Q, Thompson MA, Pippen AM, et al. Alterations in endothelial cell proliferation and apoptosis contribute to vascular remodeling following hindlimb ischemia in rabbits. Vasc Med 2002;7:87–93.

57. Iwaguro H, Yamaguchi J, Kalka C, et al. Endothelial progenitor cell vascular-endothelial growth factor gene transfer for vascular regeneration. Circulation 2002;105:732–738.

58. Luttun A, Carmeliet G, Carmeliet P. Vascular progenitors:from biology to treatment. Trends Cardiovasc Med 2002;12:84–92.

59. Tateishi-Yuyama E, Matsubara H, Murohara T, et al. Therapeutic angiogenesis for patients with limb ischaemia by autologous transplantation of bone-marrow cells: a pilot study and a randomised controlled trial. Lancet 2002;360:427–435.

10 Bone Marrow Cell Transplantation for Myocardial Regeneration and Therapeutic Angiogenesis

Hung-Fat Tse, MD, Pui-Yin Lee, MBBS, and Chu-Pak Lau, MD

CONTENTS

INTRODUCTION

Coronary artery disease remains the leading cause of death in developing countries. In the United States, up to 12 million Americans have a history of myocardial infarction, angina pectoris, or both *(1)*. Although recent advances in medical treatment and interventional procedures have reduced the mortality in patients with coronary artery disease *(2)*, the number of patients with refractory myocardial ischemia and congestive heart failure is rapidly increasing. In a significant proportion of these

From: *Contemporary Cardiology: Angiogenesis and Direct Myocardial Revasularization*
Edited by: R. J. Laham and D. S. Baim © Humana Press Inc., Totowa, NJ

patients, percutaneous coronary intervention or surgical bypass revascularization is either not feasible or incomplete as a result of patients' comorbidity, total occlusion, or poor distal vessels. After a myocardial infarction, some cardiomyocytes are lost and others hibernate because of insufficient myocardial perfusion. Therefore, therapeutic approaches aimed at promoting blood vessel formation (angiogenesis) and growing new heart muscle fibers (myocardial regeneration) are attractive alternatives. Accumulating evidence suggests that bone marrow cells have the potential of contributing to tissue revascularization and cardiac regeneration after myocardial injury. This chapter summarizes the current status of bone marrow cell transplantation for myocardial regeneration and therapeutic angiogenesis.

BONE MARROW STEM CELLS

With the recent advances in stem cell biology, it has been shown that adult bone marrow contains several stem cell populations that can transdifferentiate into various mesenchymal and nonmesenchymal cell types *(3,4)*. These stem cells can be broadly divided into two main groups based on their expression of cell marker CD34: CD34+ hematopoietic stem/progenitor cells and CD34– mesenchymal stem cells (MSCs) (Fig. 1).

The CD34+ hematopoietic stem/progenitor cells are precursors of blood and endothelial cells in adult bone marrow. The hematopoietic stem cells (HSCs) refer to those stem cell populations that can self-renew and differentiate into more mature progenitor cells in the bone marrow and provide permanent long-term reconstitution of the entire hematopoietic system. In contrast, hematopoietic progenitor cells of bone marrow have a limited capacity for self-renewal and differentiation and can only sustain hematopoiesis for a short-term period. A small population of endothelial progenitor cells (EPCs) has also been identified in the bone marrow, which can be mobilized to the circulatory system and contribute to the postnatal neovascularization process *(5)*.

The CD34– MSCs are precursors of stromal cells and appear to have multilineage differentiation capacity in vitro *(6)*. However, there is no adequate cell marker to allow selection of purified cell populations, and thus their phenotypes remain unclear. Cardiomyocytes can be differentiated from MSCs after exposure to 5-azacytidine, a cytosine analog capable of alterating gene expression that regulates differentiation *(7)*. Recently, another subset of bone marrow stromal cells, referred to as multipotent stem cells, has been described on the basis of their capacity to differentiate into multiple lineages *(8)*.

Recent studies have shown that the adult heart is not a terminally differentiated organ, although the rate of myocardial cell turnover is

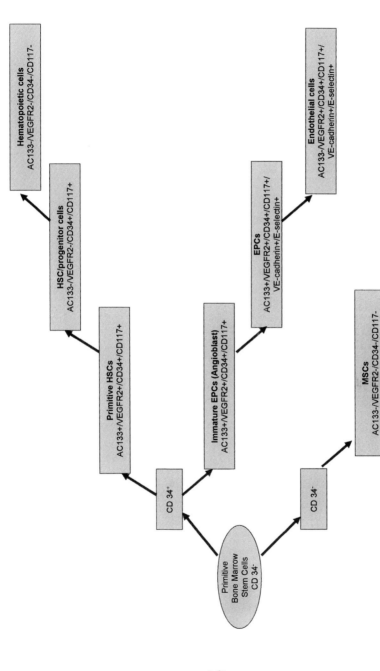

Fig. 1. Origin and differentiation of stem cells in adult bone marrow. Representative antigenicities to stem/progenitor cells are shown (+, positive; −, negative).

extremely low *(9)*. The origin of stem cells in regenerating myocardium remains unclear. Emerging data suggest that bone marrow cells have the ability to differentiate into stem and progenitor cells that mature into functional cells in a variety of tissues including myocardium *(10)*. Experimental studies have suggested that bone marrow-derived cells can transdifferentiate into liver, brain, skeletal muscle, heart, lung, kidney, gut, and skin cells *(11)*. Many such studies are based on a sex-mismatched hematopoietic stem cell transplantation model using the Y chromosome as a marker *(3,4)*. Furthermore, recent clinical studies have also demonstrated male chimerism in heart allografts from female donors *(12,13)*. It has been postulated that in addition to the effect of direct migration of cardiomyocytes from adjacent recipient tissue into the allograft, the circulating stem cells from the bone marrow may have a favorable role in ventricular remodeling after transplantation. In addition to transdifferentiation of bone marrow stem cells, cell fusion also appears to account for a proportion of the presence of cells that show donor characteristics in solid organ tissue *(14,15)*. However, the relative importance of stem cell fate transition and cell fusion is unknown.

KINETICS OF ADULT BONE MARROW STEM CELLS

It has been postulated that circulating bone marrow-derived stem cells may contribute to tissue regeneration and repair in solid organs *(4)*. Myocardial injury that causes changes in the microenvironment may play an important role in stem cell recruitment. Previous studies have demonstrated that EPCs were mobilized from the hematopoietic system after acute myocardial infarction *(16)*. However, the mechanisms by which circulating bone marrow-derived stem cells are recruited into the heart and the subsequent cardiomyocyte generation is not fully understood.

Several cytokines may regulate the proliferation, mobilization, and homing of bone marrow stem cells into the injured solid-organ. Stem cell factor (SCF) is expressed in HSCs and is a ligand of c-kit (a tyrosine kinase receptor). It may regulate the migration of HSC during embryonic development as well as in response to myocardial injury. Recent studies have demonstrated that SCF, c-kit, and metalloproteinase-9 play an important role in the mobilization of stem and progenitor cells from the bone marrow after myocardial necrosis *(17)*. Granulocyte-macrophage colony-stimulating factor (GM-CSF) is a well-known stimulator of hematopoietic stem/progenitor cells. However, experimental studies also demonstrated that GM-CSF mobilizes EPCs to severely ischemic tissue and enhances neovascularization *(18)*. Similar modulation of EPC kinetics has been observed in response to other hematopoietic cytokines, such

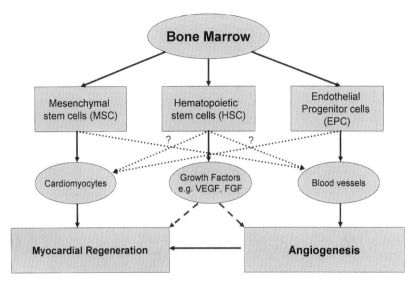

Fig. 2. Therapeutic role of different types of bone marrow stem cells in myocardial regeneration and angiogenesis.

as granulocyte colony-stimulating factor (G-CSF) and stromal-derived factor (SDF)-1 *(19,20)*. The roles of vascular endothelial growth factors (VEGFs) and the tyrosine kinase VEGF receptors in endothelial cell proliferation and differentiation during neovascularization are well described *(21)*. However, evidence is emerging that VEGF-mediated mobilization of bone marrow-derived EPCs also contributes to neovascularization *(22,23)*.

BONE MARROW AS A CELL SOURCE FOR MYOCARDIAL REGENERATION AND THERAPEUTIC ANGIOGENESIS

As discussed above, bone marrow contains multiple types of stem cells and progenitor cells, which can potentially be used for cellular therapy for myocardial regeneration and therapeutic angiogenesis (Fig. 2).

Myocardial Regeneration

Acute myocardial infarction or chronic ischemic heart disease results in the loss of cardiomyocytes and vasculature that is difficult to regenerate. Furthermore, peri-infarct tissue undergoes apoptosis as a result of ischemia and acts as a barrier to the incorporation of vascular or myocardial cells to damaged tissues. Experimental studies have shown that bone

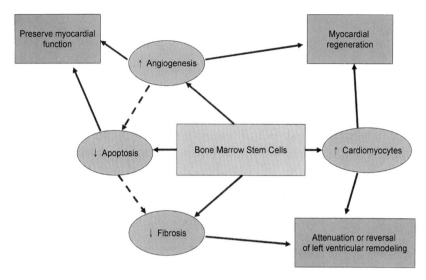

Fig. 3. Potential beneficial mechanisms of bone marrow cell therapy after myocardial infarction. Angiogenesis, decreased apoptosis, myocardial regeneration, and reduced fibrosis can preserve the myocardial function and diminish or reverse negative left ventricular remodeling after myocardial infarction.

marrow-derived stem cells can be transdifferentiated into cardiomyocytes in vitro and in vivo. Treatment of bone marrow cells with 5-azacytidine resulted in the formation of a cell line that, upon further differentiation, gave rise to cells with spontaneous electrical and contractile activity and other molecular attributes of differentiated cardiomyocytes (7). In animal models of myocardial infarction, direct intramyocardial injection of c-kit expressing bone marrow stem cells into the sites of myocardial infarcts formed myocardium comprised of new myocytes as well as endothelial and smooth muscle cells (24,25). Myocardial regeneration was not observed in hearts that were transplanted with the subpopulation of c-kit– bone marrow cells known to be devoid of stem cells. A concomitant improvement of cardiac hemodynamic and angiogenesis, and reduction in fibrosis and apoptosis were observed in hearts transplanted with c-kit+ bone marrow stem cells compared with negative control mice (25) (Fig. 3). Furthermore, bone marrow-derived myocytes and endothelial cells were observed in the infarcted mouse heart following bone marrow reconstitution with CD34– side-population bone marrow hematopoietic stem cells (26). In fact, this subpopulation of stem cells may represent a more primitive type of stem cell that can differentiate into either mesenchymal stem cells or endothelial progenitor cells.

MCSs isolated from bone marrow also appeared to undergo differentiation into cardiomyocytes *(27)*. Furthermore, cardiomyocytes derived from mesenchymal stem cells transplanted into ventricular scar tissue have shown to integrate with the myocardium and improve left-ventricular function *(28,29)*. Several studies also supported the notion that adult bone marrow stem cells can migrate into the heart for myocardial regeneration. Administration of cytokines can expand and mobilize bone marrow stem cells into circulation. A 250-fold increase in circulating bone marrow stem cells was induced in mice after myocardial infarction with the combined use of SCF and G-CSF *(24)*. This cytokine therapy resulted in a new brand of myocardium, consisting of myocytes and blood vessels, occupying 70% of the infarcted area, and improving cardiac hemodynamic functions.

These experiments demonstrated the capacity of adult bone marrow stem cells to give rise to new myocytes, endothelial cells, and smooth muscle cells in ischemic myocardium. However, the population of bone marrow stem cells responsible for the generation of these several myocardial cell types remains undefined. A recent experimental study failed to show any evidence of myocardial regeneration after transplantation of autologous fresh bone marrow into infarcted myocardium *(30)*. This highlighted the potential importance of the timing as well as the composition of the bone marrow stem cells used for myocardial regeneration. The fate of the transplanted bone marrow stem cells may be affected by the local microenvironment. During the early phase of myocardial infarction or in the presence of residual ischemia at the peri-infarct tissue, the local myocardial environment may harbor the appropriate signal for driving the bone marrow stem cells toward an endothelial and/or cardiomyogenic differentiation pathway. Indeed, experimental studies have shown evidence of myocardial regeneration after transplantation of bone marrow cells early after myocardial infarction *(24–26)*. However, the local cues are likely to be lost at the late stage of chronic scarring or in the absence of active ischemia. Currently, there is no evidence of new cardiomyocyte formation after bone marrow transplantation into an old fibrous postinfarct scar. Furthermore, the composition and/or the concentration of different types of bone marrow stem cells in the fresh bone marrow may not be optimal for myocardial regeneration. A sufficient amount of cardiomyocyte/mesenchymal stem cells will also require the presence of endothelial progenitor cells to provide vascular structures for the supply of oxygen and nutrients to both the chronically ischemic, endogenous myocardium and the newly implanted cardiomyocytes (Fig. 2). Furthermore, recent studies have shown the existence of adult cardiac stem cells, which are multipotent and contribute to myocardial regeneration *(31)*.

Therapeutic Angiogenesis

Recently, EPCs were successfully isolated from circulating mononuclear cells (MNCs) using VEGFR2, CD34, and CD133 antigens shared by both embryonic EPCs and HSCs in adults. EPCs are thought to share common stem/progenitor cells with HSCs and to derive from bone marrow (Fig. 1). In the presence of sufficient density and appropriate growth factors, EPCs can differentiate into endothelial-like cells that aggregate into capillary-like structures. Experimental studies have shown that EPCs functionally contribute to neoangiogenesis during wound healing, limb ischemia, postmyocardial infarction, endothelialization of vascular grafts, and atherosclerosis *(32)*. This is consistent with vasculogenesis, a critical paradigm well described for embryonic neovascularization, but recently proposed in adults.

Recent studies with animal bone marrow transplantation models in which bone marrow donor-derived EPCs could be distinguished have shown that the contribution of EPCs to endothelialization and neovascularization *(32,33)*. In chronic hindlimb ischemic models, infusion of EPCs derived from bone marrow, cord blood, or peripheral blood enhanced the formation of new vasculature and improved perfusion *(4,32,33)*. EPCs also induced neovascularization after myocardial infarction. In a rat model of myocardial infarction, injection of EPCs isolated from rat or human peripheral blood (after treatment with G-CSF) induced neovascularization, reduced infarct size, and preserved cardiac function *(34,35)*. Furthermore, direct intramyocardial injection of autologous bone marrow cells in the swine model of chronic ischemic myocardium also induced neovascularization and improved myocardial function *(36,37)*. Although the mechanism remains unclear, these experimental studies suggest that autologous bone marrow cells could augment neovascularization in ischemic myocardium mainly through the production of angiogenic growth factors and less through the differentiation of a portion of the cells into EPCs/ECs *in situ* (Fig. 4). Furthermore, the improvement in cardiac function in these studies without evidence of myocardial regeneration was attributed to the improvement in myocardial perfusion, which in turn prevented cardiomyocyte apoptosis at the peri-infarct zone and decreased left ventricular remodeling (Fig. 3).

CLINICAL UTILIZATION OF BONE MARROW CELL TRANSPLANTATION

Clinical Approach of Transplantation

The delivery route of stem cells may have a critical role in the success of bone marrow cell therapy for myocardial regeneration and therapeutic

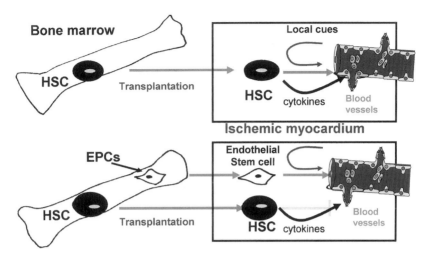

Fig. 4. Two proposed mechanisms of neovascularization by bone marrow cell transplantation. First, hematopioetic stem cells (HSCs) dfferentiate into endothelial cells due to the local cue in the ischemic myocardium and secret cytokines to induce neovascularization (upper panel). Alternatively, both the HSCs and endothelail progenitor cells (EPCs) are transplanted into ischemic myocardium. The EPCs differentiate into endothelial cells as a result of local cue in the ischemic myocardium and the HSCs secret cytokines to induce neovascularization (lower panel).

angiogenesis. There are two clinical strategies for delivering bone marrow stem cells into the ischemic and/or infarcted myocardium. One approach is based on direct delivery of bone marrow stem cells to the heart via intramyocardial or intracoronary injection. The other approach is based on the in vivo availability of a pool of systemic and circulating bone marrow stem cells that can be mobilized by cytokine therapy to the heart. The advantages and disadvantages of the two potential clinical strategies for myocardial regeneration and angiogenesis are summarized in Table 1.

It is now established that after myocardial infarction, there is spontaneous mobilization of bone marrow EPCs to the circulation *(16)*. This raises the questions of why mobilization of these cells does not automatically result in myocardial regeneration and angiogenesis and what is the role of delivering the bone marrow cells into the myocardium. It has been postulated that the EPCs mobilized during the acute phase of tissue injury have not achieved the complete maturation necessary for incorporation into the ischemic myocardium. Furthermore, the lack of blood supply to the ischemic tissue after occlusion of the coronary artery reduces

Table 1
Advantages and Disadvantage of Potential Clinical Strategies
for Bone Marrow Therapy

Strategy	Advantage	Disadvantage
Direct Delivery		
Intramyocardial		
Open heart surgery	Applicable to patients who need open heart surgery Allows direct visualization of the site of injection	Risk of mortality and morbidity of open heart surgery
Catheter-based approach	Avoids the risk of open heart surgery Short-term safety proven Clinical trials ongoing	Specialized catheters and imaging technology needed
Intracoronary	Possible wide use in catheterization laboratory	Efficacy of cell delivery to the myocardium uncertain Not applicable to patients with an occluded artery Risk of systemic administration unclear
Intravenous	Avoids the risk of cardiac catheterization procedure	Low efficacy of cell delivery Not applicable to patients with an occluded artery Risk of systemic administration unclear
Mobilization		
Cytokine therapy	Avoids the cost and risk associated with bone marrow cell harvest and preparation Widespread practicality	Uncertainty regarding risk and timing

the number of EPCs that arrive at the sites of myocardial injury. Finally, other bone marrow cells in addition to EPCs may also be required to achieve an optimal response *(32)*. Direct introduction of bone marrow stem cells into the compromised zone by direct intramyocardial injection or by intracoronary infusion may circumvent these hurdles. However, systemic delivery of bone marrow stem cells may contribute to tumorigenesis, atherosclerosis, or retinopathy and this strategy should be used with utmost caution *(38)*.

Mobilization of bone marrow stem cells with cytokine therapy is appealing as a potential therapy as it is easy to administer and applies to a larger patient population. In clinical hematological practice, short-term administration of G-CSF in healthy humans is not associated with an increased risk of a coronary event *(39)*. On the other hand, there is no suitable animal model to test the safety and feasibility of this approach in the presence of coronary artery disease. In patients with acute coronary syndrome, multiple unstable coronary plaques may exist in the coronary artery. Theoretically, these plaques might be destabilized by an increased number of circulating leukocytes after cytokine therapy. Indeed, an elevated white cell count does predict a poorer prognosis in patients with acute myocardial infarction *(40)*. Furthermore, hyperviscosity resulting from an increased number of circulating leukocytes may also lead to a worsening of the myocardial perfusion in patients with severe coronary artery disease. Therefore, the short-term safety of this treatment approach remains a concern.

Early Clinical Experience

Based on the encouraging results from the experimental models, direct introduction of bone marrow cells into the peri-infarct region has been investigated as a means to facilitate revascularization. This procedure, known as cellular cardiomyoplasty, involves either direct intramyocardial injection or intracoronary arterial delivery of stem cells into the peri-infarct area. Clinical investigation of patients with both chronic myocardial ischemia and myocardial infarction is currently in the early stage of nonrandomized testing of safety and feasibility (Table 2). In human subjects, autologous bone-marrow mononuclear cells were delivered either by using direct intramyocardial injection during coronary artery bypass surgery *(41)* or as guided by electromechanical mapping technique *(42–44)* or by intracoronary infusion into the coronary arteries feeding the infarcted and ischemic tissue *(45,46)*.

Recently, our group has reported the first human experience of catheter-based direct intramyocardial injection of autologous bone marrow mononuclear cells in eight patients with end-stage ischemic heart disease *(42)*. The procedure was guided by using three-dimensional nonfluoroscopic electromechanical mapping (NOGA™ system, Biosense-Webster) *(47)*. The use of the electromechanical system mapping can allow us to target ischemic regions for bone marrow cell injection (Fig. 5). No acute complication was observed after the procedure. After 3 mo follow-up, the number of anginal episodes and nitroglycerin tablet usage decreased. Magnetic resonance imaging (MRI) 90 d after procedure demonstrated improved wall motion, wall thickness and myocardial perfusion at the target region (Figs. 6, 7). During follow-up, none of our patients experienced ventricular arrhythmias or developed new tumors or myocardial scar on MRI. Subsequently, reports from other investigators *(43,44)* using a similar method have also suggested a beneficial effect.

Table 2
Clinical Trials of Autologous Blood- or Bone Marrow (BM)–Derived Cell Transplantation for Ischemic Heart Disease

Authors (ref.)	No. of patients	Type of BM cell	Route of administration	Clinical outcome
			Myocardial Ischemia	
Hamano et al., 2001 (41)	5	BM mononuclear cells	Direct intramyocardial injection during coronary artery bypass graft surgery	Improved in myocardial perfusion
Tse et al., 2003 (42)	8	BM mononuclear cells	Catheter-based intramyocardial injection guided by electromechanical mapping	Improved in symptoms, myocardial perfusion and function
Fuchs et al., 2003 (43)	10	Fresh aspirated BM cells	Catheter-based intramyocardial injection guided by electromechanical mapping	Improved in symptoms and myocardial perfusion
Perin et al., 2003 (44)	14	BM mononuclear cells	Catheter-based intramyocardial injection guided by electromechanical mapping	Improved in myocardial perfusion and symptoms
			Myocardial Infarction	
Strauer et al., 2002 (45)	10	BM mononuclear cells	Intracoronary injection after percutaneous coronary intervention	Decreased infarct size, improved myocardial function and perfusion
Assmus et al., 2002 (46)	20	BM mononuclear cells (n = 9) or peripheral blood-derived progenitor cells (n = 11)	Intracoronary injection after percutaneous coronary intervention	Improved myocardial function, improved regional wall motion in infarct zone; similar efficacy of blood-derived and BM-derived progenitor cells
Stamm et al., 2003 (47)	6	Purified BM–derived hematopoietic stem cells (AC133+)	Direct intramyocardial injection during coronary artery bypass graft surgery	Improved myocardial function and regional wall motion in infarct zone

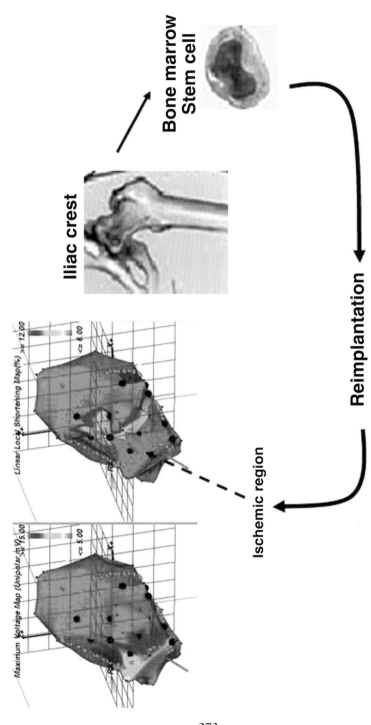

Fig. 5. Nonfluoroscopic electromechanical mapping technique-guided catheter-based intramyocardial injection of autologous bone marrow cells into the ischemic myocardium.

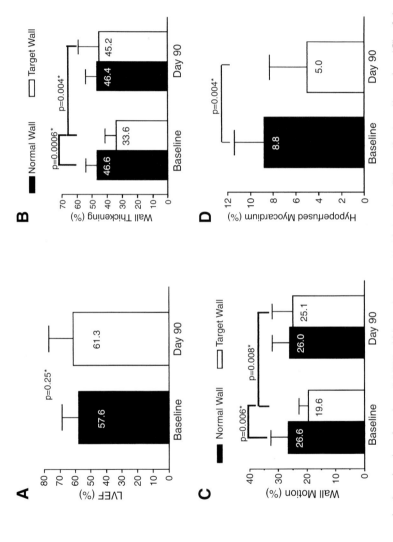

Fig. 6. Left-ventricular ejection fraction (LVEF) (**A**), regional wall thickening (**B**), radical wall motion (**C**) of the normal and target wall, and percent of hypoperfused myocardium (**D**), as determined by magnetic resonance imaging at baseline and 90 d after bone marrow cell implantation. *Statistical significance with a *p* < 0.05. From ref. *41*.

Stress MRI Perfusion Image

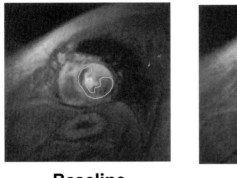 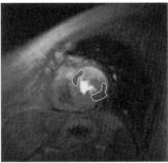

Baseline   **Day 90**

Fig. 7. An example of adenosine stress gadolinium-DTPA enhanced myocardial perfusion imaging at baseline and after 90 d. The amount of hyoperfusion myocardium at the targeted inferior site (yellow area) reduced after bone marrow cell implantation. MRI, magnetic resonance imaging.

Intracoronary infusion of bone marrow mononuclear cells was performed in 10 patients 5–9 d after acute myocardial infarction. At 3 mo, these patients had improvement in myocardial function and viability *(45)*. In the Transplantation of Progenitor Cells and Regeneration Enhancement in Acute Myocardial Infarction (TOPCARE-AMI) study, the efficacy of the ex vivo expanded peripheral blood mononuclear cells was compared to bone marrow-derived EPCs in restoring revascularization after acute myocardial infarction. In both treatment arms there was a similar improvement in myocardial function and viability *(46)*.

In all of these studies there was improved blood flow and left ventricular function, suggesting that infusion of autologous bone marrow cells appears to be feasible, safe, and may confer short-term therapeutic benefit. However, a mixture of bone marrow mononuclear cells was used, and it remains unclear which types of cells are therapeutic and whether the injected cells themselves or the cytokines produced by them contribute to the beneficial effects.

The use of purified populations of autologous bone marrow-derived CD133+ cells were investigated in six patients with acute myocardial infarction who underwent coronary bypass graft surgery *(48)*. After 9 mo, all patients were alive, with improvement in cardiac function in four patients. However, reasons for beneficial effects are confounded by the surgery.

The effect of intracoronary and systemic administration of GM-CSF was investigated using 10 patients with coronary artery disease *(49)*. An improvement in collateral flow was demonstrated in these patients by invasive measures of collateral artery blood flow (estimated by coronary artery pressure distal to balloon occlusion). However, no clinically relevant endpoint or assessment on the mobilization of bone marrow stem cells was performed. It is unclear whether the coronary vascular benefit determined in this study may have resulted from direct effects of this cytokine on angiogenesis or on collateral vascular dilator tone with improved regional blood flow.

Despite enthusiasm for these pioneering clinical trials, none of them are randomized or have sufficient efficacy data to support any conclusion. It remains to be determined in randomized clinical trials whether bone marrow cell transplantation will result in long-standing improvement in cardiac function and decrease morbidity and mortality without any long-term toxicity.

Potential Clinical Complications

In the preliminary safety and feasibility trials, no authors have reported a significant short-term safety problem. However, late-onset toxicity may emerge as a result of the use of whole populations of bone marrow mononuclear cells, which contain different organ-specific stem, progenitor, and hematopoietic cells. These nonessential cells, if incorporated into regenerating myocardium, may result in generation of noncardiac tissues as well as life-threatening arrhythmias. In particular, as bone marrow stem cells are also a rich source of different angiogenic factors, including VEGF-A, this may result in the generation of edema and aberrant angiomas *(50)*. Therefore, whole bone marrow mononuclear cells should be used with caution and close long-term clinical monitoring. As many pathophysiological conditions, including tumor growth, diabetic- or age-related retinopathies, and atheroma formation are angiogenesis dependent, intravenous introduction of proangiogenic EPCs and hematopoietic cells may have adverse effects by inducing neovascularization in other organs.

Future Perspective

In human studies, autologous bone marrow cells are used to avoid the potential issue of rejection, which necessitates the use of immunosuppressive therapy. However, this approach would deliver a much lower concentration of stem cells than those used in animal studies, especially for myocardial regeneration. Therefore, the fundamental scarcity of bone marrow stem cells (EPCs, MSCs, and HSCs) in the circulation, combined with their possible functional impairment associated with a variety of diseases such as aging and diabetes, constitute major limitations of autologous bone marrow transplantation for myogenesis. Considering autologous bone marrow stem cell therapy, certain technical improvements that may help to overcome the primary scarcity of a viable and functional stem cell population should include (1) delivery of optimal composition of types of bone marrow stem cells, (2) adjunctive strategies to promote stem cell mobilization and survival, e.g., combined with cytokines, (3) enrichment procedures, i.e., leukapheresis and ex vivo expansion, or (4) enhancement of stem cells function by gene transduction to improve survival and homing. These more complex isolation and preparation procedures for bone marrow stem cells may be associated with increased cost and regulatory hurdles. However, these procedures may be essential to avoid future complications and to substantiate the true value of bone marrow stem cell therapeutics for myocardial regeneration and angiogenesis.

Recently, bone marrow stem cells have also been applied to the field of tissue engineering as a means of improving biocompatibility. Recent studies have demonstrated that the use of bone marrow stem cells enables the establishment of tissue engineered vascular autograft *(51,52)* and heart valves *(53)*, which might reduce the complications associated with incompatible material, such as thrombosis. Alternatively, as previously reported, the cell sheets of cultured cardiomyocytes with EPCs may be effective for the improvement of cardiac function in damaged hearts, i.e., ischemic heart disease or cardiomyopathy, and induce neovascularization to maintain the viability of the cardiomyocytes *(54)*.

CONCLUSIONS

Recent advances in the understanding of the mechanisms involved in proliferation, recruitment, mobilization, and incorporation of bone marrow stem cells into the myocardium and blood vessels have prompted the development of cellular transplantation therapy for heart diseases refractory to conventional therapy. To acquire the more optimized quality and quantity of bone marrow stem cells for myocardial regeneration several issues remain to be addressed, such as the development of a more efficient method of stem cell identification, purification, and expansion. Despite the initial promising studies indicating potential clinical benefit of bone marrow therapy for therapeutic myogenesis and angiogenesis, many obstacles remain, such as long-term safety, optimal timing, and treatment strategy. Emerging, rationally designed, randomized clinical trials assessing the role of bone marrow-derived stem cells in tissue revascularization and myocardial regeneration will open new avenues of research in stem cell therapeutics.

ACKNOWLEDGMENTS

This project was supported in part by a research grant from the Hong Kong Research Grants Council (HKU 7357/02M), Sun Chieh Yeh Heart Foundation, and SK Yee Medical Foundation, (Project no. 203217) and the Research Grant Council of Hong Kong (HKU 7357/02M).

REFERENCES

1. American Heart Association. Heart and Stroke Statistical Update. Dallas, TX: American Heart Association, 2001.
2. Ryan TJ, Antman EM, Brooks NH, Califf RM, Hillis LD, Hiratzka LF, Rapaport E, Riegel B, Russell RO, Smith EE III, Weaver WD, Gibbons RJ, Alpert JS, Eagle KA, Gardner TJ, Garson A Jr, Gregoratos G, Ryan TJ, Smith SC Jr. 1999 update: ACC/AHA guidelines for the management of patients with acute myocardial infarction: report of the American College of Cardiology/American Heart Association Task Force on Practice Guidelines (Committee on Management of Acute Myocardial Infarction). J Am Coll Cardiol 1999;34:890–911.
3. Rosenthal N. Prometheus's vulture and the stem-cell promise. N Engl J Med 2003;349:267–274.
4. Körbling M, Estrov Z. Adult stem cells for tissue repair-a new therapeutic concept? N Engl J Med 2003;349:570–582.
5. Asahara T, Murohara T, Sullivan A, Silver M, van der Zee R, Li T, Witzenbichler B, Schatteman G, Isner JM. Isolation of putative progenitor endothelial cells for angiogenesis. Science 1997;275:964–967.
6. Pittenger MF, Mackay AM, Beck SC, Jaiswal RK, Douglas R, Mosca JD, Moorman MA, Simonetti DW, Craig S, Marshak DR. Multilineage potential of adult human mesenchymal stem cells. Science 1999;284:143–147.
7. Makino S, Fukuda K, Miyoshi S, Konishi F, Kodama H, Pan J, Sano M, Takahashi T, Hori S, Abe H, Hata J, Umezawa A, Ogawa S. Cardiomyocytes can be generated from marrow stromal cells in vitro. J Clin Invest 1999;103:697–705.
8. Jiang Y, Jahagirdar BN, Reinhardt RL, Schwartz RE, Keene CD, Ortiz-Gonzalez XR, Reyes M, Lenvik T, Lund T, Blackstad M, Du J, Aldrich S, Lisberg A, Low WC, Largaespada DA, Verfaillie CM. Pluripotency of mesenchymal stem cells derived from adult marrow. Nature 2002;418:41–49.
9. Beltrami AP, Urbanek K, Kajstura J, Yan SM, Finato N, Bussani R, Nadal-Ginard B, Silvestri F, Leri A, Beltrami CA, Anversa P. Evidence that human cardiac myocytes divide after myocardial infarction. N Engl J Med 2001;344:1750–1757.
10. Jackson KA, Majka SM, Wang H, Pocius J, Hartley CJ, Majesky MW, Entman ML, Michael LH, Hirschi KK, Goodell MA. Regeneration of ischemic cardiac muscle and vascular endothelium by adult stem cells. J Clin Invest 2001;107:1395–1402.
11. Burt R, Pearce W, Luo K, Oyama Y, Davidson C, Beohar N, Gheorghiade M. Hematopoietic stem cell transplantation for cardiac and peripheral vascular disease. Bone Marrow Transplant 2003;32:S29–S31.
12. Quaini F, Urbanek K, Beltrami A, Finato N, Beltrami CA, Nadal-Ginard B, Kajstura J, Leri A, Anversa P. Chimerism of the transplanted heart. N Engl J Med 2002;346:5–15.
13. Muller P, Pfeiffer P, Koglin J, Schafers HJ, Seeland U, Janzen I, Urbschat S, Bohm M. Cardiomyocytes of noncardiac origin in myocardial biopsies of human transplanted hearts. Circulation 2002;106:31–35.

14. Wang X, Willenbring H, Akkari Y, Torimaru Y, Foster M, Al-Dhalimy M, Lagasse E, Finegold M, Olson S, Grompe M. Cell fusion is the principal source of bone-marrow-derived hepatocytes. Nature 2003;422:897–901.
15. Vassilopoulos G, Wang PR, Russell DW. Transplanted bone marrow regenerates liver by cell fusion. Nature 2003;422:901–904.
16. Shintani S, Murohara T, Ikeda H, Ueno T, Honma T, Katoh A, Sasaki KI, Shimada T, Oike Y, Imaizumi T. Mobilization of endothelial progenitor cells in patients with acute myocardial infarction. Circulation 2001;103:2776–2779.
17. Heissig B, Hattori K, Dias S, Friedrich M, Ferris B, Hackett NR, Crystal RG, Besmer P, Lyden D, Moore MA, Werb Z, Rafii S. Recruitment of stem and progenitor cells from the bone marrow niche requires MMP-9 mediated release of kit-ligand. Cell. 2002;109:625–637.
18. Takahashi T, Kalka c, Masuda H, Chen D, Silver M, Kearney M, Magner M, Isner JM, Asahara T. Ischemia- and cytokine-induced mobilization of bone marrow-derived endothelial progenitor cells for neovascularization. Nat Med 1999;5:434–438.
19. Moore MA, Hattori K, Heissig B, Shieh JH, Dias S, Crystal RG, Rafii S. Mobilization of endothelial and hematopoietic stem and progenitor cells by adenovector-mediated elevation of serum levels of SDF-1, VEGF, and angiopoietin-1. Ann NY Acad Sci 2001;938:36–45.
20. Hattori K, Heissig B, Tashiro K, Honjo T, Tateno M, Shieh JH, Hackett NR, Quitoriano MS, Crystal RG, Rafii S, Moore MA. Plasma elevation of stromal cell-derived factor-1 induces mobilization of mature and immature hematopoietic progenitor and stem cells. Blood 2001;97:3354–3360.
21. Risau W, Flamme I. Vasculogenesis. Annu Rev Cell Dev Biol 1995;11:73–91.
22. Asahara T, Takahashi T, Masuda H, Kalka C, Chen D, Iwaguro H, Inai Y, Silver M, Isner JM. VEGF contributes to postnatal neovascularization by mobilizing bone marrow-derived endothelial progenitor cells. EMBO J 1999;8:3964–3972.
23. Kalka C, H. Masuda, T. Takahashi, Gordon R, Tepper O, Gravereaux E, Pieczek A, Iwaguro H, Hayashi SI, Isner JM, Asahara T. Vascular endothelial growth factor (165) gene transfer augments circulating endothelial progenitor cells in human subjects. Circ Res 2000;86:1198–1202.
24. Orlic D, Kajstura J, Chimenti S, Limana F, Jakoniuk I, Quaini F, Nadal-Ginard B, Bodine DM, Leri A, Anversa P. Mobilized bone marrow cells repair the infarcted heart, improving function and survival. Proc Natl Acad Sci USA 2001;98:10344–10349.
25. Orlic D, Kajstura J, Chimenti S, Jakoniuk I, Anderson SM, Li B, Pickel J, McKay R, Nadal-Ginard B, Bodine DM, Leri A, Anversa P. Bone marrow cells regenerate infarcted myocardium. Nature 2001;410:701–705.
26. Jackson KA, Majka SM, Wang H, Pocius J, Hartley CJ, Majesky MW, Entman ML, Michael LH, Hirschi KK, Goodell MA. Regeneration of ischemic cardiac muscle and vascular endothelium by adult stem cells. J Clin Invest 2001;107:1395–1402.
27. Jiang Y, Jahagirdar BN, Reinhardt RL, Schwartz RE, Keene CD, Ortiz-Gonzalez XR, Reyes M, Lenvik T, Lund T, Blackstad M, Du J, Aldrich S, Lisberg A, Low WC, Largaespada DA, Verfaillie CM. Pluripotency of mesenchymal stem cells derived from adult marrow. Nature 2002;418:41–49.
28. Wang JS, Shum-Tim D, Galipeau J, Chedrawy E, Eliopoulos N, Chiu RC. Marrow stromal cells for cellular cardiomyoplasty: feasibility and potential clinical advantages. J Thorac Cardiovasc Surg 2000;120:999–1005.
29. Toma C, Pittenger MF, Cahill KS, Byrne BJ, Kessler PD. Human mesenchymal stem cells differentiate to a cardiomyocyte phenotype in the adult murine heart. Circulation 2002;105:93–98.

30. Bel A, Messas E, Agbulut O, Richard P, Samuel JL, Bruneval P, Hagege AA, Menasche P. Transplantation of autologous fresh bone marrow into infarcted myocardium: a word of caution. Circulation 2003;108(Suppl 1):II247–II252.
31. Beltrami AP, Barlucchi L, Torella D, Baker M, Limana F, Chimenti S, Kasahara H, Rota M, Musso E, Urbanek K, Leri A, Kajstura J, Nadal-Ginard B, Anversa P. Adult cardiac stem cells are multipotent and support myocardial regeneration. Cell 2003;114:763–776.
32. Rafii S, Lyden D. Therapeutic stem and progenitor cell transplantation for organ vascularization and regeneration. Nat Med 2003;9:702–712.
33. Masuda H, Asahara T. Post-natal endothelial progenitor cells for neovascularization in tissue regeneration. Cardiovasc Res 2003;58:390–398.
34. Kocher AA, Schuster MD, Szabolcs MJ, Takuma S, Burkhoff D, Wang J, Homma S, Edwards NM, Itescu S. Neovascularization of ischemic myocardium by human bone-marrow-derived angioblasts prevents cardiomyocyte apoptosis, reduces remodeling and improves cardiac function. Nat Med 2001;7:430–436.
35. Kawamoto A, Gwon HC, Iwaguro H, Yamaguchi JI, Uchida S, Masuda H, Silver M, Ma H, Kearney M, Isner JM, Asahara T. Therapeutic potential of ex vivo expanded endothelial progenitor cells for myocardial ischemia. Circulation 2001;103:634–637.
36. Fuchs S, Baffour R, Zhou YF, Shou M, Pierre A, Tio FO, Weissman NJ, Leon MB, Epstein SE, Kornowski R. Transendocardial delivery of autologous bone marrow enhances collateral perfusion and regional function in pigs with chronic experimental myocardial ischemia. J Am Coll Cardiol 2001;37:1726–1732.
37. Kawamoto A, Tkebuchava T, Yamaguchi J, Nishimura H, Yoon YS, Milliken C, Uchida S, Masuo O, Iwaguro H, Ma H, Hanley A, Silver M, Kearney M, Losordo DW, Isner JM, Asahara T. Intramyocardial transplantation of autologous endothelial progenitor cells for therapeutic neovascularization of myocardial ischemia. Circulation 2003;107:461–468.
38. van Royen N, Hoefer I, Bottinger M, Hua J, Grundmann S, Voskuil M, Bode C, Schaper W, Buschmann I, Piek JJ. Local monocyte chemoattractant protein-1 therapy increases collateral artery formation in apolipoprotein E-deficient mice but induces systemic monocytic CD11b expression, neointimal formation, and plaque progression. Circ Res 2003;92:218–225.
39. Gutierrez-Delgado F, Bensinger W. Safety of granulocyte colony-stimulating factor in normal donors. Curr Opin Hematol 2001;8:155–60.
40. Sabatine MS, Morrow DA, Cannon CP, Murphy SA, Demopoulos LA, DiBattiste PM, McCabe CH, Braunwald E, Gibson CM. Relationship between baseline white blood cell count and degree of coronary artery disease and mortality in patients with acute coronary syndromes: a TACTICS-TIMI 18 (Treat Angina with Aggrastat and determine Cost of Therapy with an Invasive or Conservative Strategy—Thrombolysis in Myocardial Infarction 18 trial) substudy. J Am Coll Cardiol 2002;40:1761–1768.
41. Hamano K, Nishida M, Hirata K, Mikamo A, Li TS, Harada M, Miura T, Matsuzaki M, Esato K. Local implantation of autologous bone marrow cells for therapeutic angiogenesis in patients with ischemic heart disease: clinical trial and preliminary results. Jpn Circ J 2001;65:845–847.
42. Tse HF, Kwong YL, Lo G, Ho CL, Chan JKF, Yeung DW, Lau CP. Angiogenesis in ischemic myocardium by intramyocardial autologous bone marrow mononuclear cell implantation. Lancet 2003;361:47–49.
43. Fuchs S, Satler LF, Kornowski R, Okubagzi P, Weisz G, Baffour R, Waksman R, Weissman NJ, Cerqueira M, Leon MB, Epstein SE. Catheter-based autologous bone marrow myocardial injection in no-option patients with advanced coronary artery disease: a feasibility study. J Am Coll Cardiol 2003;41:1721–1724.

44. Perin EC, Dohmann HF, Borojevic R, Silva SA, Sousa AL, Mesquita CT, Rossi MI, Carvalho AC, Dutra HS, Dohmann HJ, Silva GV, Belem L, Vivacqua R, Rangel FO, Esporcatte R, Geng YJ, Vaughn WK, Assad JA, Mesquita ET, Willerson JT. Transendocardial, autologous bone marrow cell transplantation for severe, chronic ischemic heart failure. Circulation 2003;107:2294–2302.

45. Strauer BE, Brehm M, Zeus T, Kostering M, Hernandez A, Sorg RV, Kogler G, Wernet P. Repair of infarcted myocardium by autologous intracoronary mononuclear bone marrow cell transplantation in humans. Circulation 2002;106:1913–1918.

46. Assmus B, Schachinger V, Teupe C, Britten M, Lehmann R, Dobert N, Grunwald F, Aicher A, Urbich C, Martin H, Hoelzer D, Dimmeler S, Zeiher AM; Transplantation of Progenitor Cells and Regeneration Enhancement in Acute Myocardial Infarction. Transplantation of Progenitor Cells and Regeneration Enhancement in Acute Myocardial Infarction (TOPCARE-AMI). Circulation 2002;106:3009–3017.

47. Stamm C, Westphal B, Kleine HD, Petzsch M, Kittner C, Klinge H, Schumichen C, Nienaber CA, Freund M, Steinhoff G. Autologous bone-marrow stem-cell transplantation for myocardial regeneration. Lancet 2003;361:45–46.

48. Gepstein L, Hayam G, Ben-Haim SA. A novel method for nonfluoroscopic catheter-based electroanatomical mapping of the heart: in vitro and in vivo accuracy results. Circulation 1997;95:1611–1622.

49. Seiler C, Pohl T, Wustmann K, Hutter D, Nicolet PA, Windecker S, Eberli FR, Meier B. Promotion of collateral growth by granulocyte-macrophage colony-stimulating factor in patients with coronary artery disease: a randomized, double-blind, placebo-controlled study. Circulation 2001;104:2012–2017.

50. Epstein SE, Kornowski R, Fuchs S, Dvorak HF. Angiogenesis therapy: amidst the hype, the neglected potential for serious side effects. Circulation 2001;104:115–119.

51. He H, Shirota T, Yasui H, Matsuda T. Canine endothelial progenitor cell-lined hybrid vascular graft with nonthrombogenic potential. J Thorac Cardiovasc Surg 2003;126:455–464.

52. Matsumura G, Miyagawa-Tomita S, Shin'oka T, Ikada Y, Kurosawa H. First evidence that bone marrow cells contribute to the construction of tissue-engineered vascular autografts in vivo. Circulation 2003;108:1729–1734.

53. Perry TE, Kaushal S, Sutherland FW, Guleserian KJ, Bischoff J, Sacks M, Mayer JE. Bone marrow as a cell source for tissue engineering heart valves. Ann Thorac Surg 2003;75:761–767.

54. Zimmermann WH, Eschenhagen T. Cardiac tissue engineering for replacement therapy. Heart Fail Rev 2003;8:259–269.

11 Transplantation of Embryonic Stem Cells for Myocardial Regeneration and Angiogenesis

Yong-Fu Xiao, MD, PhD,
Jiang-Yong Min, MD,
and James P. Morgan, MD, PhD

Contents

INTRODUCTION

Congestive heart failure remains the leading cause of death in developed countries. Myocardial infarction (MI) results in the loss of heart muscle cells, which is the main contributor to the development of heart failure. Classical medical therapy and mechanical left-ventricular assist devices are available for physicians to improve the prognosis of patients with MI and heart failure, but only half of the patients with end-stage heart failure survive the following year *(1)*. At the present time, allogeneic heart transplantation to extend life span and to improve the quality of daily life is probably the preferred alternative treatment for patients with end-stage heart failure, but extreme organ shortage and chronic

From: *Contemporary Cardiology: Angiogenesis and Direct Myocardial Revasularization*
Edited by: R. J. Laham and D. S. Baim © Humana Press Inc., Totowa, NJ

cardiac rejection limit the therapy. In recent years, research on stem cells is leading scientists to investigate the possibility of cell-based therapies for cardiac repair, often referred to as regenerative or reparative medicine. Stem cell-based cellular cardiomyoplasty (CCM) for cardiomyocyte replacement/regeneration has been evaluated in animal settings *(2–6)* and clinical trials *(7–9)*. Transplantation of exogenous stem cells could regenerate damaged myocardium and improve cardiac function in failing hearts. Such efforts may offer exciting novel options for treating patients with end-stage heart failure.

The feasibility of CCM for repair of failing hearts has been examined via transplantation of exogenous stem cells into host myocardium suffering from cardiomyocyte loss *(6,7,10,11)*. Formation of intercalated disks and gap junctions between transplanted cells and the host tissue indicates functional electrical-contraction coupling *(2,10,12)*. In infarcted mice transplantation of bone marrow cells regenerated infarcted myocardium and improved heart function *(6)*. Our previous study showed that co-transplantation of human mesenchymal stem cells (hMHCs) and human fetal cardiomyocytes significantly improved cardiac function in postinfarcted pigs *(13)*. Transplantation of mouse embryonic stem cells (ESCs) or their derived cardiac-like cells also improved cardiac function in diseased animal models *(14–17)*. Perin and associates reported that transendocardial injections of autologous mononuclear bone marrow cells in patients with end-stage ischemic heart disease can safely promote neovascularization and improve regional and global left-ventricular function *(5)*. Another study shows that 3 mo after intramyocardial implantation of autologous mononuclear bone marrow cells, improvement in symptoms, myocardial perfusion, and function was observed in patients with severe ischemic heart disease *(8)*. Other clinical studies demonstrate that compared to the standard therapy group, transplantation of bone marrow stem cells significantly improved cardiac function in the cell-treated MI patients *(7,18)*. Generally speaking, tissue engineering is a potential therapy for end-stage organ disease or tissue loss. Therefore, cell therapy holds great promise for cardiac disease.

Stem cells are one of the most fascinating areas of biology today, but the big question is how they can replace damaged cells in adult organs. Most adult tissues have stem or progenitor cells, and environmental stimuli can activate and mobilize them. But adult stem cells can only form a limited number of cell types *(19,20)*. ESCs in culture have the capacity for differentiation into all of specialized somatic cell types of the body, including cardiomyocytes. Human embryonic stem cells (hESCs) in culture were isolated and cultured in 1998 by Thomson's group *(21)*. Therefore, identification, derivation, and characterization of hESCs may push the rapidly progressing field of therapeutic cell transplantation. Because of the proliferation and plasticity of differentiation to various mature tissues, ESCs are a potential valuable resource for cell therapy targeting regeneration of functional myocardium in diseased hearts. However, many ethical, political, and scientific barriers have to be overcome before hESCs or their differentiated cells can be used clinically. Here we summarize the findings on transplantation of ESCs or their derived cells in experimental animals with myocardial injury and highlight the progress in research on these particular cells.

EMBRYONIC STEM CELLS
Characterization

ESCs are pluripotent cells that are obtained from the blastocyst stage of early mammalian embryos. A blastocyst includes three structures: the trophoblast, which is the layer of cells that surrounds the blastocyst; the blastocoel, which is the hollow cavity inside the blastocyst; and the inner cell mass, which is a group of cells at one end of the blastocoel. These unique inner cells are characterized by their capacity for prolonged undifferentiated proliferation in culture and have the capability to derive descendants of all three embryonic germ layers—endoderm, mesoderm, and ectoderm. Because ESCs are derived prior to implantation and certain immune-related cell surface proteins (e.g., class I products of the major histocompatibility complex) are not yet expressed, ESCs are a potentially rich source for cell transplantation. An important test to ensure undifferentiation of ESCs is the presence of a protein called Oct-4, which is expressed in totipotent and pluripotent cells of the early embryo and the germ cell lineage. Oct-4 is a transcription factor that helps turn genes on and off at the right time (22,23). ESCs lack the growth phase 1 (G1) checkpoint in the cell cycle and do not require any external stimulus to initiate DNA replication. Mouse ESCs were successfully isolated from murine blastocysts by Evans and Kaufman (24) and Martin (25) more than two decades ago. The hESC lines were obtained in 1998 (21). The histological profile of the hESCs is (1) positive for alkaline phosphatase, stage-specific embryonic antigen (SSEA)-3, SSEA-4, tumor rejection antigen (TRA)-1-60, and TRA-1-81, (2) negative for SSEA-1, and (3) strongly positive staining of SSEA-1 after differentiation (21).

Cardiomyocyte Differentiation

If ESCs in culture are removed from conditions that maintain them in an undifferentiated state, they clump together to form embryoid bodies (EBs) and begin to differentiate spontaneously. They can form muscle cells, nerve cells, and many other cell types. During in vitro differentiation, ESCs have been shown to recapitulate many processes of early embryonic development. The heart is one of the first organs to develop during embryogenesis. The heart tube with spontaneous contractions appears at about embryonic d 8 in mice *(26)*. Cardiomyocytes derived from cultured mouse ESCs exhibit cell morphology, sarcomere formation, and cell–cell junctions similar to those observed in cardiomyocytes developing in vivo *(27,31)*. Mouse ESCs in embryoid bodies present highly specialized phenotypes of cardiac tissue with several electrophysiological characteristics similar to those in adult cardiomyocytes *(32,34)*. Figure 1A shows the hanging-drops procedure to induce cardiomyocyte differentiation of cultured mouse ESCs. These cells showed cardiac action potentials (Fig. 1B) and contractions that responded well to the change of extracellular Ca^{2+} concentrations (Fig. 1C).

If conditions in vitro allow, hESCs also spontaneously form EBs containing derivatives of all three germ layers and differentiate into various cell types, including cardiomyocytes. The phenotypic properties of cardiomyocytes derived from hESCs have been described *(35,36)*. Immunostaining against cardiac myosin heavy chain, α-actinin, desmin, cardiac troponin I, and atrial natriuretic factor was positive in cells from the spontaneously contracting areas within EBs. Electron microscopy revealed varying degrees of myofibrillar organization, consistent with early-stage cardiomyocytes. Expression of several cardiac-specific genes and transcription factors was found in human ESC-derived cardiac-like cells, which also showed electrophysiological properties as cardiomyocytes. These contracting cells showed positive and negative chronotropic responses to the stimuli of isoproterenol and carbamylcholine, respectively *(35)*. In addition, functional cardiomyocytes could efficiently be differentiated from three parent (H1, H7, and H9) hESC lines and two clonal (H9.1 and H9.2) hESC lines *(36)*, even after long-term culture (50 passages, or approx 260 population doublings). Beating cells were observed in hESCs 1 wk after culture under differentiation conditions and increased in numbers with time. The beating cells expressed several transcription factors and characteristic markers of cardiomyocytes. The dissociated and enriched population of differentiated cells reached 70% cardiomyocytes and was proliferative. Therefore, cardiomyocytes derived from ESCs can be a rich and viable source as donor cells for clinical application in heart disease.

Factors Influencing Cardiomyocyte Differentiation

To generate specific types of differentiated cells, such as heart muscle cells, scientists try to influence the direction of ESC differentiation via change in the chemical composition of the surface on which the ESCs are

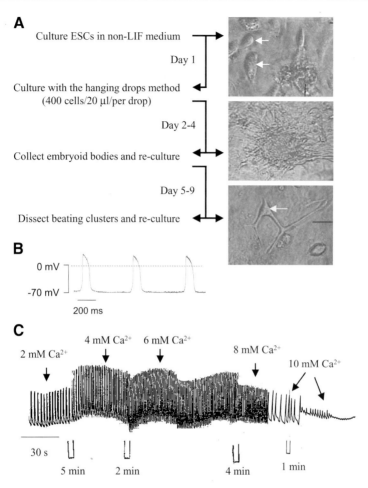

Fig. 1. Action potentials and cell contractions of cardiomyocytes differentiated from mouse embryonic stem cells (ESCs). **(A)** The protocol is shown to induce differentiation of cultured mouse ESCs (ES-D3 cell line) to cardiomyocytes. Left column is a schematic diagram of the hanging-drops method to differentiate ESCs to heart cells. Right column shows single ESCs in culture (white arrows in upper panel, ×200), an embryoid body (red arrow in middle panel, ×100), and a beating cluster of cardiac-like cells (yellow arrow in lower panel, ×200) corresponding to the time periods (black arrows) in culture after withdrawal of leukemia inhibitory factor (LIF) from the conditioned culture medium. **(B)** Cardiac action potentials were observed in a spontaneously beating cell approx 10 d after differentiation of mouse ESCs. **(C)** Cell contractions of ESC-derived cardiomyocytes are shown. Cell shortenings were detected and recorded by the edge-detection method. The amplitude and beating rate of cell contraction were increased when the levels of extracellular Ca^{2+} were raised to 4 or 6 mM. However, the amplitude of cell shortening was significantly reduced in the 8 mM Ca^{2+} solution, and the cells eventually stopped beating in the 10 mM Ca^{2+} solution.

growing, alteration of contents (growth factors) in culture medium, or insertion of specific genes. The microenvironment, known as "niche," greatly affects the fate of stem cells (37). ESCs with adequate environments have a great ability to proliferate and differentiate. During the differentiation process, ESCs have the ability to express different receptor types and release growth factors. In addition, many growth factors and cytokines or other signals from adjacent cells affect ESC proliferation and differentiation. Therefore, cross-talks are always there between ESCs and their environment or neighboring cells.

Co-culture with mouse embryonic fibroblast feeders or addition of leukemia inhibitory factor (LIF) in culture medium suppresses differentiation of mouse ESCs (38). When ESCs spontaneously differentiate, cardiomyocytes of pacemaker-, atrium-, and ventricle-like types can be generated (27). It has been shown that retinoic acid (RA) treatment during ESC differentiation increases the number of cardiomyocytes (39). RA treatment during the first 2 d or between d 2 and 5 of ESC-derived EB formation significantly inhibited cardiogenesis, whereas treatment between d 5 and 7 resulted in an increased cardiomyocyte differentiation (40). The number of differentiated cardiomyocytes with Purkinje- and ventricle-like properties was increased in the presence of RA, whereas the number of pacemaker- and atrium-like cells was reduced (39). Recently, Hidaka et al. (41) also reported that murine ESCs differentiate to chamber-specific Nkx2.5-positive cardiac precursor cells and RA modifies the differentiation potential in a time- and dose-dependent fashion. Our results demonstrate that vascular endothelial growth factor (VEGF) did not affect proliferation of mouse ESCs in vitro in the presence of LIF, but stimulated their proliferation and differentiation to cardiomyocytes in the absence of LIF (42). Our data in vivo also show that transplantation of ESCs with overexpression of VEGF produced a better improvement of heart function in MI mice, which might result from stronger stimulation of myocardial regeneration and neovascularization by ESC-released VEGF (17). A recent study demonstrates that the intact signaling pathway of transforming growth factor (TGF)-β was required for engrafted ESCs to differentiate into functional cardiomyocytes in infarcted myocardium (43). Engrafted ESCs with engineered disruption of TGF-β family failed to differentiate to cardiomyocytes after cell transplantation in infarcted animals. Additionally, Schuldiner et al. (44) reported the effects of eight factors—basic fibroblast growth factor (bFGF), TGF-β, activin-A, bone morphogenic protein (BMP)-4, hepatocyte growth factor (HGF), epidermal growth factor (EGF), β nerve growth factor (β-NGF), and RA—on the differentiation of human embryonic stem-derived cells in vitro. Human ESCs initiated development as aggregates

Table 1
Factors Influencing Differentiation of ESCs to Cardiomyocytes

Factor	Result	Ref.
Mouse ESCs		
LIF	Prevention of differentiation	*38*
Retinoic acid	Increase in number of Purkinje- and ventricle-like cells and decrease in pacemaker- and atrium-like cells	*39*
VEGF	Increase in percentage of α-MHC and cTn-I positive cells	*42*
TGF-β/BMP-2	Significant increase in beating areas and enhancement of myofibrillogenesis	*43*
HBR	Increase in the expression of GATA-4 and Nkx-2.5 and enhancement of yield of beating cardiomyocytes	*91*
PDGF-BB	Promoting cardiogenesis in vitro	*92*
Dynorphin B	Increase in gene expression of GATA-4 and Nkx-2.5 and enhancement of appearance of α-MHC and MLC-2v	*93*
Human ESCs		
Retinoic acid	No effects on cardiomyocyte differentiation	*36*
5-aza-2'-dC	Increase in percentage of cardiomyocyte differentiation	*36*
TGF-β	Enrichment of myocardial-specific cells	*44*

ESCs, embryonic stem cells; LIF, leukemia inhibitory factor; VEGF, vascular endothelial growth factor; TGF-β, transforming growth factor β; BMP-2, bone morphogenic protein 2; HBR, an ester of hyaluronan linked to both butyric and retinoic acid; PDGF-BB, platelet-derived growth factor-BB; 5-aza-2'-dC, 5-aza-2'-deoxycytidine; MHC, myosin heavy chain.

(EBs) expressed a receptor for each of these factors. Each factor had a unique effect on cell differentiation *(44)*. These results indicate that several factors, cytokines, and growth factors affect ESC differentiation. Table 1 summarizes the factors affecting cardiomyocyte differentiation of ESCs reported in literature.

Understanding the regulation of ESC proliferation and differentiation at the cellular and molecular levels may be make it possible to direct ESC differentiation to certain cell types for clinical cell therapy in the future. Specific differentiated cells may be used to treat certain diseases, including Parkinson's disease, diabetes, traumatic spinal cord injury, Purkinje cell degeneration, Duchenne's muscular dystrophy, heart disease, and vision and hearing loss. Alteration of environments of cultured human

ESCs can initiate cardiomyocyte differentiation. The percentage of hECS-derived cardiomyocytes could be enhanced by treatment of them with 5-aza-2'-deoxycytidine, but not by dimethylsulfoxide (DMSO) or RA *(36)*. Because of their combined properties of indefinite proliferation and differentiation to heart cells, hESCs can potentially provide a large number of cardiomyocytes for cell therapy aiming to regenerate functional myocardium. However, studies are required to prove the feasibility of transplantation of hESCs or their derived cells for cardiac repair before clinical utilization is possible.

TRANSPLANTATION OF EMBRYONIC STEM CELLS FOR CARDIAC REPAIR

Myocardial Infarction

Cell transplantation is a potentially novel approach to deliver viable myocytes or cells in adult hearts. In 1994, Soonpaa et al. *(2)* reported that implantation of embryonic d 15 transgenic cardiomyocytes into the myocardium of syngeneic hosts formed stable grafts for as long as the 2-mo observation period. Engrafted cardiomyocytes had no significant negative effects on the host myocardium and formed nascent intercalated disk connection with the host myocardium *(2)*. One year later, Connold and coworkers *(45)* transplanted small fragments of embryonic hearts into soleus muscles of adult rat hosts. The implanted grafts survived and grew for at least 6 mo after transplantation and established a network of blood vessels communicated with the host's circulation. The grafted tissue was rhythmically active with a contraction rate similar to that of adult rat hearts. Application of acetylcholine caused a reversible slowing of the beating rate of the grafts *(45)*. Klug et al. recently reported that transplantation of cultured cardiomyocytes differentiated from murine ESCs formed stable intracardiac grafts and gap junctions *(30)*. They genetically selected relatively pure cultures of cardiomyocytes from differentiating murine ESCs. The selected cardiomyocyte cultures were more than 99% pure and highly differentiated. Intracardiac transplantation of genetically selected cardiomyocytes formed stable grafts in adult mouse hearts for 7-wk observation after implantation *(30)*. These studies demonstrate that grafts of embryonic cardiac tissue or ESC-derived cardiomyocytes survived well in normal tissues with adequate blood supply from the host's circulation (Table 2).

In a non-MI animal model, Roell et al. *(46)* reported that embryonic murine ventricular cardiomyocytes labeled with enhanced green fluorescent protein (GFP) were transplanted into mouse left ventricular walls 2 wk after cryoinfarction. GFP-positive cardiomyocytes isolated from cell-engrafted hearts had postnatal ventricular action potentials and in-

Table 2
Transplantation of ESCs or Embryonic Cardiomyocytes into the Heart in Animal Models

Cell type	Cell delivery	Animal model	Observation period	Result	Ref.
Rat cells					
Small fragment of rE-heart	ism	Rat	6 mo	Forming gap junction CX-43, neovascularization	45,
Small pieces of rE-hearts	im	Rat with cut-injured heart	2 d to 7 mo	Forming gap junction, migration to injured area	47
Dissected rE-cardiomyocytes	im	MI rat	1–8 wk	Graft formation, functional improvement, positive staining aginst α-MHC and CX-43	48
Mouse cells					
Dissected mE-cardiomyocytes	im	Mouse	2 mo	Graft formation, intercalated disks	2
Dissected ESC beating cells	im	MI rat	30 d	Survival, positive staining gainst sarcomeric myosin	15
ESC-derived cardiomyocytes	im	Mouse	7 wk	Formation of stable grafts	30
ESC-derived cardiomyocytes	im	Mouse with cryoinjured heart	1–8 wk	New cardiomyocytes, functional improvement, positive staining against cTn-I	46
ESC-derived cells	im	MI mouse	6 wk	Neovascularization, functional improvement, positive staining against α-MHC, cTn-I, and CX-43	17
ESCs	im	MI rat	6–32 wk	Neovascularization and cardiogenesis, funcional improvement	14,16,43
ESCs	iv	Myocarditic mouse	2–4 wk	New cardiomyocytes, reduction of mortality	52

rE, rat embryonic; mE, mouse embryonic; im, intramyocardial injection or implantation; ism, intraskeletal muscle implantation; MHC, myosin heavy chain; cTn-I, cardiac troponin I; CX-43; connexin-43; mESC, mouse embryonic stem cells; MI, myocardial infarction.

tact β-adrenergic modulation. Analysis of echocardiography showed a significant improvement of force generation and heart function in cell-transplanted hearts. These results show that the grafted embryonic cardiac tissue or myocytes survived in adult host myocardium and expressed characteristics typical of heart cells, which improved damaged heart function (Table 2).

Similarly, two studies show that transplantation of pieces of embryonic ventricular myocardium or cardiomyocytes isolated from early embryos survived in infarcted myocardium and improved damaged heart function. In an early study, Connold et al. *(47)* transplanted pieces of embryonic ventricular myocardium (prelabeled with 4',6-diamindino-2-phenylindole) into a damaged area of the host myocardium and examined the grafts between 2 d and 5–7 mo later. Initially the 4'-6-diamindino-2-phenylindole–labeled cells were localized only at the site of grafting, but by 2–5 wk they migrated along the ventricular surface of the heart. The greatest density of grafted cells was always found in the damaged area. The 4'-6-diamindino-2-phenylindole-labeled cells contained myosin heavy chains and stained positively with antibodies against cardiac gap junction proteins. Recently, Etzion and colleagues *(48)* transplanted cardiomyocytes isolated from 15-d-old embryos into rat MI hearts. Embryonic cardiac cells were labeled with 5-bromo-2'-deoxyuridine (BrdU) or the reporter gene *LacZ*. They found that cell-transplanted MI animals had attenuated left ventricular dilatation, infarct thinning, and myocardial dysfunction. Immunostaining for several cardiac proteins revealed grafts in various stages of differentiation in cell-treated hearts.

Transplanted mouse ESCs have survived and differentiated in infarcted mouse or rat myocardium *(14,16,17)*. ESCs tagged with GFP were transplanted locally into injured myocardium in a rat model with ligation of the left coronary artery. Compared with the control MI animals, cardiac function was significantly improved in ESC-implanted MI rats 6 wk after cell transplantation. Double immunostaining against GFP and cardiac sarcomeric α-actin, α-myosin heavy chain, or troponin I confirmed the survival and differentiation of engrafted cells in MI hearts with ESC transplantation. Additionally, isolated single cells showed rod-shaped GFP-positive myocytes with clear striations in ESC-transplanted animals. GFP-positive myocytes were 7.3% of total cells isolated from each MI left ventricle. The shape and size of mature GFP-positive myocytes did not significantly differ from those of host cardiomyocytes. In contrast, no GFP-positive cells were detected in cells isolated from the sham-operated or MI control hearts *(14)*. Recently, Naito et al. reported similar findings in rats with ligation of the left coronary artery *(15)*. Cells dissected from beating regions of GFP-tagged mouse ESCs were injected into the border zone between the infarcted myocardium and normal myocardium. Thirty days after transplantation, GFP-expressed cells were detected and stained positively by the antibody against sarcomeric myosin *(15)*. These results indicate that transplanted ESCs survived and differentiated in injured myocardium and improved cardiac function in MI animals (Table 2).

More recently, the long-term effects of ESC transplantation on cardiac function were investigated in postinfarcted rats *(16)*. Mouse ESCs were implanted into the border area and infarcted myocardium. During the observation period of 32 wk, the survival rate was significantly increased in MI rats with ESC transplantation. Hemodynamic and echocardiographic data showed significant improvement of cardiac function in the cell-transplanted MI group. GFP-positive tissue was identified in the injured myocardium and stained positively by the antibodies against several specific cardiac proteins *(16)*. The data demonstrate that ESC engrafts exhibit long-term survival in a myocardial infarct model and contribute to long-term improvement of injured heart function (Table 2).

Genetic manipulation of ESCs may produce better turnout after cell transplantation. The effects of transplantation of mouse ESCs transfected with cDNA of VEGF were investigated in a MI mouse model *(17)*. Compared to the MI control mice, left ventricular function was significantly improved in the MI mice with ESC transplantation. In addition, the improvement of heart function was significantly greater in the MI mice engrafted with ESCs overexpressing VEGF. Histological analysis of the sections of infarcted hearts with cell transplantation showed GFP-positive spots which immunostained positively against cardiac troponin I and α-myosin heavy chain. Double staining for GFP and connexin-43 was positive in injured myocardium with ESC transplantation.

Myocarditis

Myocarditis predominantly results from infection by viruses *(49)*, and has a disease process of viral infection, immunoreaction, and microvascular spasm *(50,51)*. Myocardial necrosis and inflammation occur during the acute stage. Development of myocardial fibrosis, calcification, cardiac dilatation, hypertrophy, and heart failure are characterized in the chronic stage. It is a great challenge to prevent or reverse the structural and functional injuries that may cause death or debility of myocarditic patients. In a recent study, Wang and colleagues *(52)* investigated whether infused ESCs could migrate to the injured area of myocarditic mouse hearts and, if so, whether migrated ESCs could differentiate and proliferate in the damaged myocardium. Mice were inoculated with encephalomyocarditis virus (EMCV) immediately following an intravenous infusion of mouse ESCs tagged with GFP. The mortality of mice during the 30-d observation period was significantly reduced, from 37% for the viral control group to 16% for the viral plus ESC-treated group ($p < 0.05$). Compared with the viral control mice, the animals with ESC infusion had a significantly lower incidence of inflammatory cell infiltration and myocardial lesions. In addition, immunostaining against GFP and cardiac α-actin showed that part of infused ESCs migrated to the hearts and differentiated into myocytes there in viral inoculated mice. These results demonstrate that infusion of ESCs significantly reduced mortality and global injury of the hearts in viral myocarditis mice (Table 2). The beneficial effect of engrafted ESCs may have resulted from attenuation of myocardial necrosis and inflammation and from regeneration of damaged myocardium in viral myocarditic animals (52).

Aging Heart

Biogerontology has become attractive to biologists in the past decade. Normal human and animal cells have a finite capacity to replicate and function whether they are cultured in vitro or transplanted as grafts in vivo. This phenomenon has been interpreted to be aging at the cellular level. Alterations in the organization and mobility of cell membrane constituents of cultured rat heart myocytes (53) appear a general phenomenon of aging cells. The aging heart exhibits diastolic dysfunction and increased stiffness. Evidence shows that aging affects the passive mechanical properties of single cardiac myocytes isolated from the hearts of 4-mo young and 30-mo old rats (54). Progressive loss of cardiomyocytes occurs during the aging process and may cause heart failure. A recent study showed that intramyocardial transplantation of mouse ESCs improved cardiac function in aging old rats (55). Mouse ESCs labeled with GFP were injected into myocardium of aged rat hearts. Compared with the young adult rats, cardiac function in aging rats was significantly decreased accompanied by a significant reduction in the number of left ventricular cardiomyocytes and regional blood flow. Six weeks after ESC transplantation, the aged hearts partially restored the blood flow and the number of myocytes and improved their function. In addition, the aged hearts receiving ESCs showed positive response to isoproterenol stimulation, but not in untreated aged hearts. Histological data showed that GFP-positive cells in myocardium that received cell transplantation were positively stained by the antibody against α-myosin heavy chain. Therefore, stem cell therapy may slow down the occurrence of cardiac dysfunction during aging process.

Myocardial Regeneration

The studies presented above show that transplantation of ESCs or embryonic cardiac cells improves injured cardiac function and reduces mortality in experimental animal models. However, the underlying mechanisms of the beneficial effects remain to be delineated. Generation of new functional cardiomyocytes and formation of functional connections between engrafts and host cells are critical for restoration of cardiac function in diseased hearts. ESCs have the ability to differentiate into cardiomyocytes in vitro. Our recent results demonstrate that compared to untreated MI hearts, ESC transplantation significantly reduced the infarct size in MI rats by 5% at 6 wk *(14)* and by 7% at 32 wk *(16)* after MI induction and cell implantation. Calculation of enzymatically isolated single cells shows that 7.3% of isolated left-ventricular cardiomyocytes were GFP positive in the post-MI hearts 6 wk after ESC transplantation *(14)*. The percentage of GFP-positive cells was increased to 11.9% in MI rat hearts 32 wk after ESC engraftment *(16)*. These results suggest that engrafted cells differentiated to cardiomyocytes in MI animals and generated more heart cells if experiments lasted longer.

TGF-β and BMP-2 increased ESC cardiomyocyte differentiation in vitro and in vivo *(43)*. Engrafted mouse ESCs differentiated into functional cardiomyocytes, integrated with surrounding myocardium, beat in synchrony with host cells, and improved contractile performance in infarcted rat myocardium *(43)*. This process was significantly enhanced by TGF-β or BMP-2. Differentiation of engrafted mouse ESCs into cardiomyocytes also occurred in normal *(43)*, infarcted *(17,43)*, and viral myocarditic *(52)* myocardium in mice. Therefore, the improvement of cardiac function in injured hearts of animal models mainly results from myocardial regeneration of engrafted cells.

It has been reported that mouse ESC-derived cardiomyocytes used for cell transplantation in vivo withdrew from the cell cycle by the manifestation of multinucleation, a feature of terminally differentiated cardiomyocytes *(29)*. However, our studies showed that the number of GFP-positive cells isolated from the MI hearts at 6 or 32 wk after ESC transplantation increased by 6- to 38-fold over those of the original ESCs initially transplanted *(14,16)*. This result indicates that differentiation and proliferation continuously occurred in injured myocardium after ESC transplantation. Continuous proliferation in vitro was also observed in cultured ESCs under differentiation conditions. Additionally, spontaneously beating cells differentiated from human ESCs increased in numbers with time and retained contractility for over 70 d *(36)*. More recently, Perez-Terzic et al. *(56)* reported that compared to postmitotic cardiac cells from heart muscle, cardiomyocytes or contracting cells differentiated from mouse ESCs were proliferative and underwent structural adaptation during commitment to mature cardiac lineage. The difference related to proliferative termination of ESC-differentiated cardiomyocytes among the above studies may results from using an early or late stage of ES-derived cells or from different cell lines, types of ESCs (human vs murine), and culture conditions. Indeed, one study showed that the capacity of different mouse ES lines to differentiate to cardiomyocytes is variable *(57)*.

Angiogenesis

It has been shown that ESCs are able to differentiate in vitro to endothelial cells, and if injected, they can contribute to the developing vasculature in vivo *(58–61)*. The number of capillaries in the scar tissue was significantly larger in the bone marrow cell-transplanted group than the control untreated group. Recently, we evaluated the effects of ESC transplantation on myocardial angiogenesis in MI rats *(16)*. Rich blood vessels were observed in damaged myocardium with engrafted cells. Compared with the control MI hearts, the number of capillaries was almost doubled in injured myocardium at 32 wk after ESC transplantation. In another study we used an anti-von Willebrand Factor (vWF, a marker of endothelial cells) antibody to evaluate the effects of engrafted cells on neovascularization in infarcted areas in mice *(17)*. Compared to normal myocardium, the amount of vWF staining dramatically decreased in infarct myocardium treated with the cell-free medium. However, transplantation of mouse ESCs markedly increased the amount of vWF staining in infarcted myocardium. Additionally, calculation of capillary density showed that compared to the control MI hearts, the number of capillaries was significantly increased in injured myocardium with ESC transplantation and even much greater in the MI hearts transplanted with ESCs overexpressing VEGF (Fig. 2). The better outcome on cardiac function in MI mice transplanted with ESCs overexpressing VEGF might result from the stronger angiogenesis effect.

Transplantation with other cell types in injured myocardium also causes neovascularization. The growth of new blood vessels in MI pigs has been observed in graft area with transplantation of either human atrial cardiomyocytes or fetal human ventricular cardiomyocytes *(62,63)*. In addition, Tomita et al. observed that transplanted bone marrow cells participated the formation of new blood vessels in cryoinjured rat myocardium *(11)*. Recently, 5-azacytidine-treated bone marrow stromal cells were transplanted into injured myocardium in a porcine MI model. The cell-transplanted sites induced angiogenesis and improved regional and global contractile function *(64)*. Moreover, direct trans-

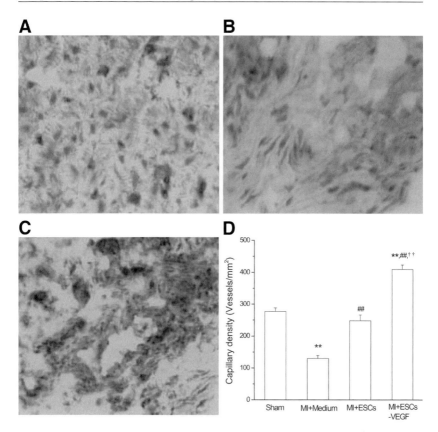

Fig. 2. Immunostaining for blood vessel endothelial cells by the anti-von Willebrand Factor (vWF) antibody in mouse myocardial sections. **(A)** vWF staining (red) in a normal myocardial section demonstrates normal blood vessel distribution in a sham-operated mouse heart. **(B)** The density of positive vWF staining was significantly reduced in the infarcted myocardium injected with the cell-free medium. Sporadic vWF staining indicates few blood vessels in myocardial infarction (MI) region. **(C)** Transplantation of mouse embryonic stem cells (ESCs) with overexpression of vascular endothelial growh factor (VEGF) significantly increased the amount of positive vWF staining in infarcted myocardium. (Magnification is ×400 in panels **A**, **B**, and **C**.) Transplantation of ESCs enhanced capillary densities in infarcted myocardium (panel **D**). The average numbers of blood vessels are shown for sham (n = 8), MI + medium (n = 7), MI + ESCs (n = 8), and MI + ESCs-VEGF (n = 7). **, p < 0.001 vs sham; ##, p < 0.001 vs MI + Medium; ††, p < 0.001 vs MI + ESCs.

plantation of aortic endothelial cell into myocardial scars in cryoinjured rats significantly increased vascular density and regional blood flow at 6 wk after cell transplantation *(65)*. Regional myocardial blood flow measured by neutron microspheres was significantly increased in postinfarcted pigs with stem cell transplantation *(13)*.

These results suggest that engrafted stem cells can be a cell source for forming new blood vessels or stimulate angiogenesis in damaged myocardium around the engrafted area. The increase in regional blood supply provides more nutrition to implanted cells, helps to remove cellular debris from infarction, and probably rescues host myocytes injured during ischemia. Therefore, neovascularization is critical in the survival of transplanted cells and plays an important role in the improvement of cardiac function in MI hearts with cell transplantation.

HOMING AND IMMUNE TOLERANCE

Homing

ESC migration is very important for tissue repair. Transplanted pieces of embryonic ventricular myocardium were initially localized only in the site of grafting, but by 2–5 wk engrafted cells migrated along the ventricular surface of the damaged heart *(47)*. A recent report showed that in the presence of an acute MI, cytokine-mediated translocation of bone marrow stem cells resulted in a significant degree of tissue regeneration *(6)*. In addition, multiple injections of the cytokines stem cell factor (SCF) and granulocyte colony-stimulating factor (G-CSF) increased the number of circulating hematopoietic stem cells traffic to the injured site in ischemic hearts and give rise to cardiomyocytes and blood vessels *(66)*. In our myocarditis study, we observed that intravenously infused ESCs were able to migrate to damaged myocardium and repair injured hearts *(52)*. It is known that tumor necrosis factor (TNF)-α plays an important role in the pathogenesis of myocardial injury and heart failure *(67)*. Clinical data show that TNF-α generation and release occur in patients with acute MI *(68)*. There is a correlation between infarct size and TNF-α concentration in infarcted patients *(69)*. High concentrations of TNF-α appear in the circulation of patients with heart failure, and the levels are directly proportional to a patient's functional class and prognosis. In rat experiments, TNF-α production of infarcted myocardium started on d 1 and was sustained for 35 d *(70)*. To test ESC migration to the heart in vivo, we intravenously infused undifferentiated mouse ESCs in cardiac ischemia-reperfusion mice. Migration was assessed in MI mice 3 d after cell infusion. Figure 3 shows that TNF-α was highly expressed in infarcted myocardium and that GFP-labeled ESCs migrated to the infarcted area of the mouse heart treated with ESC infusion.

Our recent study in vitro also show that TNF-α was able to enhance migration of mouse ESCs in vitro *(71)*. This enhancement of TNF-α-

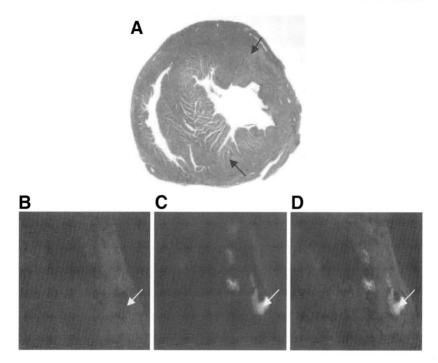

Fig. 3. Antibody immunostaining against tumor necrosis factor (TNF)-α (red) and green fluorescent protein (GFP) (green) in infarcted myocardium. The myocardial sections were made consecutively from a mouse heart on the d 3 after myocardial infarction (MI) induction and intravenous infusion of mouse ESCs (1 × 107 cells in 0.5 mL) labeled with GFP. **(A)** myocardial infarction (between two blue arrows, ×10) of a heart 3 d after MI induction. **(B–D)** Positive TNF-α **(B)** and GFP **(C)** immunostaining, and the merge **D** of **B** and **C** (×100). The yellow arrows point out a blood vessel **(B–D)** with a large cluster of migrated GFP-positive cells **(C,D)**.

induced migration of ESCs was blocked by the antibody against the Type II TNF-α receptor, but not by the antibody against the Type I TNF-α receptor. Western blot analysis showed that the phosphorylated protein levels of p38 and c-Jun N-terminal kinase (JNK) were significantly increased in TNF-α-treated ESCs. Inhibition of the activity of p38 or JNK significantly attenuated TNF-α-induced ESC migration in vitro (Fig. 4).

To further assess the signaling pathway of TNF-α-induced ESC migration, we used high-speed optical sectioning microscopy to record the migratory pattern of ESCs in the presence of TNF-α. A direct viewing chemotaxis chamber with two concentric wells (Dunn chamber) allowed

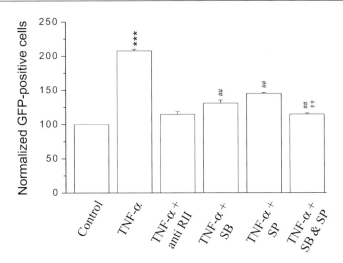

Fig. 4. Tumor necrosis factor (TNF)-α-induced enhancement of migration of mouse embryonic stem cells (ESCs). Migration of green fluorescent protein (GFP)-positive ESCs was evaluated with flow cytometry assay. ESCs were cultured with the Transwell method. Control: the lower compartments were plated with control cardiomyocytes and the upper chambers were added ESCs ($n = 23$); TNF-α: the lower compartments plated with cardiomyocytes transfected with TNF-a cDNA and the upper chambers were added ESCs ($n = 5$); TNF-α+ anti-RII: the lower compartments were plated with TNF-α-transfected cardiomyocytes and the upper chambers were added ESCs with preincubation with the antibody against TNF-RII ($n = 9$); TNF-α + SB: the lower compartments plated with TNF-α-transfected cardiomyocytes and the upper chambers were added ESCs pretreated with the p38 inhibitor SB203580 ($10\,\mu M$, $n = 5$); TNF-α + SP: the lower compartments plated with TNF-α-transfected cardiomyocytes and the upper chambers were added ESCs pretreated with the c-Jun N-terminal kinase (JNK) inhibitor SP600125 ($10\,\mu M$, $n = 5$); TNF-α + SB & SP: the lower compartments plated with TNF-α–transfected cardiomyocytes and the upper chambers were added ESCs pretreated with the inhibitors SB203580 and SP600125 ($10\,\mu M$ each, $n = 5$). ***, $p < 0.001$ vs the control and inhibitor-treated groups; ##, $p < 0.01$ vs the control; ††, $p < 0.01$ vs the single inhibitor–treated groups.

us to establish a concentration gradient of TNF-α. ESCs migrated towards the side with a higher concentration of TNF-α. TNF-α-induced formation of proteopodia might play an important role in the migration. An increase in intracellular Ca^{2+} was observed during TNF-α-induced migration of ESCs. Raising the extracellular Ca^{2+} level had a positive effect on the migration (72). These results demonstrate that ESCs are highly motivated for migration in the presence of TNF-α and increases in intracellular Ca^{2+} levels enhance the migration of ESCs. These data provide important information for understanding stem cell homing to injured myocardium, which is critical for stem cell therapy and tissue repair. The effects of other cytokines, growth factors, adhesion molecules, or cytoskeleton on stem cell migration also need to be evaluated in vitro and in vivo.

Immune Tolerance to Cellular Xenotransplantation

Tolerance of xenotransplanted mouse ESCs was evaluated in infarcted animal models. Min and coworkers locally transplanted ESCs tagged with GFP into injured myocardium in a rat MI model *(14)*. Compared with the control MI animals, cardiac function was significantly improved in ESC-grafted MI rats at 6 wk after cell transplantation. Double immunostaining against GFP and cardiac sarcomeric α-actin, α-myosin heavy chain, or troponin I showed the survival and differentiation of xenografts in MI hearts. Additionally, isolated single cells showed rod-shaped GFP-positive myocytes with clear striations in ESC-transplanted animals. The shape and size of GFP-positive myocytes did not significantly differ from those of host cardiomyocytes *(14)*. The long-term survival of mouse ESCs xenotransplanted into injured myocardium was also observed in MI rats without treatment of immunosuppression *(16)*. The similar finding was also reported by other groups in rats with ligation of the left coronary artery. Cells dissected from beating regions of EBs formed by GFP-tagged mouse ESCs were injected into the border zone between the infarcted myocardium and normal myocardium or infarcted tissue. Thirty days after transplantation, GFP-expressed cells were detected and stained positively by the antibody against sarcomeric myosin *(43,55)*. Engrafted fluorescent cells displayed a typical cardiac phenotype, including sarcomeric striations, and immunostaining positively for the ventricle-specific myosin light chain MLC2v and gap junction protein connexin *(43)*. Echocardiography showed significant improvement of left-ventricular ejection fraction of stem cell-transplanted hearts *(43)*. These results indicate that xenotransplanted mouse ESCs survived in rat host myocardium and expressed the typical characteristics of heart cells. The intriguing point of these studies is that the recipients with xenotransplantation of mouse ESCs did not receive any immunosuppressive treatment (Table 2).

Successful xenotransplantation of adult stem cells without immunosuppression *(73)* raises an interesting possibility whether bone marrow stem cells share the privilege of immune tolerance as ESCs *(74)*. Saito et al. cited the "danger model" hypothesis *(75–77)* as part of the explanation for their intriguing results *(73)*. However, it is not clear whether species between donor cells and recipients play a role in the immune tolerance of xenotransplantation of adult stem cells. The survival of xenografted hMSCs has been demonstrated in murine animals (78), but the mice were genetically immunodeficient. Rejection of the xenografted mouse ESCs in the host rats without immunosuppression was not noted in the experiments mentioned above (14–16,43) (Table 3). This xenograft acceptance presumably resulted from the nature of the stem cells used and could be due to nonexpression of major histocompatibility complex (MHC) antigen in ESCs (79) or due to the relatively privileged site, myocardium, where presentation and recognition of MHC antigen may not take place because of the lack of a lymphatic drainage system (80). It is known that ESCs do not express many membrane surface antigens (81) and share immune-privileged features relevant for tolerance induction (74). Embryonic tissue also possesses a range of proteins that efficiently counteract maternal T-cell responses (74). Therefore, the survival and tolerance of cellular xenografts in immunocompetent animals are probably correlated with the degree of differentiation of the donor cells. ESCs are the most plastic cells and presumably more easily adaptable to a new environment, even in a xeno-host.

Another question is why the recipients do not reject the xenografted ESCs after their differentiation, even if the stem cells are immune-privileged. One possibility is that the establishment of chimerism might occur at the early stage after cell transplantation. Cross talks may occur between engrafted cells and host cells, which modulates the expression of antigens of donor cells and also the immunoresponse of a host. It has been demonstrated that after cell transplantation, stem cells can downregulate the host immune response and induce mixed immune chimerism favoring long-term graft acceptance (79,82,83). Engrafted stem cells can also suppress the function of mature T-cells, either directly or by stimulating suppressor T-cells, and thus are tolerogenic (84). ESCs xenotransplanted in the above studies probably contained a smaller pool size of T-cells, which is critical in the induction of transplant tolerance (85,86). Experiments show that suppression of T-cells results in long-term survival of mouse hearts xenografts in C6-deficient rats (87). The other explanation for xenotransplant tolerance of stem cells is that engrafted ESCs in myocardium undergo cardiomyocyte differentiation. During the differential process, the expression of surface antigens of grafted cells is influenced or determined by the local microenvironment of a host heart. Indeed, it has been observed that differentiating stem cell–derived cardiomyocytes undergo structural adaptation and mobilize nuclear transport regulator in support of nucleocytoplasmic communication during commitment to mature cardiac lineage (56). In addition, natural selection of implanted cells may occur after stem cell transplantation, which results in the possibility that the surviving cells in a recipient heart are less immunogenic. More careful experiments are clearly required to confirm these possibilities or speculations.

FUTURE PERSPECTIVES AND SUMMARY

Perspectives

Research on ESCs will eventually derive cells for the regeneration of diseased or damaged tissue. To date mouse ESC preparations have been grafted successfully into adult myocardium in different animal models *(14–16,43)*. These transplanted ESCs are able to differentiate into new functional cardiomyocytes in injured myocardium and restore damaged heart function. However, there is no study using hESCs or their derived cells to test cardiac repair in vivo. Besides ethical and political concerns, other obstacles and questions need to be overcome or answered before hESCs or their derived cells can be studied in clinical trials. One question is whether undifferentiated or differentiated cells should be used. If differentiated cells are used for cardiac repair, pure cardiomyocytes or mixtures of cardiomyocytes with other cell types, such as endothelial cells and vascular smooth muscle cells, are better for transplantation. The optimal stage(s) of differentiation may also be critical for the efficacy of cell therapy. Undifferentiated ESCs have the greatest plasticity, but they also have tumorigenic potential. Therefore, studies on the feasibility of using hESCs in vivo are required, otherwise removing any undifferentiated hESCs is necessary prior to transplantation. Additionally, it is possible to devise a fail-safe mechanism—i.e., to insert into transplanted ES-derived cells suicide genes that can trigger the death of the cells should they become tumorigenic. Another obstacle is immune rejection. Scientists are experimenting with different research strategies to understand whether ESCs or their derived cells are rejected after transplantation. Successful xenotransplantation of stem cells without immunosuppression therapy has been reported in animal models *(14–16,43,73,86)*. The underlying mechanism of less immunorejection of engrafted stem cells remains to be delineated *(88)*, but ESCs have fewer membrane surface antigens *(81)* and share immune-privileged features relevant for tolerance induction *(74)*. However, whether the host rejects donor hESCs or their differentiated cells has not been examined in human trials. To solve the problem of immune incompatibility and to produce cells or tissues for human autologous transplantation, one study *(89)* transferred human somatic nuclei into rabbit oocytes and produced nuclear transfer ESCs (ntESCs). The derived ntES cells were human based on karyotype and retained phenotypes similar to those of conventional human ES cells, including the ability to undergo multilineage cellular differentiation (89). More recently, a pluripotent ESC line (SCNT-hES-1) was derived from cloned human blastocysts by somatic cell nuclear transfer (SCNT) technology (90). The SCNT-hES-1 cells displayed typical ESC morphology and cell surface markers. They were capable of differentiating into embryoid bodies in vitro and forming teratomas in vivo containing cell derivatives from all three embryonic germ layers. After continuous proliferation for more than 70 passages, SCNT-hES-1 cells maintained normal karyotypes and were genetically identical to the somatic nuclear donor cells. Therefore, SCNT-hESCs would be immunocompatible with a patient if the somatic cell comes from that patient. The SCNT-cloned hESCs may greatly advance the progress of the opportunity using hESC-derived cells in clinical cell therapies. Other approaches, such as genetic manipulation of donor cells, chimerism to induce donor-specific tolerance, and immunosuppressive therapy, are also options to enhance the success of stem cell transplantation.

At the present time, the timing of cell transplantation for cardiac repair of injured hearts is unclear. Most cell transplantation experiments in animals have been carried out at the stage of acute MI. It remains to be determined whether stem cell transplantation is also feasible in chronically infarcted hearts and whether engrafted cells are able to survive, differentiate, integrate, and communicate with the host tissue and improve the function of chronically damaged hearts. Scientists are still searching for the optimal number of cells and the best ways to deliver stem cells for cardiac repair. It is critical to know whether implanted stem cells are able to differentiate into the desired cell types and proliferate to sufficient quantities of functional cells in damaged myocardium and whether multiple transplantations are required for a diseased heart. Another big question is how transplanted stem cells integrate into the surrounding host tissue and function appropriately during the recipient's life, because engrafted ESCs or their derived cells have the potential to form arrhythmogenic sites or teratomas.

Conclusions

ESC transplantation for cardiac repair has demonstrated restoration of myocardial structure and improvement of cardiac function in experimental animal settings. Several previous reports showed that transplantation of bone marrow stem cells could regenerate heart tissue in infarcted animal models (2–7). However, we found that transplantation of human mesenchymal stem cells alone did not repair infarcted myocardium well.

Co-transplantation with human fetal cardiomyocytes significantly improved heart function in postinfarcted pigs *(13)*. More recently, two research groups have found that stem cells taken from bone marrow did not readily become heart cells in injured myocardium after intramyocardial injection *(19,20)*. Two clinical trials also suggest that improvement of heart function in heart failure patients with transplantation of bone marrow stem cells might come not from new heart muscle cells but from new blood vessel growth *(8,9)*. Therefore, the great plasticity and proliferative capacity of ESCs are their most valuable advantages and make them one of the best cell sources for cell therapy. Clearly, the use of hESCs or their derived cells is potentially more versatile for cell therapies, but ethical, political, and scientific barriers have to be overcome before clinical trials in patients can be conducted.

ACKNOWLEDGMENTS

This study was supported in part by research grants 9930254N (Y.-F.X) from the American Heart Association, DA11762 and DA12774 (J.P.M) from the National Institute of Drug Abuse, and The Cardiovascular Division Endorsement Research Fund of Beth Israel Deaconess Medical Center.

REFERENCES

1. Kessler PD, Byrne BJ. Myoblast cell grafting into heart muscle: cellular biology and potential applications. Annu Rev Physiol 1999;61:219–242.
2. Soonpaa MH, Koh GY, Klug MG, et al. Formation of nascent intercalated disks between grafted fetal cardiomyocytes and host myocardium. Science 1994;264:98–101.
3. Chiu RCJ, Zibaitis A, Kao RL. Cellular cardiomyoplasty: myocardial regeneration with satellite cell implantation. Ann Thorac Surg 1995;60:12–18.
4. Li RK, Jia ZQ, Weisel RD, et al. Cardiomyocyte transplantation improves heart function. Ann Thorac Surg 1996;62:654–661.
5. Leor J, Patterson M, Quinones MJ, et al. Transplantation of fetal myocardial tissue into the infarcted myocardium of rat: a potential method for repair of infarcted myocardium. Circulation 1996;94(Suppl II):II332–II336.
6. Orlic D, Kajstura J, Chimenti S, et al. Bone marrow cells regenerate infarcted myocardium. Nature. 2001;410:701-706.
7. Strauer BE, Brehm M, Zeus T, et al. Repair of infarcted myocardium by autologous intracoronary mononuclear bone marrow cell transplantation in humans. Circulation 2002;106(15):1913–1918.
8. Tse HF, Kwong YL, Chan JK, et al. Angiogenesis in ischaemic myocardium by intramyocardial autologous bone marrow mononuclear cell implantation. Lancet 2003;361(9351):47–49.
9. Perin EC, Dohmann HF, Borojevic R, et al. Transendocardial, autologous bone marrow cell transplantation for severe, chronic ischemic heart failure. Circulation 2003;107(18):2294–2302.

10. Koh GY, Soonpaa MH, Klug MG, et al. Long-term survival of AT-1 cardiomyocyte grafts in syngeneic myocardium. Am J Physiol 1993;264(5 Pt 2):H1727–H1733.

11. Tomita S, Li RK, Weisel RD, et al. Autologous transplantation of bone marrow cells improves damaged heart function. Circulation 1999;100(Suppl II):II247–II256.

12. Chedrawy EG, Wang JS, Nguyen DM, et al. Incorporation and integration of implanted myogenic and stem cells into native myocardial fibers: anatomic basis for functional improvements. J Thorac Cardiovasc Surg 2002;124(3):584–590.

13. Min JY, Sullivan MF, Yang Y, et al. Significant improvement of heart function by co-transplantation of human mesenchymal stem cells and fetal cardiomyocytes in postinfarcted pigs. Ann Thorac Surg 2002;74(5):1568–1575.

14. Min JY, Yang Y, Converso KL, et al. Transplantation of embryonic stem cells improves cardiac function in postinfarcted rats. J Appl Physiol 2002;92:288–296.

15. Naito H, Taniguchi S, Kawata T. Embryonic stem cell-derived cardiomyocyte transplantation into the infarcted myocardium. Heart Surg Forum 2002;6(1):1.

16. Min JY, Yang Y, Sullivan MF, et al. Long-term improvement of cardiac function in rats after infarction by transplantation of embryonic stem cells. J Thorac Cardiovasc Surg 2003;25(2):361–369.

17. Yang Y, Min JY, Rana JS, et al. VEGF enhances functional improvement of postinfarcted hearts by transplantation of ESC-differentiated cells. J Appl Physiol 2002;93(3):1140–1151.

18. Strauer BE, Brehm M, Zeus T, et al. Intracoronary, human autologous stem cell transplantation for myocardial regeneration following myocardial infarction. Dtsch Med Wochenschr 2001;126(34–35):932-938.

19. Murry CE, Soonpaa MH, Reinecke H, et al. Haematopoietic stem cells do not transdifferentiate into cardiac myocytes in myocardial infarcts. Nature 2004;428(6983):664–668.

20. Balsam LB, Wagers AJ, Christensen JL, Kofidis T, Weissman IL, Robbins RC. Haematopoietic stem cells adopt mature haematopoietic fates in ischaemic myocardium. Nature 2004;428(6983):668–673.

21. Thomson JA, Itskovitz-Eldor J, Shapiro SS, et al. Embryonic stem cell lines derived from human blastocysts. Science 1998;282(5391):1145–1147.

22. Scholer HR, Ciesiolka T, Gruss P. A nexus between Oct-4 and E1A: implications for gene regulation in embryonic stem cells. Cell 1991;66(2):291–304.

23. Pesce M, Scholer HR. Oct-4: gatekeeper in the beginnings of mammalian development. Stem Cells 2001;19(4):271–278.

24. Evans MJ, Kaufman MH. Establishment in culture of pluripotential cells from mouse embryos. Nature 1981;292(5819):154–156.

25. Martin GR. Isolation of a pluripotent cell line from early mouse embryos cultured in medium conditioned by teratocarcinoma stem cells. Proc Natl Acad Sci USA 1981;78(12):7634–7638.

26. Sissman NJ. Developmental landmarks in cardiac morphogenesis: comparative chronology. Am J Cardiol 1970;25(2):141–148.

27. Wobus AM, Wallukat G, Hescheler J. Pluripotent mouse embryonic stem cells are able to differentiate into cardiomyocytes expressing chronotropic responses to adrenergic and cholinergic agents and Ca^{2+} channel blockers. Differentiation 1991;48:173–182.

28. Maltsev VA, Rohwedel J, Hescheler J, et al. Embryonic stem cells differentiate in vitro into cardiomyocytes representing sinusnodal, atrial and ventricular cell types. Mech Dev 1993;44(1):41–50.

29. Klug MG, Soonpaa MH, Field LJ. DNA synthesis and multinucleation in embryonic stem cell-derived cardiomyocytes. Am J Physiol 1995;269:H1913–H1921.
30. Klug MG, Soonpaa MH, Koh GY, Field LJ. Genetically selected cardiomyocytes from differentiating embryonic stem cells form stable intracardiac grafts. J Clin Invest 1996;98:216–224.
31. Westfall MV, Samuelson LC, Metzger JM. Troponin I isoform expression is developmentally regulated in differentiating embryonic stem cell-derived cardiac myocytes. Dev Dyn 1996;206:24–38.
32. Westfall MV, Pasyk KA, Yule DI, et al. Ultrastructure and cell-cell coupling of cardiac myocytes differentiating in embryonic stem cell cultures. Cell Motil Cytoskeleton 1997;36:43–54.
33. Kilborn MJ, Fedida D. A study of the developmental changes in outward currents of rat ventricular myocytes. J Physiol (Lond) 1990;430:37–0.
34. Rohwedel J, Maltsev V, Bober E, et al. Muscle cell differentiation of embryonic stem cells reflects myogenesis in vivo: developmentally regulated expression of myogenic determination genes and functional expression of ionic currents. Dev Biol 1994;164(1):87–101.
35. Kehat I, Kenyagin-Karsenti D, Snir M, et al. Human embryonic stem cells can differentiate into myocytes with structural and functional properties of cardiomyocytes. J Clin Invest 2001;108(3):407–414.
36. Xu C, Police S, Rao N, et al. Characterization and enrichment of cardiomyocytes derived from human embryonic stem cells. Circ Res 2002;91(6):501–508.
37. Spradling A, Drummond-Barbosa D, Kai T. Stem cells find their niche. Nature 2001;414(6859):98–104.
38. Smith AG. Culture and differentiation of embryonic stem cells. J Tissue Culture Methods 1991;13:89–94.
39. Wobus AM, Kaomei G, Shan J, et al. Retinoic acid accelerates embryonic stem cell-derived cardiac differentiation and enhances development of ventricular cardiomyocytes. J Mol Cell Cardiol 1997;29(6):1525–1539.
40. Boheler KR, Czyz J, Tweedie D, et al. Differentiation of pluripotent embryonic stem cells into cardiomyocytes. Circ Res 2002;91(3):189–201.
41. Hidaka K, Lee JK, Kim HS, et al. Chamber-specific differentiation of Nkx2.5-positive cardiac precursor cells from murine embryonic stem cells. FASEB J 2003;17(6):740–742.
42. Chen Y, Yang Y, Rana JS, et al. Effects of vascular endothelial growth factor on proliferation and differentiation of embryonic stem cells. J Am Coll Cardiol 2003;41(6, Suppl A):273A.
43. Behfar A, Zingman LV, Hodgson DM, et al. Stem cell differentiation requires a paracrine pathway in the heart. FASEB J 2002;16(12):1558–1566.
44. Schuldiner M, Yanuka O, Itskovitz-Eldor J, et al. From the cover: effects of eight growth factors on the differentiation of cells derived from human embryonic stem cells. Proc Natl Acad Sci USA 2000;97(21):11307–11312.
45. Connold AL, Frischknecht R, Vrbova G. Survival of embryonic cardiac myocytes transplanted into host rat soleus muscle. J Muscle Res Cell Motil 1995;16(5):481–489.
46. Roell W, Lu ZJ, Bloch W, et al. Cellular cardiomyoplasty improves survival after myocardial injury. Circulation 2002;105(20):2435–2441.
47. Connold AL, Frischknecht R, Dimitrakos M, et al. The survival of embryonic cardiomyocytes transplanted into damaged host rat myocardium. J Muscle RESC Motil 1997;18(1):63–70.

48. Etzion S, Battler A, Barbash IM, et al. Influence of embryonic cardiomyocyte transplantation on the progression of heart failure in rat model of extensive myocardial infarction. J Mol Cell Cardiol 2001;33:1321–1330.
49. Feldman AM, McNamara D. Myocarditis. N Engl J Med 2000;343:1388–1398.
50. Silver MA, Kowalczyk D. Coronary microvascular narrowing in acute murine Coxsackie B3 myocarditis. Am Heart J 1989;118:173–174.
51. Kawai C. From myocarditis to cardiomyopathy: mechanisms of inflammation and cell death-learning from the past for the future. Circulation 1999;99:1091–1100.
52. Wang JF, Yang Y, Wang G, et al. Embryonic stem cells attenuate viral myocarditis in murine model. Cell Transplant 2002;11(8):753–758.
53. Yechiel E, Barenholz Y, Henis YI. Lateral mobility and organization of phospholipids and proteins in rat myocyte membranes. Effects of aging and manipulation of lipid composition. J Biol Chem 1985;260(16):9132–9136.
54. Lieber S, Pain J, Diaz G, et al. Aging increases stiffness of cardiac myocytes measured by atomic force microscopy. Circulation 2003;108(17):IV-276.
55. Min JY, Malek S, Chen Y, et al. Stem cell therapy in aging hearts: myogenesis vs angiogenesis. Circulation 2003;108(17):IV-276.
56. Perez-Terzic C, Behfar A, Mery A, et al. Structural adaptation of the nuclear pore complex in stem cell-derived cardiomyocytes. Circ Res 2003;92(4):444–452.
57. Mummery C, Ward D, van den Brink CE, et al. Cardiomyocyte differentiation of mouse and human embryonic stem cells. J Anat 2002;200(Pt 3):233–242.
58. Vittet D, Prandini MH, Berthier R, et al. Embryonic stem cells differentiate in vitro to endothelial cells through successive maturation steps. Blood 1996;88(9):3424–3431.
59. Hirashima M, Kataoka H, Nishikawa S, et al. Maturation of embryonic stem cells into endothelial cells in an in vitro model of vasculogenesis. Blood 1999;93(4):1253–1263.
60. Yamashita J, Itoh H, Hirashima M, et al. Flk1-positive cells derived from embryonic stem cells serve as vascular progenitors. Nature 2000;408(6808):92–96.
61. Yurugi-Kobayashi T, Itoh H, Yamashita J, et al. Effective contribution of transplanted vascular progenitor cells derived from embryonic stem cells to adult neovascularization in proper differentiation stage. Blood 2003;101(7):2675–2678.
62. Van Meter CH, Claycomb WC Jr, Delcarpio JB, et al. Myoblast transplantation in the porcine model: a potential technique for myocardial repair. J Thorac Cardiovasc Surg 1995;110:1142–1148.
63. Watanabe E, Smith DM Jr, Delcarpio JB, et al. Cardiomyocyte transplantation in a porcine myocardial infarction model. Cell Transplant 1998;7:239–246.
64. Tomita S, Mickle DA, Weisel RD, et al. Improved heart function with myogenesis and angiogenesis after autologous porcine bone marrow stromal cell transplantation. J Thorac Cardiovasc Surg 2002;123(6):1132–1140.
65. Kim EJ, Li RK, Weisel RD, et al. Angiogenesis by endothelial cell transplantation. J Thorac Cardiovasc Surg 2001;122(5):963–971.
66. Orlic D, Kajstura J, Chimenti S, et al. Mobilized bone marrow cells repair the infarcted heart, improving function and survival. Proc Natl Acad Sci USA 2001;98(18):10344–10349.
67. Li D, Zhao L, Liu M, et al. Kinetics of tumor necrosis factor alpha in plasma and the cardioprotective effect of a monoclonal antibody to tumor necrosis factor alpha in acute myocardial infarction. Am. Heart J 1999;137:1145–1152.
68. Maury CP, Teppo AM. Circulating tumour necrosis factor-alpha (cachectin) in myocardial infarction. J Intern Med 1989;225:333–336.
69. Halawa B, Salomon P, Jolda-Mydlowska B, et al. Levels of tumor necrosis factor (TNF-alpha) and interleukin 6 (IL-6) in serum of patients with acute myocardial infarction. Pol. Arch Med Wewn 1999;101:197–203.

70. Irwin MW, Mak S, Mann DL, et al. Tissue expression and immunolocalization of tumor necrosis factor-alpha in postinfarction dysfunctional myocardium. Circulation 1999;99:1492–1498.
71. Chen Y, Ke Q, Yang Y, et al. Cardiomyocytes overexpressing TNF-alpha attract migration of embryonic stem cells via activation of p38 and c-Jun amino-terminal kinase. FASEB J 2003;17(15):2231–2239.
72. Kaplan E, Chen Y, Min JY, et al. Intracellular calcium regulates tumor necrosis factor-alpha-induced embryonic stem cell migration. Circulation 2004;43(5-Suppl A):270A.
73. Saito T, Kuang JQ, Bittira B, et al. Xenotransplant cardiac chimera: immune tolerance of adult stem cells. Ann Thorac Surg 2002;74(1):19–24.
74. Fandrich F, Dresske B, Bader M, et al. Embryonic stem cells share immune-privileged features relevant for tolerance induction. J Mol Med 2002;80(6):343–350.
75. Matzinger P. An innate sense of danger. Ann NY Acad Sci 2002;961:341–342.
76. Matzinger P. The danger model: a renewed sense of self. Science 2002;296(5566):301–305.
77. Anderson CC, Matzinger P. Danger: the view from the bottom of the cliff. Semin Immunol 2000;12(3):231–238.
78. Toma C, Pittenger MF, Cahill KS, et al. Human mesenchymal stem cells differentiate to a cardiomyocyte phenotype in the adult murine heart. Circulation 2002;105:93–98.
79. Fandrich F, Lin X, Chai GX, et al. Preimplantation-stage stem cells induce long-term allogeneic graft acceptance without supplementary host conditioning. Nat Med 2002;8:171–178.
80. Morris PJ. The immunobiology of cell transplantation. Cell Transplant 1993;2:7–12.
81. O'Shea KS. Embryonic stem cell models of development. Anatom Rec 1999;257:32–41.
82. Beschorner WE, Sudan DL, Radio SJ, et al. Heart xenograft survival with chimeric pig donors and modest immune suppression. Ann Surg 2003;237:265–272.
83. Billingham RE, Brent L, Medawar PB. Actively acquired tolerance of foreign cells. Nature 1953;172:603–606.
84. Bartholomew A, Sturgeon C, Siatskas M, et al. Mesenchymal stem cells suppress lymphocyte proliferation in vitro and prolong skin graft survival in vivo. Exp Hematol 2002;30:42–48.
85. Strom TB, Field LJ, Ruediger M. Allogeneic stem cells, clinical transplantation, and the origins of regenerative medicine. Transplant Proc 2001;33:3044–3049.
86. Ildstad ST, Wren SM, Boggs SS, et al. Cross-species bone marrow transplantation: evidence for tolerance induction, stem cell engraftment, and maturation of T lymphocytes in a xenogeneic stromal environment (rat–mouse). J Exp Med 1991;174:467–478.
87. Wu G, Korsgren O, van Rooijen N, et al. Suppression of T cells results in long-term survival of mouse heart xenografts in C6-deficient rats. Xenotransplantation 2001;8:303–309.
88. Xiao YF, Min JY, Morgan JP. Immunosuppression and xenotransplantation of cells for cardiac repair. Ann Thorac Surg 2004;77(2):737–744.
89. Chen Y, He ZX, Liu A, et al. Embryonic stem cells generated by nuclear transfer of human somatic nuclei into rabbit oocytes. Cell Res 2003;13(4):251–263.
90. Hwang WS, Ryu YJ, Park JH, et al. Evidence of a pluripotent human embryonic stem cell line derived from a cloned blastocyst. Science 2004;303(5664):1669–1674.
91. Ventura C, Maioli M, Asara Y, et al. Butyric and retinoic mixed ester of hyaluronan: A novel differentiating glycoconjugate affording a high-throughput of cardiogenesis in embryonic stem cells. J Biol Chem 2004;279:23574–23579.

92. Sachinidis A, Gissel C, Nierhoff D, et al. Identification of plateled-derived growth factor-BB as cardiogenesis-inducing factor in mouse embryonic stem cells under serum-free conditions. Cell Physiol Biochem 2003;13(6):423–429.

93. Ventura C, Zinellu E, Maninchedda E, et al. Dynorphin B is an agonist of nuclear opioid receptors coupling nuclear protein kinase C activation to the transcription of cardiogenic genes in GTR1 embryonic stem cells. Circ Res 2003;92(6):623–629.

12 Skeletal Myoblast Transplantation for Cardiac Repair

Audrey Rosinberg, MD,
Jamal S. Rana, MD,
and Roger J. Laham, MD

CONTENTS

INTRODUCTION

Coronary heart disease remains the single largest killer of American men and women. The American Heart Association statistics show that approx 1.1 million Americans suffer a myocardial infarction (MI) annually. Of those who survive, 22% of men and 46% of women are disabled with heart failure *(1)*. Although cardiomyocytes of infarcted or failing human hearts have been shown to undergo mitoses *(2,3)*, this regenerative capacity is by far too limited to compensate for the loss of cardiac cells resulting from a large infarct. In areas of ischemia, cell death ensues and scar forms in the place of myocardium. The remaining myocardial cells respond to mitotic signals by hypertrophy rather than hyperplasia. Necrotized myocardial cells are replaced by fibroblasts. If no viable

From: *Contemporary Cardiology: Angiogenesis and Direct Myocardial Revasularization*
Edited by: R. J. Laham and D. S. Baim © Humana Press Inc., Totowa, NJ

myocardium is present, scar formation ensues with ventricular wall thinning and dilation of the ventricular cavity. This leads to symptoms of heart failure in a significant number of patients. For conventional coronary revascularization to be beneficial, viable myocardium must be present. The prognosis for these patients is poor, with a 1-yr mortality rate of 20% and a 5-yr mortality rate of close to 50% *(1)*.

Current treatment options for patients with advanced heart failure are limited. Pharmacological treatment attempts to slow left-ventricular (LV) remodeling. The disease is progressive, and when pharmacological therapy fails, heart transplantation remains the only definitive treatment for end-stage heart failure. However, donor hearts for transplants are in limited supply, and demand far outweighs the supply. At the end of 2001, there were 4096 registrants on the heart transplant waiting list. Of those, 1897 had been waiting for more than 2 yr, and a total of only 2208 heart transplants were performed in 2001 *(4)*. Cardiac transplantation is also fraught with the problem of immunosuppression. Alternative options include LV assist devices and devices aimed at surgically reshaping the left ventricle. Despite recent improvements in ventricular assist devices, their use as destination therapy remains investigational *(5)*.

Currently, no known treatment exists to replace scar tissue with contracting myocardium. Experimental therapeutic strategies for treatment of heart failure are focusing on the transplantation of cells into regions of nonviable myocardium. Cell types that have been transplanted include skeletal myoblasts, fetal cardiomyocytes, embryonic stem cells, and mesenchymal stem cells. The goals of cell therapy are to replace scar tissue with contractile cells to restore function and to induce angiogenesis into regions of ischemia. Both skeletal myoblasts and cardiomyocytes are contractile cells. Although initial studies focused on and showed improvement with fetal cardiomyocyte transplantation in rats *(6–8)*, these studies were useful as initial proof-of-concept studies. Fetal cardiomyocytes have limited clinical value for therapeutic purposes for a variety of reasons. Cardiomyocytes cannot be expanded in culture, and it would likely be difficult to obtain a sufficient number of cells from an autologous donor to repair a myocardial infarct in humans. Additionally, cardiomyocytes are very sensitive to ischemic injury. The use of fetal cardiomyocytes in humans raises ethical issues as well. The remainder of this chapter will focus exclusively on skeletal myoblasts.

SKELETAL MYOBLASTS

Adult cardiomyocytes are terminally differentiated and are incapable of division and proliferation in response to injury. Although some stud-

Table 1
Advantages of Using Skeletal Myoblasts for Cardiac Transplantation

No ethical issues and safe transplantation
High proliferative potential under appropriate culture conditions and the
    possibility of undifferentiated myoblast amplification in vitro
Autologous origin, which overcomes problems related to availability
Grafted myoblasts have been shown to develop into functioning muscle fiber
Commitment to a well-differentiated myogenic lineage, thus eliminating the
    risk of tumoreginicity
High resistance to ischemia
No graft rejections, thus no need for immunosuppression
Possibly that grafted myoblasts will make satellite reserves to protect against
    subsequent injury

ies have shown that some cardiomyocytes can reenter the cell cycle in response to ischemic injury, this number is likely too small to significantly repair the damaged tissue *(9,10)*. Skeletal muscle, unlike cardiac muscle, retains the ability to regenerate and repair after injury. Although this capacity is not unlimited, as seen in diseases such as Duchenne's muscular dystrophy, it far outweighs the regenerative ability of cardiac muscle. During embryological development skeletal myoblasts proliferate by mitosis. Subsequently, the myoblasts fuse to form multinucleated myotubes. These mature muscle cells have a limited capacity for regeneration. However, some myoblasts persist and retain their myogenic potential. First described by Mauro in 1961, these myogenic precursors are known as satellite cells and can be found under the basal membrane of skeletal muscle fibers *(11)*. Following tissue injury, satellite cells are mobilized, proliferate, and fuse, resulting in repair and regeneration of the damaged tissue. Myoblasts have been maintained proliferating in culture for extended periods of time while maintaining their ability to fuse to form muscle cells *(14)*.

The advantages of skeletal myoblasts for cell therapy are summarized in Table 1. Because skeletal myoblasts retain the ability to regenerate, are easily accessible, and are easily cultured, they are an attractive cell type for transplantation. They are easily harvested and expanded in culture. Because an adequate number of autologous cells can be obtained, there is no need for immunosuppression to prevent rejection. Additionally, the cells are already committed to a myogenic lineage, and thus tumorigenicity is not a problem. When properly conditioned, skeletal muscle can adapt a fatigue-resistant slow-twitch phenotype capable of performing a cardiac-type workload *(12,13)*. More resistant to ischemia than cardiac muscle, skeletal muscle can withstand many hours of ischemia, whereas irreversible injury begins in cardiac muscle within 20 min *(15–17)*. Finally, satellite cells can be genetically modified in vitro to deliver angiogenic cytokines and growth factors to encourage angiomyogenesis.

Skeletal myoblasts differ from cardiomyocytes in their electromechanical properties. Cardiomyocytes have gap junctions consisting of proteins such as connexin-43 and *N*-cadherin, which are responsible for the electrical and mechanical support of the cardiomyocytes, respectively *(18)*. The skeletal myoblasts express gap junction proteins earlier on. However, this expression is downregulated during the process of differentiation, and skeletal muscle cells are electrically isolated *(19)*. Hence, grafted mature skeletal muscle should not be expected to develop electromechanical junctions with the host myocardium, resulting in the possibility of reentry arrhythmias.

PRECLINICAL DATA

Extensive preclinical data in a variety of animal models support the feasibility, safety, and efficacy of skeletal myoblast implantation into regions of myocardial infarction. The preclinical trials are summarized in Table 2. Overall, preclinical trials demonstrate that transplanted cells survive and form well differentiated myofibers with a contractile apparatus as well as contribute to significant functional improvement in injured hearts. However, the ability of skeletal myoblasts to differentiate into cardiomyocytes or form cell-to-cell junctions with host cardiomyocytes remains controversial.

Cell Survival

Investigators have used a variety of techniques to track transplanted cells, including fluorescent cell-tracking dyes, metabolic labeling such as tritiated thymidine or bromodeoxyuridine, and transfection of donor cells with reporter genes, among others. Initial reports of skeletal myoblast transplantation for cardiac repair were published by Marelli et al. in 1991 *(20)*. Although it has since been shown that more than 90% of transplanted cells die within 24 h after transplantation *(21,22)*, many studies have shown that myoblasts do survive and continue to divide *(13,23–25)*. Murry et al. evaluated cryoinjured rat hearts at 1 d, 3 d, 2 wk, 7 wk, and 3 mo after skeletal myoblast transplantation *(13)*. At 1 and 3 d after transplantation, grafted cells were seen to have fused and form multinucleated myotubes. Moreover, the cells were noted to express myosin heavy chain (MHC)-fast, a skeletal muscle marker. Some cells incorporated BrdU, indicating that some cells were dividing. At 2 wk,

Table 2
Summary of Preclinical Trials

Authors (ref.)	Animal	Type of model	Delivery	Duration	Results
Marelli et al., 1992 (20)	Dog	Cryoinjury	Intramyocardial	8 wk	Muscle present in implant area and scar present in control areas
Chiu et al., 1995 (25)	Dog	Cryoinjury	Intramyocardial	18 wk	Striated muscle at implant sites with histological appearance similar to cardiac cells
Yoon et al., 1995 (24)	Dog	Cryoinjury	Intramyocardial	8 wk	Muscle cells present in the implant channels but not in control channels
Murry et al., 1996 (13)	Rat	Cryoinjury	Intramyocardial	3 mo	Cells adopt slow fiber phenotype, no cardiac markers present
Taylor et al., 1997 (55)	Rabbit	Normal	Intracoronary	3 wk	Cells present throughout the tissue distribution of the coronary artery infused
Taylor et al., 1998 (56)	Rabbit	Cryoinjury	Intramyocardial	6 wk	Striated cells in region of cryoinfarct, improved cardiac performance by sonomicrometry
Dorfman et al., 1998 (57)	Rat	Normal	Intramyocardial	4 wk	Differentiation of myoblasts to fully developed striated muscle
Atkins et al., 1999 (29)	Rabbit	Cryoinjury	Intramyocardial	3 wk	Successful engraftment of cells in 9 of 15 animals, skeletal muscle markers present, improved diastolic performance
Scorsin et al., 2000 (43)	Rat	Occlusion	Intramyocardial	1 mo	Improved LVEF, no connexin-43
Reinecke et al., 2000 (19)	Rat	Cryoinjury	Intramyocardial	3 mo	No detectable N-cadherin or connexin-43
Hutcheson et al., 2000 (58)	Rabbit	Cryoinjury	Intramycardial	3 wk	Myoblast compared with fibroblast implantation; both improved diastolic function, but only skeletal myoblasts improved systolic function

continued

315

Table 2 (*Continued*)
Summary of Preclinical Trials

Authors (ref.)	Animal	Type of model	Delivery	Duration	Results
Jain et al., 2001 (30)	Rat	Occlusion with reperfusion	Intramyocardial	6 wk	No change in infarct size, improved exercise capacity, improved systolic pressures
Rajnoch et al., 2001 (58)	Sheep	Snake cardiotoxin	Intramyocardial	2 mo	Cells survived, improved global and regional function by Echo
Pouzet et al., 2001 (46)	Rat	Ligation	Intramyocardial	2 mo	Improved function by echo, linear relation between number of cells and improvement in LVEF
Suzuki et al., 2001 (54)	Rat	Occlusion	Intramyocardial	1 mo	Animals implanted with cells transfected with VEGF had reduced infarct size and improved cardiac function
Reinecke et al., 2002 (2)	Rat	Normal	Intramyocardial	12 wk	No expression of cardiac markers, connexin-43 or *N*-cadherin, mature skeletal muscle present
Dib et al., 2002 (59)	Pig	Occlusion	Endoventricular	10 d	Myotubes present in infarcted area
Ghostine et al., 2002 (23)	Sheep	Occlusion	Intramyocardial	1 yr	Skeletal muscle present in scar region, co-expression of fast and slow isoforms, improved systolic regional function
Leobon et al., 2003 (28)	Rat	Ligation	Intramyocardial	1 mo	No eletromechanical coupling between cells

LVEF, left-ventricular ejection fraction; VEGF, vascular endothelial growth factor.

316

maturing myofibers with well-formed sarcomeres were noted. However, no nuclei were BrdU positive, indicating that cell division had ceased. At 7 wk, islands of mature skeletal muscle within the scar tissue were evident. At 3 mo after transplantation, the investigators demonstrated mature skeletal muscle with peripheral nuclei and fiber diameters greater than that at 7 wk. In a sheep model of myocardial infarction, Ghostine et al. demonstrated the long-term viability of transplanted skeletal myoblast cells. At 1 yr, histological analysis revealed large areas of grafted cells within the scars. These cells had histological features of well-differentiated skeletal muscle cells *(23)*.

Myoblast Differentiation Into Cardiomyocytes

Although some authors have reported differentiation into cardiomyocyte-like cells, the vast preponderance of evidence to date indicates that skeletal myoblasts injected into ischemic or infracted myocardium do not differentiate to cardiomyocytes. None of the cells transplanted by Murry et al. into cryoinjured rat hearts stained for cardiac-specific α-MHC, cardiac troponin I, or atrial natriuretic peptide at any time point *(13,26)*. However, cells that were transplanted 1 wk after injury did demonstrate conversion to slow-twitch fibers by staining positive for β-MHC. Slow-twitch fibers are similar to cardiac fibers with a high capacity for oxidative phosphorylation and fatigue resistance *(13)*. Similarly, Ghostine et al. found that 30% of transplanted skeletal muscle cells expressed the slow and fast MHC isoforms *(23)*.

Cell Integration Into Host Myocardium

Cardiac muscle cells are electrically coupled by specialized cell-cell junctions called intercalated discs. *N*-Cadherin and connexin-43 are the major proteins found in these junctions. Skeletal muscle differs in that the cells are electrically isolated from one another. In adult skeletal muscle cells *N*-cadherin and connexin-43 are downregulated *(27)*. Regions of skeletal muscle grafts in cryoinjured myocardium and normal myocardium of rats did not demonstrate any detectable *N*-cadherin and connexin-43 by immunostaining at 3 mo after transplantation *(27)*. Ghostine et al. used electron microscopy to examine the transplanted skeletal myoblasts at 4 mo after transplantation. They observed a well-differentiated skeletal myocyte pattern without any junctions or intercalated disks *(23)*. Leobon and colleagues harvested the grafts at 1 mo post skeletal myoblast transplantation and used intracellular recordings coupled to video microscopy to analyze the electrical and contractile activity of transplanted cells. They did not observe any electromechanical coupling of transplanted myoblasts to host cardiomyocytes *(28)*. Integration of transplanted cells into host myocardium with the formation of electrical connections via gap junctions is important for synchronous contraction. Thus far, studies indicate that transplanted skeletal myoblasts do not form gap junctions with host cardiomyocytes.

Functional Improvement

Several groups have demonstrated that skeletal myoblasts transplanted into regions of injured myocardium not only form stable grafts but also improve cardiac functioning and limit post-MI remodeling. Various investigators have used a variety of methods to examine cardiac function. Atkins et al. implanted skeletal myoblasts in cryoinjured rabbit hearts *(29)*. Using micromanometry and sonomicrometry, they found an improvement in diastolic compliance as well as a reduction in diastolic creep in animals that received myoblast implantation. Using a coronary artery ligation model in adult male rats, Jain and colleagues transplanted 10^6 skeletal myoblasts into the infarct region *(30)*. They assessed in vivo cardiac function by maximum exercise capacity testing. Control animals demonstrated a gradual decline in exercise capacity, whereas animals that had received skeletal myoblast transplantation did not. Additionally, rats that received cell therapy showed significantly less ventricular dilation. Ghostine et al. used tissue Doppler imaging (TDI) to analyze the long-term efficacy of myoblast transplantation on cardiac function after myocardial infarction in sheep *(23)*. At 4 mo, several indices of myocardial function cardiac function showed significant improvement in transplanted animals versus control animals. Animals that received skeletal myoblast transplants had significantly less deterioration of ejection fraction (EF) as well as reduced increase in end-diastolic volume. These results persisted at 1 yr.

CLINICAL DATA

Based on the encouraging results of preclinical studies, Menasche and colleagues reported the first patient to receive autologous skeletal myoblast implantation *(31)*. The patient was a 72-yr-old man with New York Heart Association (NYHA) class III heart failure resulting from an extensive inferior MI and anterolateral ischemia. He had a mean ejection fraction of 21% with akinesia of the posterior wall and anterior and lateral dyskinesia. Positron emission tomography (PET) scanning was performed as well, demonstrating a lack of viability of the posterior wall only. Bypass to the posterior wall would therefore not be expected to improve cardiac function. The patient received bypass to the diagonal and left anterior descending arteries only and autologous skeletal myoblasts injection into the posterior wall. The patient had an uneventful postoperative course. At 5-mo follow-up, the patient's clinical status had improved to NYHA class II and his mean EF was 30%. Additionally,

PET scanning now showed new metabolic activity in the posterior wall where previously there was nonviable scar, and echocardiography demonstrated contractility of the posterior wall that had previously been akinetic. The patient did not experience any arrhythmias or complications at 5-mo follow-up. The improvement seen in the posterior wall would not have been expected from bypass alone. The patient died as a result of a stroke 1.5 yr after the procedure *(32)*. On postmortem exam of the heart, myotubes were found in the region of fibrosis. The contractile apparatus of the cells was preserved and immunohistochemical staining was positive for skeletal muscle markers but negative for cardiac specific markers. More than half of the cells were noted to express the slow MHC isoform that is characteristic of skeletal muscle. Based on this, the authors concluded that the grafts maintained long-term viability and had adapted to a cardiac workload.

The success of myoblast therapy in this patient laid the groundwork for phase I clinical trials. Menasche and colleagues reported a series of 10 patients in a phase I trial *(33)*. All patients had skeletal myoblast transplantation into regions of akinetic, nonrevascularizable, nonviable scar in conjunction with coronary artery bypass to remote areas. The patients were followed for an average of 10.9 mo postoperatively. Four patients experienced delayed episodes of sustained ventricular tachycardia (VT) requiring implantation of an internal defibrillator. None of these patients exhibited myocardial ischemia with the episodes of VT. All four patients did well after implantation of the defibrillator. The patients experienced significant improvement in NYHA class as well as ejection fraction. The authors reported that 63% of the cell-implanted scars showed improved systolic thickening by blinded echocardiographic analysis. This first phase I trial established the safety and feasibility of autologous skeletal myoblast transplantation in patients with severe ischemic heart disease.

Although demonstrating promising results, the phase I trial reported by Menasche is confounded by the concomitant coronary artery bypass grafting (CABG). Pagani and colleagues transplanted autologous skeletal myoblasts in five patients concurrently with LV device implantation *(34)*. Four patients underwent explantation for heart transplant, thus enabling histological analyisis for evidence of myoblast engraftment, survival, and differentiation. They found that less than 1% of injected cells survived. However, surviving myofibers were evident in regions of fibrosis. These myofibers were confirmed to be of skeletal muscle origin by staining for skeletal muscle-specific MHC. Additionally, they found significantly more CD-31-stained vessels present in the area of surviving grafts when compared to adjacent nongrafted scar tissue.

Smits and colleagues were the first to assess the safety and feasibility of catheter-based transendocardial delivery of autologous skeletal myoblasts *(35)*. Five patients with a previous anterior wall infarction <4 wk old, left-ventricular ejection fraction (LVEF) of <45%, and symptoms of heart failure were selected to undergo the procedure. The presence and location of the scar was assessed by akinesia or dyskinesia at rest during echocardiography, LV angiography and magnetic resonance imaging (MRI), no contractile reserve during dobutamine stress echo (DSE), and hyperenhancement by gadolinium on MRI. All of the patients were discharged from the hospital without complications within 24 h. One patient required implantation of a cardioverter-defibrillator because of asymptomatic runs of nonsustained ventricular tachycardia at 6 wk. The patients were followed for 6 mo with ECG, DSE, and pulsed-wave TDI, LV angiography, technetium-99m-labeled erythrocyte radionuclide scintigraphy, and MRI. Although no conclusions can be drawn from this pilot study as to the efficacy of treatment, analysis of these studies showed a trend toward increased LVEF, increased wall thickness, and increased contraction velocity at 6-mo follow-up compared with baseline.

Several other pilot and phase I clinical trials have been carried out in the United States as well as abroad (Table 3) *(36–41)*. The major adverse event noted in these trials is arrhythmia requiring the implantation of a cardioverter-defibrillator. It remains unclear, however, whether such arrhythmias are truly the result of the myoblast implantation or rather the increased monitoring of this high-risk patient population. The likelihood of finding nonsustained ventricular arrhythmia recording on serial Holter monitoring is 40% in patients with heart failure *(42)*. The patients as a whole in these phase I trials have demonstrated improvement in cardiac function as evidenced by improvement in NYHA class, increased LVEF, improved regional wall motion, reduced infarct size, and increased perfusion. As these phase I trials are not controlled blinded studies and the sample sizes are small, no definite conclusions regarding the efficacy of myoblast transplantation can be drawn. However, these promising results have laid the groundwork for large multicenter phase II trials currently underway.

MECHANISMS OF ACTION

Although myoblasts survive in regions of fibrosis, it is debatable whether they actually contribute to the functional improvement seen in these studies. Several theories have been proposed as to the mechanism by which skeletal myoblasts improve cardiac function. These mechanisms are not mutually exclusive, and several may contribute in concert. The preponderance of evidence suggests that although skeletal myo-

Table 3
Summary of Clinical Trials

Authors (ref.)	Source	Type of study	No. of patients	Results	Complications
Menasche et al., 2001 (31)	Autologous	Adjunct to CABG	1	Improved LVEF, segmental contractility and perfusion	None
Siminiak et al., 2002 (60)	Autologous	Adjunct to CABG	1	Improved segmental contractility	Sustained VT
Siminiak et al., 2002 (36)	Autologous	Adjunct to CABG	10	Improved segmental contractility	Sustained VT in 2 patients; 1 death not related to cell implantation
Dib et al., 2002 (37)	Autologous	Adjunct to CABG	11	Improved LVEF, evidence of viability on MRI and PET scan	None
Pagani et al., 2003 (34)	Autologous	Adjunct to LVAD	5	Increased blood vessel count, myofiber staining for MHC parallel to host myocardial fibers	AF in 2 patients, VT in 2 patients
Zhang et al., 2003 (38)	Autologous	Adjunct to CABG	3	Improved LVEF and left ventricular wall thickness, improvement on perfusion scan	Occasional arrhythmias
Menasche et al., 2003 (33)	Autologous	Adjunct to CABG	10	Improved LVEF and NYHA class	VT in 4 patients
Chachques et al., 2003 (61)	Autologous	Adjunct to CABG	5	Improvement in NYHA class and regional fractional shortening,	None
Smits et al., 2003 (35)	Autologous	Sole therapy catheter based	5	Improved LVEF, increased wall thickness on MRI	Nonsustained VT in 1 patient
Law et al., 2003 (39)	Allogenic	Adjunct to CABG	2	Improvement LVEF, improvement on perfusion scan	None

continued

321

Table 3 (*Continued*)
Summary of Clinical Trials

Authors (ref.)	Source	Type of study	No. of patients	Results	Complications
Siminiak et al., 2003 (40)	Autologous	Sole therapy catheter based	2	Improved heart function	None
Herreros et al., 2003 (41)	Autologous	Adjunct to CABG	12	Improved LVEF, improvement in the viability of cardiac tissue in the infarct area	None
Sim et al., 2004 (62)	Autologous	Adjunct to CABG on beating heart	1	Improvement LVEF, improvement on perfusion scan	None

CABG, coronary artery bypass grafting; LVAD, left ventricle assist device; LVEF, left-ventricular ejection fraction; MRI, magnetic resonance imaging; PET, positron emission tomography; VT, ventricular tachycardia; VF, ventricular fibrillation; MHC, myosin heavy chain; NYHA, New York Heart Association.

322

blasts can undergo phenotypic conversion to slow-twitch myosin isoforms, it is unlikely that they undergo transdifferentiation to cardiomyocytes or that they form gap junctions and electromechanical coupling with host cardiomyocytes. Comparison of cardiomyocyte with skeletal myoblast transplantation did not show any difference in functional improvement (43). Because propagation of electrical impulses through these specialized intercellular junctions is unlikely, it is possible that skeletal myoblasts could respond to mechanical stimulation of contracting host cardiomyocytes through which they are bound by the extracellular matrix, thereby contributing to systolic function. The elastic property of the implanted cells may have a scaffolding effect limiting postinfarction remodeling. The cells may also limit remodeling by inhibiting matrix metalloproteinases (44). Engrafted myoblasts may release growth factors, such as insulin growth factor (IGF)-1, hepatocyte growth factor (HGF), and fibroblast growth factor (FGF), promoting angiogenesis, preventing fibrosis, or recruiting cardiac stem cells (45). Some studies have demonstrated increased angiogenesis in regions of myoblast transplantation as compared to control (34). Hibernating myocardium in regions at the periphery of the infarct is therefore rescued.

FUTURE PERSPECTIVES

Although phase II clinical trials are already underway, additional preclinical work remains to be done. Optimization of parameters such as dose, cell type, and mode of delivery as well as mechanisms to improve cell survival and maximize the functional effectiveness of cell transplantation are important areas of intense investigation.

The dose of cells transplanted varies significantly among various studies. The optimal dose is yet to be determined, and dose escalation trials are required. Several investigators have determined, in rats that a relationship exists between the number of myoblasts injected and the improvement in EF (46,47). The dose of cells administered in human trials varies, as does the cell selection process. Clinical dose-escalation trials are currently underway. In addition, the purity of the cells to be implanted varies between studies from 43% to 98%. Some studies are implanting a mixture of myoblasts and fibroblasts that may affect both the efficacy as well as the complications that result. Beauchamp et al. showed that there are two distinct subpopulations of skeletal myoblasts and that only the minority of cells that are slowly growing in culture actually survive and proliferate after grafting (48).

Another important consideration is how skeletal myoblasts compare with other forms of cell therapy. Bone marrow-derived stem cells are also autologous, easy to harvest, and expandable in culture. The potential of these cells to differentiate into cardiomyocytes is an area of intense debate. A direct comparison of autologous skeletal myoblasts and bone marrow stem cells in a rabbit cryoinjury model demonstrated a similar degree of improvement in systolic function in both treatment groups *(49)*.

To date, the majority of preclinical and clinical trials have used direct injections of skeletal myoblasts via epicardial injections. Smits et al. showed promising results in a pilot study of percutaneous endoventricular delivery of skeletal myoblast *(35)*. This is also the single trial to date examining the effects of myoblast therapy without concomitant CABG or ventricular assist device. Extensive work remains to be done in the field of delivery. Improved devices for the delivery of cells to the myocardium with minimal invasiveness to the patient are currently being developed. A significant problem with all current devices is leakage of cells from the implant site *(50)*. Additionally, devices that minimize trauma to the cells upon implantation may improve cell survival.

Cell death can be attributed to trauma from the manipulation and injection of cells, inflammation, hypoxia, and incompatibility with the surrounding host tissue. Alternative strategies to improve cell survival include genetic manipulation of the cells to express a variety of proteins. Qu et al. engineered skeletal myoblasts to express an inhibitor of interleukin (IL)-1, an inflammatory cytokine thought to play an important role in the immune response to transplanted cells *(51)*. Cells expressing the inhibitor of IL-1 had significantly improved survival when compared to nontransfected cells. Zhang et al. showed that cells that overexpressed Akt, a cytoprotective protein, had increased survival compared to untreated cells when grafted into acutely injured hearts *(52)*. Another promising strategy used heat shock treatment of the cells to significantly increase their survival *(52)*. Suzuki et al. transformed myoblasts with a gene to overexpress connexin-43, the major protein present in gap junctions of cardiomyocytes, with the hopes of improving the integration of myoblasts with the host myocardium *(53)*. They showed improved gap junction intercellular communication in vitro. Another strategy to improve cell survival has been to increase angiogenesis to the transplanted myoblasts. A variety of cytokines have been shown to improve angiogenesis including vascular endothelial growth factor (VEGF), FGF, and HIF-1α. Myoblasts could be used as a vehicle for gene therapy. Suzuki et al. transfected rat skeletal myoblasts with the human VEGF$_{165}$ gene *(54)*. These cells were injected into syngeneic rat hearts 1 h after left coronary artery occlusion. Myocardial VEGF expression increased for 2 wk in the VEGF group, resulting in enhanced angiogenesis without the formation of tumors. Additionally, grafted myoblasts had differentiated into multinucleated myotubes within host myocardium. Infarct size was significantly reduced with VEGF treatment, and cardiac function improved in the VEGF. Importantly, a gradation of improvement was seen, with the combined VEGF and cell therapy group showing significant improvement over the cell therapy alone group, and the cell therapy-alone was significantly better than control injections.

The growing field of cell therapy holds enormous promise for the growing number of patients with few options. Early preclinical and clinical trials are encouraging; however, this optimism must be tempered with caution as extensive research remains before the reality of the therapeutic value of cell therapy is realized. It is likely that the answer for these patients will not be a simplistic approach, but rather a combination of cell transplantation and angiogenic and gene therapy.

REFERENCES

1. 2003 Heart and Stroke Statistical Update. American Heart Association, 2003.
2. Kajstura J, Leri A, Finato N, Di Loreto C, Beltrami CA. Myocyte proliferation in end-stage cardiac failure in humans. Proc Natl Acad Sci 1998;95:8801–8805.
3. Beltrami AP, Urbanek K, Kajstura J, et al. Evidence that human cardiac myocytes divide after myocardial infarction. N Engl J Med 2001;344:1750–1757.
4. URREA; UNOS. 2002 Annual Report of the U.S. Organ Procurement and Transplantation Network and the Scientific Registry of Transplant Recipients: Transplant Data 1992-2001 [Internet]. Rockville (MD): HHS/HRSA/OSP/DOT; 2003 [modified 2003 Feb 18]. Available from: http://www.optn.org/data/annualReport.asp.
5. Rose EA, Gelijns AC, Moskowitz AJ, et al. Long term mechanical left ventricular assist device for endstage heart failure. N Engl J Med 2001;345:1435–1443.
6. Li R-K, Jia Z-Q, Weisel RD, et al. Cardiomyocyte transplantation improves heart function. Ann Thorac Surg 1996;62:654–661.
7. Scorsin M, Hagège A.A, Marotte F, et al. Does transplantation of cardiomyocytes improve function of infarcted myocardium. Circulation 1997;96(Suppl II):188–193.
8. Müller-Ehmsen J, Peterson KL, Kedes L, et al. Long term survival of transplanted neonatal rat cardiomyocytes after myocardial infarction and effect on cardiac function. Circulation 2002;105:1720–1726.
9. Beltrami AP, Barlucchi L, Torella D, et al. Adult cardiac stem cells are multipotent and support myocardial regeneration. Cell 2003;114:763–776.
10. Beltrami AP, Urbanek K, Kajstura J, et al. Evidence that human cardiomyocytes divide after myocardial infarction. N Engl J Med 2001;344:1750–1757.
11. Mauro A. Satellite cell of skeletal muscle fibers. J Biophys Biochem Cytol 1961;9:493–495.
12. Mannion JD, Bitto T, Hammond NA, et al. Histochemical and fatigue characteristics of conditioned canine latissimus dorsi muscle. Circ Res 1986;58:298–304.
13. Murry CE, Wiseman RW, Schwartz SM, et al. Skeletal myoblast transplantation for repair of myocardial necrosis. J Clin Invest 1996:98:2512–2523.
14. Alberts B, Bray D, Lewis J, et al. Differentiated cells and the maintenance of tissues. In: Molecular Biology of the Cell, 3d ed. Garland, New York:1994;1161–1175.
15. Eckert P, Schnackerz K. Ischemic tolerance of human skeletal muscle. Ann Plast Surg 1991;26:77–84.

16. Wolff KD, Stiller D. Ischemic Tolerance of free-muscle flaps: an NMR-spectroscopic study in the rat. Plast Reconstr Surg 1993;91:485–491.
17. Jennings RB, Reimer KA. Lethal myocardial ischemic injury. Am J Pathol 1981;102:241–255.
18. Verheule S, van Kempen MJ, Welscher PH, et al. Characterization of gap junction channels in adult rabbit atrial and ventricular myocardium. Circ Res 1997;80:673–681.
19. Reinecke H, Macdonald GH, Hauschka SD, et al. Electromechanical coupling between skeletal and cardiac muscle: Implications for infarct repair. J Cell Biol 2000;149:731–740.
20. Marelli D, Desrosiers C, el-Alfy M, et al. Cell Transplantation for myocardial repair: an experimental approach. Cell Transplant 1992;1(6):383–390.
21. Irintchev A, Zweyer M, Wernig A. Cellular and molecular reactions in mouse muscles after myoblast transplantation. J Neurocytol 1995;24:319–331.
22. Fan Y, Maley M, Beilharz M, et al. Rapid death of injected myoblasts in myoblast transfer therapy. Muscle Nerve 1996;19:853–860.
23. Ghostine S, Carrion C, Souza LCG, et al. Long-term efficacy of myoblast transplantation on regional structure and function after myocardial infarction. Circulation 2002;106(Supp 1):I131–I136.
24. Yoon PD, Kao RL, Magovern GJ. Myocardial regeneration: transplanting satellite cells into damaged myocardium. Texas Heart Inst J 1995;22:119–125.
25. Chiu RCJ, Zibaitis A, Kao RL. Cellular cardiomyoplasty: myocardial regeneration with satellite cell implantation. Ann Thorac Surg 1995;60:12–18.
26. Reinecke H, Poppa V, Murry CE. Skeletal muscle stem cells do not transdifferentiate into cardiomyocytes after cardiac grafting. J Mol Cell Cardiol 2002;34:241–249.
27. Reinecke H, Macdonald GH, Hauschka SD, et al. Electromechanical coupling between skeletal and cardiac muscle: implications for infarct repair. J Cell Biol 2000;149:731–740.
28. Leobon B, Garcin I, Menasche P, et al. Myoblasts transplanted into rat infracted myocardium are functionally isolated from their host. PNAS 2003;100:7808–7811.
29. Atkins BZ, Hueman MT, Meuchel J, et al. Cellular cardiomyoplasty improves diastolic properties of injured hearts. J Surg Res 1999;85:234–242.
30. Jain M, DerSimonian H, Brenner DA, et al. Cell therapy attenuates deleterious ventricular remodeling and improves cardiac performance after myocardial infarction. Circulation 2001;103:1920–1927.
31. Menasche P, Hagege AA, Scoesin M, et al. Myoblast transplantation for Heart failure. Lancet 2001;357:279–280.
32. Hagege AA, Carrion C, Menasche P, et al. Viabiliy and differentiation of autologous skeletal myoblast grafts in ischemic cardiomyopathy. Lancet 2003;361:491–492.
33. Menasche P, Hagege AA, Vilquin JT, et al. Autologous skeletal myoblast transplantation for severe postinfarction left ventricular dysfunction. J Am Coll Cardiol 2003;41:1078–1083.
34. Pagani FD, DerSimonian H, Zawadzka A, et al. Autologous skeletal myoblast transplanted to ischemia-damaged myocardium in humans. J Am Coll Cardiol 2003;41:879–888.
35. Smits PC, van Geuns RJM, Poldermans D, et al. Catheter-based intramyocardial injection of autologous skeletal myoblasts as a primary treatment of ischemic heart failure. J Am Coll Cardiol 2003;42:2063–2069.
36. Siminiak T, et al. Transplantation of autologous skeletal myoblasts in the treatment of patients with post infarction heart failure. Circulation 2002;106:II636 (Abstract 3137).

37. Dib N, et al. Safety and feasibility of autologous myoblast transplantation in patients with ischemic cardiomyopathy: interim results from the United States experience. Circulation 2002;106(Suppl II):II463 (Abstract 2291).
38. Zhang FM, et al. Clinical cellular cardiomyoplasty: technical considerations. J Cardiovasc Surg 2003;18:268–273.
39. Law PK, Fang G, Chua F, Kakuchaya T, Bockeria LA. First-in-man myoblast allografts for heart degeneration. Int J Med Implants Devices 2003;1:100–155.
40. Siminiak T, Fiszer D, Jerzykowska O, et al. Percutaneous autologous myoblast transplantation in the treatment of post-infarction myocardial contractility impairment—report on two cases. Kardiol Pol 2003;59(12):492–501.
41. Herreros J, Prosper F, Perez A, et al. Autologous intramyocardial injection of cultured skeletal muscle-derived stem cells in patients with non-acute myocardial infarction. Eur Heart J 2003;(22):2012–2020.
42. Cleland JGF, Chattopaddhyay S, Khand A, et al. Prevalence and incidence of arrhythmias and sudden death in heart failure. Hear Fail Rev 2002;7:229–242.
43. Scorsin M, Hagege AA, Vilquin JT, et al. Comparison of the effects of fetal cardiomyocytes and skeletal myoblast transplantation on post-infarction left ventricular function. J Thorac Cardiovasc Surg 2000;119:1169–1175.
44. Spinale FG, Coker ML, Krombach D, et al. Matrix metalloproteinase inhibition during the development of congestive heart failure. Circ Res 1999;85:364–376.
45. Tatsumi R, Anderson JE, Nevoret CJ, et al. HGF/SF is present in normal adult skeletal muscle and is capable of activating satellite cells. Dev Biol 1998;194:114–128.
46. Pouzet B, Vilquin JT, Hagege AA, et al. Factors affecting functional outcome after autologous skeletal myoblast transplantation. Ann Thorac Surg 2001;71:844–851.
47. Tambara K, Sakakibara Y, Sakaguchi G, et al. Transplanted skeletal myoblasts can fully replace the infracted myocardium when they survive in the host in large numbers. Circulation 2003;108(Suppl II):II259–II263.
48. Beauchamp RJ, Morgan JE, Pagel CN, et al. Dynamics of myoblast transplantation reveal a discrete minority of recursors with stem cell like properties as the myogenic source. J Cell Biol 1999;144:1113–1121.
49. Thompson RB, Emani SM, Davis BH, et al. Comparison of Intracardiac Cell transplantation: Autologous skeletal myoblasts versus bone marrow cells. Circulation 2003;108(Suppl II):II264–II271.
50. Grossman PM, Han ZG, Palasis M, Barry JJ, Lederman RJ. Incomplete retention after direct myocardial injection. Cath Cardiovasc Intervent 2002;55:392–397.
51. Qu Z, Balkir L, van Deutekom JCT, et al. Development of approaches to improve cell survival in myoblast transfer therapy. J Cell Biol 1998;142:1257–1267.
52. Zhang M, Methot D, Poppa V, et al. Cardiomyocyte grafting for cardiac repair: graft cell death and anti-death strategies. J Mol Cell Cardiol 2001;33:907–921.
53. Suzuki K, Brand NJ, Allen S, et al. Overexpression of connexin 43 in skeletal yoblasts: relevance to cell transplantation to the heart. J Thorac Cardiovasc Surg 2001;122:759–766.
54. Suzuki K, Murtuza B, Smolenski RT, et al. Cell transplantation for the treatment of acute myocardial infarction using vascular endothelial growth factor-expressing skeletal myoblasts. Circulation 2001;104(Suppl 1):I207–I212.
55. Taylor DA, Silvestry SC, Bishop SP, et al. Delivery of primary autologous skeletal myoblasts into rabbit heart by coronary infusion: a potential approach to myocardial repair. Proc Assoc Am Phys 1997;109(3):245–253.
56. Taylor DA, Atkins BZ, Hungspreugs P, et al. Regenerating functional myocardium: improved performance after skeletal myoblast transplantation. Nat Med 1998;4:929–933.

57. Dorfman J, Duong M, Zibaitis A et al. Myocardial tissue engineering with autologous myoblast implantation. J Thorac Cardiovasc Surg 1998;116:744–751.

58. Rajnoch C, Chachques JC, Berrebi A, et al. Cellular therapy reverses myocardial dysfunction. J Thorac Cardiovasc Surg 2001;121:871–878.

59. Dib N, Diethrich EB, Campbell A. Endoventricular transplantation of allogeneic skeletal myoblasts in a porcine model of myocardial infarction. J Endovasc Ther 2002;9:313–319.

60. Siminiak T, Kalawski R, Kurpisz M. Myoblast transplantation in the treatment of post infarction myocardial contractility impairment—a case report. Kardiol Pol 2002;53:131.

61. Chachques JC, Gonzalez JH, Trainini JC. Cardiomioplastia celular. Rev Arg Cardiol 2003;71:138–145.

62. Haider HKh, Tan AC, Aziz S, Chachques JC, Sim EK. Myoblast transplantation for cardiac repair: a clinical perspective. Mol Ther 2004;9:14–23.

13 Transmyocardial Laser Revascularization

Keith A. Horvath, MD

CONTENTS

INTRODUCTION
METHODS
RESULTS
MECHANISMS
SUMMARY

INTRODUCTION

History

Numerous patients with coronary artery disease have been successfully treated with conventional methods, such as coronary artery bypass grafting (CABG) or percutaneous coronary intervention (PCI), but a significant and increasing number of patients have exhausted the ability to undergo these procedures repeatedly because of the diffuse nature of their coronary artery disease. As a result, they have chronic disabling angina that is often refractory to medical therapy. Transmyocardial laser revascularization (TMR) was developed to treat these patients. Although Mirhoseini et al. *(1,2)* and Okada et al. *(3,4)* pioneered the use of a laser to perform this type of revascularization in conjunction with CABG in the early 1980s, the use of a laser as sole therapy required advancements in the technology to establish its efficacy. Since then, more than 15,000 patients have been treated with TMR around the world and results from individual institutions, multicenter studies, and prospective randomized control trials have been reported *(5–18)*.

From: *Contemporary Cardiology: Angiogenesis and Direct Myocardial Revasularization*
Edited by: R. J. Laham and D. S. Baim © Humana Press Inc., Totowa, NJ

Clinical Results

The significant angina relief seen in such patients enrolled in nonrandomized trials led to prospective randomized studies to further demonstrate the efficacy of TMR. In these pivotal trials more than 1000 patients were enrolled and randomized to receiving TMR or medical management for their severe angina *(12–17)*. The six trials employed a 1:1 randomization in which one-half of the patients were treated with laser and the other half continued on maximal medical therapy. All patients were followed for 12 mo.

METHODS

Patients

The entry criteria for these studies are as follows: patients had refractory angina that was not amenable to standard methods of revascularization as verified by a recent angiogram. They had evidence of reversible ischemia based on myocardial perfusion scanning, and their left-ventricular ejection fractions were greater than 25%.

The typical patient profile of TMR patients is listed in Table 1. Because the patients were equally randomized to the medical management group, there were no significant demographic differences between the TMR and the control groups for any of these trials. Three studies *(12–14)* employed a holmium:yttrium-aluminum-garnett (Ho:YAG) laser, and three *(15–17)* used a carbon dioxide (CO_2) laser. Two of the trials *(12,15)* permitted a crossover from the medical management group to laser treatment for the presence of unstable angina that necessitated intravenous (iv) anti-anginal therapy for which they were unweanable over a period of at least 48 h. By definition, these crossover patients were less stable and significantly different from those who had been initially randomized to TMR or medical management alone.

Operative Technique

For sole therapy TMR, patients undergo a left anterior thoracotomy in the fifth intercostal space (Fig. 1). Once the ribs are spread by a retractor, the lung is deflated and the pericardium is opened to expose the epicardial surface of the heart (Fig. 2). Channels are created starting near the base of the heart and then serially in a line approx 1 cm apart toward the apex, starting inferiorly and working superiorly to the anterior surface of the heart. The number of channels created depends on the size of the heart and the size of the ischemic area.

The handpiece in Fig. 2 is from a CO_2 laser and illustrates one of differences between the two lasers employed for TMR. The CO_2 laser energy is delivered via hollow tubes and is reflected by mirrors to reach

Table 1
Baseline Characteristics of Transmyocardial Revascularization Patients

Average age	62
Women	14%
CCS Angina Class III	39%
CCS Angina Class IV	61%
Ejection fraction (mean ±SD)	48 ± 10%
Previous myocardial infarction	72%
Previous coronary artery bypass grafting	83%
Previous percutaneous transluminal coronary angioplasty	37%
Insulin-dependent diabetes mellitus	32%

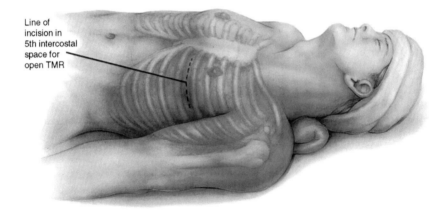

Fig. 1. Sole therapy transmyocardial laser revascularization performed as an open surgical procedure is typically done through a left anterolateral thoracotomy in the 5th intercostal space. Exposure of the heart through this incision can typically be achieved without division of the ribs or costal cartilages.

the epicardial surface. One-millimeter channels are made with a 20–30-J pulse. The firing of the laser is synchronized to occur on the r wave of the electrocardiograph to avoid arrhythmias. The transmural channel is created by a signal pulse in 40 ms and can be confirmed by transesophageal echocardiography (TEE). The vaporization of blood by the laser energy as the laser beam enters the ventricle creates an obvious and characteristic acoustic effect as noted on TEE. The Ho:YAG laser achieves a similar 1-mm channel by manually advancing a fiber through the myocardium while the laser fires. Typical pulse energies are 2 J for this laser, with 20–30 pulses being required to traverse the myocardium. Detection of transmural penetration is primarily by tactile and auditory feedback.

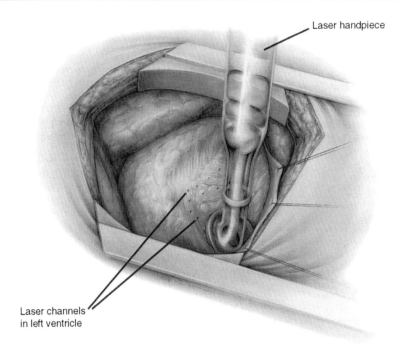

Fig. 2. Channels are created in a distribution of one per square centimeter, starting inferiorly and then working superiorly to the anterior surface of the heart. The number of channels created depends on the size of the heart and on the size of the ischemic area.

Endpoints

The principal subjective endpoint for all of the trials was a change in angina symptoms. This was assessed by the investigator and/or a blinded independent observer. In addition to assigning an angina class, other tools such as the Seattle Angina Questionnaire, the Short Form Questionnaire 36 (SF-36), and the Duke Activity Status Index were employed. Objective measurements consisted of repeated exercise tolerance testing as well as repeat myocardial perfusion scans. Patients were reassessed at 3, 6, and 12 mo postrandomization.

RESULTS

Mortality

Prior to the randomized studies, mortality rates in the 10–20% *(5–11)* range were reported for TMR patients. In the randomized trials, lower perioperative mortality rates were reported ranging from 1 to 5% *(12–17)*. One of the important lessons learned from these controlled trials that differ from the earlier studies was a decrease in the mortality when patients taken to the operating room were not unstable, specifically not on iv heparin or nitroglycerin. When patients were allowed to recover from their most recent episode of unstable angina and were able to be weaned from iv medications such that their operation could be performed 2 wk later, the mortality dropped to 1% *(15)*. The 1-yr survival for TMR patients was 85–95% and for medical management patients was 79–95%. Meta-analysis of the 1-yr survival demonstrated no statistically significant difference between the patients treated with a laser and those who continued with medical therapy.

Morbidity

Unlike mortality, the exact definition of various complications varied from one study protocol to the next, and therefore, morbidity data are difficult to pool. Nevertheless, the typical postoperative course had a lower incidence of myocardial infarction, heart failure, and arrhythmias than was documented in a similar cohort of patients, those that have reoperative CABG *(12–17)*.

Angina Class

The principal reason for performing TMR is to reduce the patient's anginal symptoms. This can be quantified by assessing the angina class pre- and postprocedure. Angina class assessment was performed by a blinded independent observer in all studies. Significant symptomatic improvement was seen in all studies for patients treated with the laser. Using a definition of success as a decrease of two or more angina classes, all of the studies demonstrated a significant success rate after TMR with success rates ranging from 25 to 76% (Table 2). Significantly fewer patients in the medical management group experienced symptomatic improvement, and the success rate for these patients ranged from 0 to 32%. The seemingly broad range of success is due to differences between the baseline characteristics of the studies. It is more difficult to achieve a two angina class improvement if the baseline angina class is III. Studies that started with most of their patients in angina class III, not surprisingly, showed the lowest success rate. In contrast, the largest success rate for TMR was seen in the trial in which all of the patients were in class IV at enrollment. Of note, the medical management group in this study also showed the largest success rate *(12)*. This underscores some of the baseline differences between the studies.

Quality of Life and Myocardial Function

Quality of life indices as assessed by the Seattle Angina Questionnaire, the SF-36, and Duke Activity Status Index demonstrated signifi-

Table 2
One-Year Success Rate for Randomized Trials of Transmyocardial
Revascularization (TMR) vs Medical Management (MM)

Study	Laser	MM	TMR
Aaberge et al. *(17)*	Co_2	0%	39%
Schofield et al. *(16)*	CO_2	4%	25%
Burkhoff et al. *(13)*	Ho:YAG	11%	61%
Frazier et al. *(15)*	CO_2	13%	72%
Allen et al. *(80)*	Ho:YAG	32%	76%

Success rate = proportion of patients who experienced a decrease of two or more angina classes.

cant improvement for TMR-treated patients vs medical management in every study. Global assessment of myocardial function by ejection fraction using echocardiography or radionuclide multigated acquisition scans showed no significant change in the overall ejection fraction for any of the patients, regardless of group assignment or study.

Hospital Admission

Another indicator of the efficacy of TMR was a reduction in hospital admissions for unstable angina or cardiac-related events postprocedure. A meta-analysis of the data provided indicates that the 1-yr hospitalization rate of patients in the laser-treated group was statistically significantly less then for those treated medically. Medical management patients were admitted four times more frequently than TMR patients over the year of follow-up *(19)*.

Exercise Tolerance

Additional functional test assessment using exercise tolerance was also performed in three of the trials *(3,16,17)*. Although the method of treadmill testing differed between the trials, the results demonstrate an improvement in exercise tolerance for TMR-treated patients. Two studies showed an average of 65- to 70-s improvement in the TMR group at 12 mo compared to baseline, while the medical management group had either an average of 5-s improvement or a 46-s decrease in exercise time over the same interval *(16,17)*. One additional trial demonstrated that the time to chest pain during exercise increased significantly and fewer patients were limited by chest pain in the TMR group, whereas the medical management group showed no improvement *(17)*.

Medical Treatment

All of the studies employed protocols that continued all of the patients on maximal medical therapy. TMR patients, as a result of their symptomatic improvement, had a reduction in their medication use over the year of follow-up. The overall medication use decreased or remained unchanged in 83% of the TMR patients, and conversely the use of medications increased or remained unchanged in 86% of the medical management patients (15).

Myocardial Perfusion

As previously stated, myocardial perfusion scans were obtained preoperatively to verify the extent and severity of reversible ischemia. The four largest randomized trials included follow-up scans as part of their study (12,13,15,16). These results reflect over 800 of the patients randomized. The methodology of recording and analyzing these results differed in each study, so it is difficult to pool the data. Nevertheless, review of the results demonstrated an improvement in perfusion for CO_2 TMR-treated patients. Fixed (scar) and reversible (ischemic defects) were tallied for both the TMR-treated patients and the medical management groups. A CO_2 study demonstrated a significant decrease in the number of reversible defects for both the TMR and the medical management patients (16). This improvement in the reversible defects in the TMR group was seen without a significant increase in the fixed defects at the end of the study. However, the number of fixed defects in the medical management group had nearly doubled over the same interval. Similarly, there was a 20% improvement in the perfusion of previously ischemic areas in the CO_2 TMR group of another trial, and in that same trial there was a 27% worsening of the perfusion of the ischemic areas in the medical management group at 12 mo (15). There was no difference in the number of fixed defects between the groups at 12 mo, nor was there a significant change in the number of fixed defects for each patient compared with their baseline scans. The remaining two Ho:YAG studies that obtained follow-up scans showed no significant difference between the TMR and the medical management groups at 12 mo and no significant improvement in perfusion in the TMR-treated patients over the same interval (12,13).

Long-Term Results

Long-term results of Ho:YAG and CO_2 TMR also differ. As noted, after Ho:YAG TMR, significant short-term angina relief was demonstrated at one year, as the average angina class fell from 3.5 ± 0.5 at baseline to 1.8 ± 0.8 at 1 yr ($p < 0.01$). However the average angina class

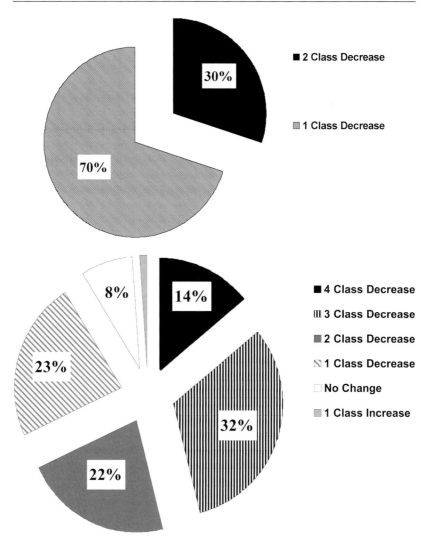

Fig. 3. (A) Distribution of holmium:yttrium-aluminum-garnett (Ho:YAG) transmyocardial laser revascularization treated patients by decrease in Canadian Cardiovascular Society (CCS) angina class; baseline vs 3 yr. (B) Distribution of CO_2 transmyocardial laser revascularization treated patients by decrease in Canadian Cardiovascular Society (CCS) angina class; baseline vs 5 yr.

at 3 yr after Ho:YAG TMR was reported to increase significantly to 2.2 ± 0.7 ($p = 0.003$ vs 1 yr) (20,21). Additionally, at 3 yr only 30% of the patients had a two-class improvement in angina compared to their baseline, and 70% had a one-class improvement (Fig. 3A). Long-term results with the CO_2 laser were markedly different. As reported, these results demonstrate a decrease in angina class from 3.7 ± 0.4 at baseline to 1.6 ± 1.0 at 5 yr ($p = 0.0001$) *(22)*. This was unchanged from the 1.5 ± 1.0 average angina class at 1 yr of follow-up ($p = $ ns vs 5 yr). Additionally, 68% of the patients at 5 yr had a two or more angina class improvement, and 17% had no angina with a length of follow-up out to 7 yr (Fig. 3B). As would be expected, the patient's quality-of-life improvements were also maintained long-term. Additionally, one report of late clinical follow-up of another of the randomized control trials also demonstrated continued symptomatic improvement with CO_2 TMR *(23)*. This study is noteworthy in that the medical management arm of the original randomized trial was also followed long-term. In this study with up to 5 yr of follow-up, the average angina class for CO_2 TMR-treated patients decreased from 3.3 at baseline to 2.0 at follow-up. Over the same interval, the medical management group average angina class increased from 3.2 to 3.7. Only 3% of the medical management group showed a two-class angina reduction at ≥ 5 yr, whereas 24% of the TMR-treated patients maintained a two or greater class reduction in angina. Additionally, medical management patients were hospitalized twice as frequently for unstable angina as those treated with CO_2 TMR.

MECHANISMS

Understanding the mechanism of TMR starts with understanding the laser tissue interaction. While numerous devices *(24,25)*, including ultrasound *(26)*, cryoablation *(27)*, radio frequency *(28,29)*, heated needles *(30,31)*, as well as the aforementioned hollow and solid needles have been used; none have engendered the same response that is seen with a laser. Additionally, numerous wavelengths of laser light have also been employed *(32,36)*. Only CO_2 and Ho:YAG are used clinically for TMR. The result of any laser tissue interaction is dependent on both laser and tissue variables *(35–37)*. CO_2 has a wavelength of 10,600 nm, whereas Ho:YAG has a wavelength of 2120 nm. These infrared wavelengths are primarily absorbed in water and therefore rely on thermal energy to ablate tissue. One significant difference, however, is that the Ho:YAG laser is pulsed and the arrival of two successive pulses must be separated by time to allow for thermal dissipation, otherwise the accumulated heat will cause the tissue to explode under pressure. Such explosions create acoustic waves, which travel along the planes of lower resistance between muscle fibers and cause structural trauma as well as thermocoagulation *(38)*. The standard operating parameters for the Ho:YAG laser are pulse energies of 1–2 Js and 6–8 W/pulse. The energy is delivered at a rate of 5 pulses/s through a flexible 1-mm optical fiber. It takes approx 20 pulses to create a transmural channel. Despite the low energy level and short pulse duration, very high levels of peak power are delivered to the tissue so that with each pulse there is an explosion (Fig. 4). Additionally, the fiber is advanced manually through the myocardium, and it is therefore impossible to know whether the channel is being created by the kinetic energy delivered via the mechanical effects of the fiber or whether there has been enough time for thermal dissipation prior to the next pulse.

In contrast, the CO_2 was used at an energy level of 20–30 J/pulse with a pulse duration of 25–40 ms. At this level the laser photons do not cause explosive ablation and the extent of structural damage is limited. Additionally, a transmural channel can be created with a single pulse (Fig. 4). Confirmation of this transmurality is obtained by observing the vaporization of blood within the ventricle using TEE.

Finally, the CO_2 laser is synchronized to fire on the r wave, and with its short pulse duration arrhythmic complications are minimized. The Ho:YAG device is unsynchronized and, because of the motion of the fiber through the myocardium over several cardiac cycles, is more prone to ventricular arrhythmias.

Patent Channels

As noted, the original concept of TMR was to create perfusion via channels connecting the ventricle with the myocardium. Clinical work demonstrated some evidence of long-term patency *(39,40)*. Additional experimental work showed some evidence of patency as well *(41–44)*. There are also significant reports from autopsy series and laboratories that indicate that the channels do not remain patent *(45–49)*. What evidence there is that channel patency may be a mechanism was only following CO_2 TMR (Fig. 5). There has never been any evidence that Ho:YAG TMR channels stay patent.

Denervation

In contrast to the open channel mechanism, damage to the sympathetic nerve fibers may explain the angina relief noted in clinical trials. The nervous system of the heart can function independent of inputs from extracardiac neurons to regulate regional cardiac function by reflex action. This intrinsic system contains afferent neurons, sympathetic efferent, postganglionic neurons, and parasympathetic efferent, postganglionic neurons. Because of this complex system, it is difficult to demonstrate true denervation. However, several experimental studies have demonstrated that denervation may indeed play a role in Ho:YAG TMR *(50–52)*. Experimental evidence to the contrary was reported in a

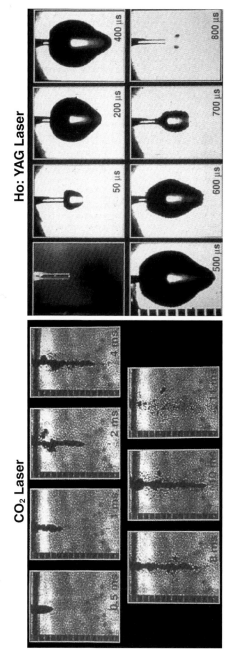

Fig. 4. Sequential photography of the firing of a single pulse from a CO$_2$ laser (left) and a holmium:yttrium-aluminum-garnett (Ho:YAG) laser (right) into water. The pulse duration and energy levels are the same as those being used clinically.

339

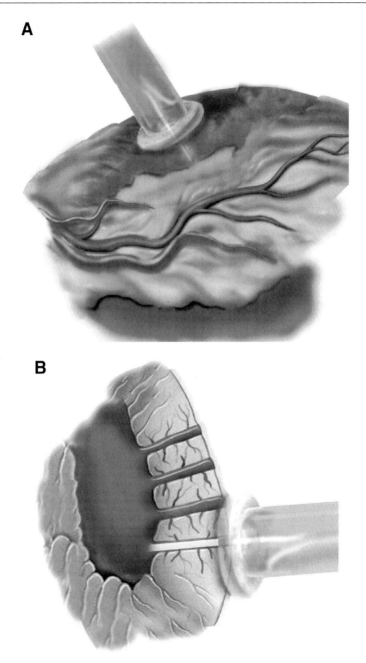

Fig. 5. The CO_2 laser creates a transmural channel in a single 20-J pulse. Conceptually direct perfusion may occur via the channel. Evidence indicates that the laser stimulates angiogenesis in and around the channel and leads to improved perfusion.

nonischemic animal model *(53)*. Regardless of the methodology employed in the laboratory, there is significant evidence of sympathetic denervation following positron emission tomography (PET) of Ho:YAG TMR-treated patients *(54)*. Although the studies were carefully carried out, it is difficult to isolate the sympathetic afferent nerve fibers, and the experiments were in the acute setting and only address the short-term effects.

Angiogenesis

The likely underlying mechanism for the clinical efficacy of TMR is the stimulation of angiogenesis. This mechanism fits the clinical picture of significant improvement in symptoms over time as well as a concomitant improvement in perfusion, as seen with the CO_2 laser. Numerous reports have demonstrated a histological increase in neovascularization as a result of TMR channels *(46,48,55–61)*. More molecular evidence of this angiogenic phenomenon was derived from work that demonstrated an upregulation of vascular endothelial growth factor (VEGF), messenger RNA, expression of fibroblast growth factor (FGF)-2, as well as matrix metalloproteinases following TMR *(62–64)*. Histologically, similar degrees of neovascularization have been noted after mechanical injury of various types. Needle injury has been demonstrated by immunohistochemistry to also stimulate growth factor expression and angiogenesis. The conclusion is that TMR-induced angiogenesis is a nonspecific response to injury *(65–67)*. Investigation of this using hot and cold needles, radiofrequency energy, and laser energy to perform TMR clearly demonstrates a spectrum of tissue response to the injury *(30)*. The results in a model of chronic myocardial ischemia to mimic the clinical scenario indicate that indeed neovascularization can occur after mechanical TMR, but if these new blood vessels grow in the midst of a scar, there will be little functional contribution from blood flow through these new vessels. The recovery of function with laser TMR was the result of a minimization of scar formation and a maximization of angiogenesis.

If TMR induces angiogenesis, is there an ensuing improvement in function? Clinically, this has been demonstrated subjectively with quality-of-life assessments, but, more importantly, it has been demonstrated objectively with multiple techniques, including dobutamine stress echocardiography *(68)*, PET *(69)*, and cardiac magnetic resonance imaging *(70,71)*. As further evidence of the angiogenic response, experimental data have mirrored the clinical perfusion results noted, with improvements in perfusion in porcine models of chronic ischemia where the ischemic zone was treated with CO_2 TMR *(72–75)*. This improved perfusion led to an improvement in myocardial function as well.

SUMMARY

Myocardial laser revascularization has been performed percutaneously *(76–78)*, thoracoscopically *(79)*, via thoracotomy *(12–18)*, and via sternotomy *(80–82)*. Aside from the percutaneous approach, the other surgical approaches have yielded similar symptomatic improvement. A recent double-blind, randomized, controlled trial showed no benefit to the percutaneously treated patients compared to the untreated control group *(78)*. As the patients were blinded to their treatment, the possibility of a significant placebo effect for pecutaneous TMR (PMR) has been raised. Of note, the morbidity and mortality of PMR is reportedly similar to that seen with TMR. As a result, the US Food and Drug Administration recently rendered PMR unapprovable. The failure of PMR to achieve the same clinical results that have been seen with TMR may be a result of several significant limitations, the first of which is the partial thickness treatment of the left ventricle. Even at the maximal estimated depth of 6 mm reported with PMR, this is significantly less than the full thickness treatment of the myocardium achieved with an open TMR approach. Furthermore, fewer of these partial thickness channels are typically created with PMR. The exact location of the channel and the establishment of a wide distribution of the channels from inside a moving ventricle is also problematic. Finally, the limitations of the Ho:YAG TMR—the wavelength of light that has been employed—are also applicable to PMR.

While the results of sole TMR therapy are encouraging and were necessary to confirm the efficacy of the procedure, the future of TMR is in combination therapy *(80–82)*. Mirhoseini's description of using TMR with CABG provides the likely clinical scenario for the future. As PCI techniques improve and evolve, patients who undergo coronary artery bypass grafting will more likely than not have more diffuse disease and more occluded coronary arteries. As a result, some territories may be bypassable, but others may be better suited for TMR. A combination of both of these methods will provide a more complete revascularization. Early results with a randomized trial comparing CABG to CABG plus TMR indicated a mortality benefit to undergoing the combined procedure *(80)*. Unfortunately, the mortality rate for the CABG-only patients in the study was high at 7.5% and may be the key contributing factor in the results. Additionally, the patients were randomized based on their angiograms and prior to investigation in the operating room. Nevertheless, these results indicate that the combined procedure is feasible, and in fact, longer-term outcomes of CABG plus TMR patients indicate that significant angina relief and low morbidity and mortality can be achieved in such high-risk patients *(81,82)*.

Other applications include the use of TMR in the treatment of cardiac transplant graft atherosclerosis. Although performed on a small number of patients, the results have indicated a benefit following TMR *(83,84)*. Finally, the combination of TMR plus other methods of angiogenesis may provide an even more robust response. Experimental work investigating these combinations has verified a synergistic effect with regard to histological evidence of significant angiogenesis and, perhaps more importantly, an improvement in myocardial function with a combination of TMR and gene therapy vs either therapy alone *(85,89)*.

REFERENCES

1. Mirhoseini M, Muckerheide M, Cayton MM. Transventricular revascularization by laser. Lasers Surg Med 1982;2(2):187–198.
2. Mirhoseini M, Fisher JC, Cayton M. Myocardial revascularization by laser: A clinical report. Lasers Surg Med 1983;3(3):241–245.
3. Okada M, Ikuta h, Shimizu OK, Horii H, Nakamura K. Alternative method of myocardial revascularization by laser: experimental and clinical study. Kobe J Med Sci 1986;32:151–161.
4. Okada M, Shimizu K, Ikuta H, Horii H, Nakamura K. A new method of myocardial revascularization by laser. Thorac Cardiovasc Surg 1991;39(1):1–4.
5. Horvath KA, Mannting F, Cummings N, Shernan SK, Cohn LH. Transmyocardial laser revascularization: operative techniques and clinical results at two years. J Thorac Cardiovasc Surg 1996;111(5):1047–1053.
6. Cooley DA, Frazier OH, Kadipasaoglu KA, Lindenmeir MH, Pehlivanoglu S, Kolff JW, Wilansky S, Moore WH. Transmyocardial laser revascularization: clinical experience with twelve-month follow-up. J Thorac Cardiovasc Surg 1996;111(4):791–797.
7. Horvath KA, Cohn LC, Cooley DA, Crew JR Frazier OH, Griffith BP, Kadipasaglu K, Lansing A, Mannting FR, March R, Mirhoseini MR, Smith C. Transmyocardial laser revascularization: results of a multi-center trial using TLR as sole therapy for end stage coronary artery disease. J Thorac Cardiovasc Surg 1997;113:645–654.
8. Krabatsch T, Tambeur L, Lieback E, Shaper F, Hetzer R. Transmyocardial laser revascularization in the treatment of end-stage coronary artery disease. Ann Thorac Cardiovasc Surg 1998;4(2):64–71.
9. Hattler BG, Griffith BP, Zenati MA, Crew JR, Mirhoseini M, Cohn LH, Aranki SF, Frazier OH, Cooley DA, Lansing AM, Horvath KA, Fontana GP, Landolfo KP, Lowe JE, Boyce SW. Transmyocardial laser revascularization in the patient with unmanageable unstable angina. Ann Thor Surg 1999;68:1203–1209.
10. Milano A, Pratali S, Tartarini G, Mariotti R, DeCarlo M, Paterni G, Boni G, Bortolotti U. Early results of transmyocardial revascularization with a holmium laser. Ann Thorac Surg 1998;65:700–704.
11. Dowling RD, Petracek MR, Selinger SL, Allen KB. Transmyocardial revascularization in patients with refractory, unstable angina. Circulation 1998;98(Suppl II):II73–II75.
12. Allen KB, Dowling RD, Fudge TL, Schoettle GP, Selinger SL, Gangahar DM, Angell WW, Petracek MR, Shaar CJ, O'Neill WW. Comparison of transmyocardial revascularization with medical therapy in patients with refractory angina. N Engl J Med 1999;341:1029–1036.

13. Burkhoff D, Schmidt S, Schulman SP, Myers J, Resar J, Becker LC, Weiss J, Jones JW. Transmyocardial laser revascularization compared with continued medical therapy for treatment of refractory angina pectoris: a prospective randomized trial. Lancet 1999;354:885–890.

14. Jones JW, Schmidt SE, Richman BW, Miller CC, Sapire KJ, Burkhoff D, Baldwin JC. Holmium: YAG laser transmyocardial revascularization relieves angina and improves functional status. Ann Thorac Surg 1999;67:1596–1602.

15. Frazier OH, March RJ, Horvath KA. Transmyocardial revascularization with a carbon dioxide laser in patients with end-stage coronary artery disease. N Engl J Med 1999;341:1021–1028.

16. Schofield PM, Sharples LD, Caine N, Burns S, Tait S, Wistow T. Transmyocardial laser revascularization in patients with refractory angina: a randomized controlled trial. Lancet 1999;353:519–524.

17. Aaberge L, Nordstrand K, Dragsund M, Saatvedt K, Endresen K, Golf S, Geiran O, Abdelnoor M, Forfang K. Transmyocardial revascularization with CO_2 laser in patients with refractory angina pectoris. Clinical results from the Norwegian randomized trial. J Am Coll Cardiol 2000;35(5):1170–1177.

18. Agarwal R, Ajit M, Kurian VM, Rajan S, Arumugam SB, Cherian KM. Transmyocardial laser revascularization: early results and 1-year follow-up. Ann Thor Surg 2000;69(6):1993–1995.

19. Horvath KA. Results of prospective randomized controlled trials of transmyocardial laser revascularization. Heart Surg Forum 2002;5(1):33–40.

20. De Carlo M, Milano AD, Pratali S, Levantino M, Mariotti R, Bortolotti U. Symptomatic improvement after transmyocardial laser revascularization: how long does it last? Ann Thorac Surg 2000;70(3):1130–1133.

21. Schneider J, Diegeler A, Krakor R, Walther T, Kluge R, Mohr FW. Transmyocardial laser revascularization with the holmium:YAG laser: loss of symptomatic improvement after 2 years. Eur J Cardiothorac Surg 2001;19(2):164–169.

22. Horvath KA, Aranki SF, Cohn LH, Frazier OH, Kadipasaoglu KA, Boyce SW, Lytle BW, Lansing AM. Sustained angina relief 5 years after transmyocardial laser revascularization with a CO_2 laser. Circulation 2001;104(Suppl I):I81–I84.

23. Aaberge L, Rootwelt K, Blomhoff S, Saatvedt K, Abdelnoor M, Forfang K. Continued symptomatic improvement three to five years after transmyocardial revascularization with CO_2 laser. JACC 2002;39(10):1588–1593.

24. Shawl FA, Kaul U, Saadat V. Percutaneous myocardial revascularization using a myocardial channeling device: first human experience using the AngioTrax system. J Am Coll Cardiol 2000;35:61A.

25. Malekah R, Reynolds C, Narula N, Kelley ST, Suzuki Y, Bridges CR. Angiogenesis in transmyocardial laser revascularization—a nonspecific response to injury. Circulation 1998;98:II62–II65.

26. Smith NB, Hynynen K. The feasibility of using focused ultrasound for transmyocardial revascularization. Ultrasound Med Biol 1998;24:1045–1054.

27. Khairy P, Dubuc M, Gallo R. Cryoapplication induces neovascularization: a novel approach to percutaneous myocardial revascularization. J Am Coll Cardiol 2000;35:5A–6A.

28. Yamamoto N, Gu AG, Derosa CM, Shimizu J, Zwas DR, Smith CR, Burkhoff D. Radio frequency transmyocardial revascularization enhances angiogenesis and causes myocardial denervation in a canine model. Lasers Surg Med 2000;27:18–28.

29. Dietz U, Darius H, Eick O, Buerke M, Ed Odeh R. Transmyocardial revascularization using temperature controlled HF energy creates reproducible intramyocardial channels. Circulation 1998;98:3770.

30. Horvath KA, Belkind N, Wu I, Greene R, Lomasney JW, McPherson DD, Fullerton DA. Functional comparison of transmyocardial revascularization by mechanical and laser means. Ann Thorac Surg 2001;72:1997–2002.
31. Whittaker P, Rakusan K, Kloner RA. Transmural channels can protect ischemic tissue. Assessment of long-term myocardial response to laser- and needle-made channels. Circulation 1996;93:143–152.
32. Hughes GC, Kypson AP, Annex BH, et al. Induction of angiogenesis after TMR: a comparison of holmium: YAG, CO_2, and excimer lasers. Ann Thorac Surg 2000;70(2):504–509.
33. Martin JS, Sayeed-Shah U, Byrne JG, Danton MH, Flores KQ, Laurence RG, Cohn LH. Excimer versus carbon dioxide transmyocardial laser revascularization: effects on regional left ventricular function and perfusion. Ann Thorac Surg 2000;69:1811–1816.
34. Whittaker P, Spariosu K, Ho ZZ. Success of transmyocardial laser revascularization is determined by the amount and organization of scar tissue produced in response to initial injury: results of ultraviolet laser treatment. Lasers Surg Med 1999;24:253–260.
35. Genyk IA, Frenz M, Ott B, Walpoth BH, Schaffner T, Carrel TP. Acute and chronic effects of transmyocardial laser revascularization in the nonischemic pig myocardium by using three laser systems. Lasers Surg Med 2000;27:438–450.
36. Jeevanandam V, Auteri JS, Oz MC, Watkins J, Rose EA, Smith CR. Myocardial revascularization by laser-induced channels. Surg Forum 1990;41:225–227.
37. Kadipasaoglu K, Frazier OH. Transmyocardial laser revascularization: effect of laser parameters of tissue ablation and cardiac perfusion. Sem Thor Cardiovasc Surg 1999;11:4–11.
38. Kadipasaoglu KA, Sartori M, Masai T, Cihan HB, Clubb FJ Jr, Conger JL, Frazier OH. Intraoperative arrhythmias and tissue damage during transmyocardial laser revascularization. Ann Thorac Surg 1999;67(2):423–431.
39. Cooley DA, Frazier OH, Kadipasaoglu KA, Pehlivanoglu S, Shannon RL, Angelini P. Transmyocardial laser revascularization. Anatomic evidence of long-term channel patency. Tex Heart Inst J 1994;21(3):220–224.
40. Mirhoseini M, Shelgikar S, Cayton M. Clinical and histological evaluation of laser myocardial revascularization. J Clin Laser Med Surg 1990;8(3):73–77.
41. Hardy RI, James FW, Millard RW, Kaplan S. Regional myocardial blood flow and cardiac mechanics in dog hearts with CO_2 laser-induced intramyocardial revascularization. Basic Res Cardiol 1990;85(2):179–197.
42. Horvath KA, Smith WJ, Laurence RG, Schoen FJ, Appleyard RF, Cohn LH. Recovery and viability of an acute myocardial infarct after transmyocardial laser revascularization. J Am Coll Cardiol 1995;25:258–263.
43. Krabatsch T, Schaper F, Leder C, Tulsner J, Thalmann U, Hetzer R. Histologic findings after transmyocardial laser revascularization. J Card Surg 1996;11(5):326–331.
44. Lutter G, Martin J, Ameer K, Heilmann C, Sarai k, Beyersdorf F. Microperfusion enhancement after TMLR in chronically ischemic porcine hearts. Cardiovasc Surg 2001;9(3):281–291.
45. Gassler N, Wintzer HO, Stubbe HM, Wullbrand A, Helmchen U. Transmyocardial laser revascularization: histological features in human nonresponder myocardium. Circulation 1997;95(2):371–375.
46. Khomoto T, Fisher PE, Gu A, Smith CR, De Rosa C, Burkhoff D. Physiology, histology, and two week morphology of acute myocardial channels made with a CO_2 laser. Ann Thorac Surg 1997;63:1275–1283.

47. Kohmoto T, Fisher PE, Gu A, Shu-Ming Z, Yano OJ, Spotnitz HM, Smith CR, Burkhoff D. Does blood flow through holmium:YAG transmyocardial laser channels? Ann Thoracic Surg 1996;61(3):861–868.

48. Burkhoff D, Fisher PE, Apfelbaum M, Kohmoto T, DeRosa CM, Smith CR. Histologic appearance of transmyocardial laser channels after 4 1/2 wk. Ann Thor Surg 1996;61(5):1532–1535.

49. Sigel JE, Abramovitch CM, Lytle BW, Ratliff NB. Transmyocardial laser revascularization: three sequential autopsy cases. J Thorac Cardiovasc Surg 1998;115:1381–1385.

50. Kwong KF, Kanellopoulos GK, Nikols JC, Sundt TR III. Transmyocardial laser treatment denervates canine myocardium. J Thorac Cardiovasc Surg 1997;114:883–890.

51. Kwong KF, Schuessler RB, Kanellopoulos GK, Saffitz JE, Sundt TM. Nontransmural laser treatment incompletely denervates canine myocardium. Circulation 1998;98:1167–1171.

52. Hirsch GM, Thompson GW, Arora RC, Hirsch KJ, Sullivan JA, Armour JA. Transmyocardial laser revascularization does not denervate the canine heart. Ann Thorac Surg 1999;68(2):460–468.

53. Minisi AJ, Topaz O, Quinn MS, Mohanty LB. Cardiac nociceptive reflexes after tansmyocardial laser revascularization: implications for the neural hypothesis of angina relief. J Thorac Cardiovasc Surg 2001;122:712–719.

54. Al-Sheikh T, Allen KB, Straka SP, Heimansohn DA, Fain RL, Hutchins GD, Sawada SG, Zipes DP, Engelstein ED. Cardiac sympathetic denervation after transmyocardial laser revascularization. Circulation 1999;100(2):135–140.

55. Yamamoto N, Kohmoto T, Gu A, DeRosa C, Smith CR, Burkhoff D. Angiogenesis is enhanced in ischemic canine myocardium by transmyocardial laser revascularization. J Am Coll Cardiol 1998;31(6):1426–1433.

56. Fisher PE, Khomoto T, DeRosa CM, Spotnitz HM, Smith CR, Burkhoff D. Histologic analysis of transmyocardial channels: comparison of CO_2 and Holmium:YAG lasers. Ann Thorac Surg 1997;64:466–472.

57. Zlotnick AY, Ahmad RM, Reul RM. Neovascularization occurs at the site of closed laser channels after transmyocardial laser revascularization. Surg Forum 1996;48:286–287.

58. Kohmoto T, Fisher PE, DeRosa, C, Smith CR, Burkhoff D. Evidence of angiogenesis in regions treated with transmyocardial laser revascularization. Circulation 1996;94:1294.

59. Spanier T, Smith CR, Burkhoff D. Angiogenesis. A possible mechanism underlying the clinical benefits of transmyocardial laser revascularization. J Clin Laser Med Surg 1997;15:269–273.

60. Mueller XM, Tevaearai HT, Chaubert P, Genton CY, von Segesser LK. Does laser injury induce a different neovascularization pattern from mechanical or ischemic injuries? Heart 2001;85:697–701.

61. Hughes GC, Lowe JE, Kypson AP, St Louis JD, Pippen AM, Peters KG, Coleman RE, DeGrado TR, Donovan CL, Annex BH, Landolfo KP. Neovascularization after transmyocardial laser revascularization in a model of chronic ischemia. Ann Thorac Surg 1998;66:2029–2036.

62. Horvath KA, Chiu E, Maun DC, Lomasney JW, Greene R, Pearce WH, Fullerton DA. Up-regulation of VEGF mRNA and angiogenesis after transmyocardial laser revascularization. Ann Thorac Surg 1999;68:825–859.

63. Li W, Chiba Y, Kimura T, Morioka K, Uesaka T, Ihaya A, Muraoka R. Transmyocardial laser revascularization induced angiogenesis correlated with the expression

of matrix metalloproteinase and platelet-derived endothelial cell growth factor. Eur J Cardiothorac Surg 2001;19:156–163.

64. Pelletier MP, Giaid A, Sivaraman S, Dorfman J, Li CM, Philip A, Chiu RC. Angiogenesis and growth factor expression in a model of transmyocardial revascularization. Ann Thorac Surg 1998;66:12–18.

65. Chu V, Kuang J, McGinn A, Giai A, Korkola S, Chiu RC. Angiogenic response induced by mechanical transmyocardial revascularization. J Thorac Cardiovasc Surg 1999;118:849–856.

66. Chu VF, Giaid A, Kuagn JQ, McGinn AN, Li CM, Pelletier MP, Chiu RC. Angiogenesis in transmyocardial revascularization: comparison of laser versus mechanical punctures. Ann Thor Surg 1999;68(2):301–307.

67. Malekan R, Reynolds C, Narula N, Kelley ST, Suzuki Y, Bridges CR. Angiogenesis in transmyocardial laser revascularization: a nonspecific response to injury. Circulation. 1998;98(Suppl II):II62–II66.

68. Donovan CL, Landolfo KP, Lowe JE, Clements F, Coleman RB, Ryan T. Improvement in inducible ischemic during dobutamine stress echocardiography after transmyocardial laser revascularization in patients with refractory angina pectoris. J Am Coll Cardiol 1997;30:607–612.

69. Frazier OH, Cooley DA, Kadipasaoglu KA, Pehlivanoglu S, Lindenmeir M, Barasch E, Conger JL, Wilansky S, Moore WH. Myocardial revascularization with laser. Preliminary findings. Circulation 1995;92(Suppl):II58–II65.

70. Laham RJ, Simons M, Pearlman JD, Ho KKL, Baim DS. Magnetic resonance imaging demonstrates improved regional systolic wall motion and thickening and myocardial perfusion of myocardial territories treated by laser myocardial revascularization. J Am Coll Cardiol 2002;39:1–8.

71. Kim RJ, Rafael A, Chen E, Wu E, Parker MA, Horvath KA, Simonetti O, Finn P, Bonow RO, Klocke FJ, Judd RM. Contrast-enhanced MRI predicts wall motion improvement after coronary revascularization. Circulation 1999;100(Suppl):I-797.

72. Horvath KA, Greene R, Belkind N, Kane B, McPherson D, Fullerton DA. Left ventricular functional improvement after transmyocardial laser revascularization. Ann Thor Surg 1998;66:721–725.

73. Hughes GC, Kypson AP, St Louis JD, Annex BH, Coleman RE, DeGrado TR, Donovan CL, Lowe JE, Landolfo, KP. Improved perfusion and contractile reserve after transmyocardial laser revascularization in a model of hibernating myocardium. Ann Thor Surg 1999;67(6):1714–1720.

74. Krabatsch T, Modersohn D, Konertz W, Hetzer R. Acute changes in functional and metabolic parameters following transmyocardial laser revascularization: an experimental study. Ann Thorac Cardiovasc Surg 2000;6(6):383–388.

75. Lutter G, Martin J, von Samson P, Heilmann C, Sarai K, Beyersdorf F. Microperfusion enhancement after TMLR in chronically ischemic porcine hearts. Cardiovasc Surg 2001;9:281–291.

76. Oesterle SN, Sanborn TA, Ali N, Resar J, Ramee SR, Heuser R, Dean L, Knopf W, Schofield P, Schaer GL, Reeder G, Masden R, Yeung AC, Burkoff D. Percutaneous transmyocardial laser revascularization for severe angina: the PACIFIC randomized trial. Lancet 2000;356:1705–1710.

77. Stone GW, Teirstein PS, Rubenstein R, Schmidt D, Whitlow PL, Kosinski EJ, Mishkel G, Power JA. A prospective, multicenter, randomized trial of percutaneous transmyocardial laser revascularization in patients with nonrecanalizable chronic total occlusions. J Am Coll Cardiol 2002;39:1581–1587.

78. Leon MB, Baim DS, Moses JW, Laham R, Knopf W, Reisman M, McCormick D, Cohen H, Fischell T, Cohen B, Kuntz RE, Kornowski R. A randomized blinded

clinical trial comparing percutaneous laser myocardial revascularization vs. placebo in patients with refractory coronary ischemia. Circulation 2000;102:II-565.

79. Horvath KA. Thoracoscopic transmyocardial laser tevascularization. Ann Thorac Surg 1998;65:1439–1441.

80. Allen KB, Dowling RD, DelRossi AJ, Realyvasques F, Lefrak EA, Pfeffer TA, Fudge TL, Mostovych M, Schuch D, Szentpetery S, Shaar CJ. Transmyocardial laser revascularization combined with coronary artery bypass grafting; a multicenter, blinded, prospective, randomized, controlled trial. J Thorac Cardiovasc Surg 2000;119:540–549.

81. Trehan N, Mishra Y, Mehta Y, Jangid DR. Transmyocardial laser as an adjunct to minimally invasive CABG for complete myocardial revascularization. Ann Thorac Surg 1998;66:1113–1118.

82. Stamou SC, Boyce SW, Cooke RH, Carlos BD, Sweet LC, Corso PJ. One-year outcome after combined coronary artery bypass grafting and transmyocardial laser revascularization for refractory angina pectoris. Am J Cardiol 2002;89:1365–1368.

83. Mehra MR, Uber PA, Prasad AK, Park MH, Scott RL, McFadden PM, Van Meter CH. Long-term outcome of cardiac allograft vasculopathy treated by transmyocardial laser revascularization early rewards, late losses. J Heart Lung Transplant 2000;19:801–804.

84. Frazier OH, Kadipasaoglu KA, Radovancevic B, Cihan HB, March RJ, Mirhoseini M, Cooley DA. Transmyocardial laser revascularization in allograft coronary artery disease. Ann Thorac Surg 1998;65:1138–1141.

85. Fleischer KJ, Goldschmidt-Clermont PJ, Fonger JD, Hutchins GM, Hruban RH, Baumgartner WA. One-month histologic response of transmyocardial laser channels with molecular intervention. Ann Thorac Surg 1996;62:1051–1058.

86. Sayeed-Shah U, Mann MJ, Martin J, Grachev S, Reimold S, Laurence R, Dzau V, Cohn LH. Complete reversal of ischemic wall motion abnormalities by combined use of gene therapy with transmyocardial laser revascularization. J Thorac Cardiovasc Surg 1998;116:763–768.

87. Doukas J, Ma CL, Craig D. Therapeutic angiogenesis induced by FGF-2 gene delivery combined with laser transmyocardial revascularization. Circulation 2000;102:1214.

88. Lutter G, Dern P, Attmann T, Handke M, Ameer K, Schreiber J, Buerkle M, Martin J, Marme D, Beyersdorf F. Combined use of transmyocardial laser revascularization with basic fibroblastic growth factor in chronically ischemic porcine hearts. Circulation 2000;102:3693.

89. Horvath KA, Doukas J, Lu CJ, Belkind N, Greene R, Pierce GF, Fullerton DA. Myocardial functional recovery after FGF2 gene therapy as assessed by echocardiography and MRI. Ann Thorac Surg 2002;74:481–487.

INDEX